CLEFT LIP AND PALATE

To my wife, Colette, and to our children, who patiently suffered through the all too time-consuming preparation of this book.

With all my love

CLEFT LIP AND PALATE
LESIONS, PATHOPHYSIOLOGY AND PRIMARY TREATMENT

René Malek
Chirurgien des Hôpitaux de Paris
France

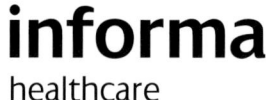

© 2001 Informa UK Ltd

First published in the United Kingdom in 2001 by Martin Dunitz, now part of Informa Healthcare.

Reprinted in 2008 by Informa Healthcare, Telephone House, 69-77 Paul Street, London EC2A 4LQ. Informa Healthcare is a trading division of Informa UK Ltd. Registered Office: 37/41 Mortimer Street, London W1T 3JH. Registered in England and Wales number 1072954.

Tel: +44 (0)20 7017 5000
Fax: +44 (0)20 7017 6699
Website: www.informahealthcare.com

A CIP record for this book is available from the British Library.
Library of Congress Cataloging-in-Publication Data

Data available on application

ISBN-10: 1-85317-491-2
ISBN-13: 978-1-85317-491-9

Distributed in the United States and Canada by:

Thieme New York
333 Seventh Avenue
New York, NY 10001

Book orders in the rest of the world

Paul Abrahams
Tel: +44 (0)20 7017 4036
Email: bookorders@informa.com

Composition by Scribe Design, Ashford, UK

Printed and bound in India by Replika Press Pvt. Ltd

Contents

Contributors

Patrice Oger
Surgeon

Hervé Martinez
Orthodontist

Marie-Rose Mousset
Speech Therapist

Chantal Trichet
Speech Therapist

All are at the Cleft Lip and Palate Unit, Hôpital Robert Debré, Paris, France.

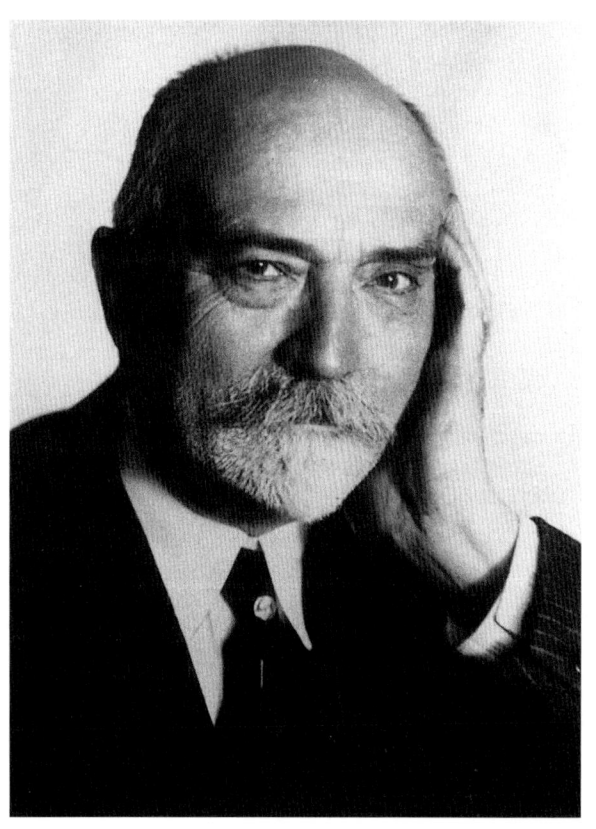

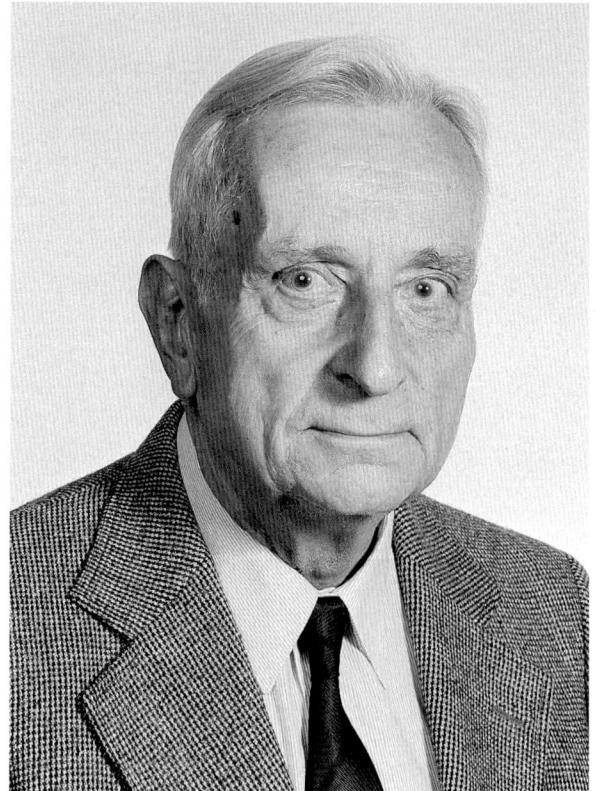

Victor Veau   *Pierre Petit*

F oreword

After a year of internship in my department, René Malek accepted my offer to join the staff at St Vincent de Paul and collaborate in the development of pediatric surgery. He remained there until my departure. Since then, he has headed the Department of Surgery at the Hospital of Sèvres, and later ended his public career as Surgeon at Robert Debré Hospital in Paris.

A large number of facial cleft cases were referred to me as the successor of Victor Veau. René Malek immediately took an active interest in them.

At the time, I continued to apply the treatment recommended by Victor Veau – in other words, repair of the lip and palate by simple approximation of the borders of the cleft where all the anatomical elements were present. A few minor innovations had been added to avoid any risk of separation: for the lip, suturing of the muscle layer with a very fine wire, which was left in place; and for the palate, fracture of the hamular processes to permit better mobility of each side of the cleft soft palate.

In those days, the palatal mucoperiosteum was completely undermined and detached along the alveolar ridge on both sides. This was then easily sutured together along the midline, and provided efficient protection for the more fragile suture of the nasal layer. The procedure was virtually risk-free, and breakdown of the palatal

closure was extremely uncommon. However, there were still two major defects:

1. The height deficiency of the white or cutaneous lip.
2. As far as palatal surgery was concerned, displacement of the fibro-mucosae towards the midline left a raw area. This was quickly covered, not by reconstituted mucosa, but by scar tissue. The two bony borders, due to their extreme pliability in early infancy, tended to draw together, thus causing secondary maxillary collapse.

René Malek immediately concentrated on these two problems. He had an excellent background in plastic surgery, and soon found a solution to the problem of lip correction. He devised a highly accurate method of calculating the dimensions of the necessary Z-plasty. His geometric construction is easy to work with during the operation, and has been consistently applied ever since.

For hard and soft palate repair, René Malek was highly conscious of the important role played by the tongue in the development of the maxilla – a role of which I had become aware thanks to my orthodontist, Jean Psaume – and realized that primary velar repair performed at a very early age could prevent the tongue from moving backward, restoring its essential role in moulding the bone structures. With this aim in mind, he radically transformed the surgical agenda established by Victor Veau (lip and anterior palate repair at the age of 3 months, bony vault and soft palate reconstruction at 18 months).

René Malek performs primary veloplasty at 3 months, and corrects the lip and hard palate at 6 months. He successfully sutures the borders of the cleft without extensive use of the mucoperiosteum, which was the source of maxillary deformities, and has proved that these early operations are perfectly feasible. However, I must add that the technique involved is far more demanding than it once was. It takes the skill and experience of a surgeon like René Malek to carry out his program with such efficiency, and he has done so with great success. The results of over 20 years of surgery are there to prove that he made the right choices. He amply deserves our congratulations.

Pierre Petit

Preface

A book written by a single author may seem to contradict the present trend of medical publications. Virtually all recent editions tend to compile articles by specialists, who deal with the various aspects of the volume's main topic. Such a selection of papers may guarantee that the text is of current interest, yet the caliber of the whole is often uneven. Some articles date more quickly than others, and prospective contributors are not always able to convey the sum of their experience or add a personal note in a domain that others present in a totally different light.

I believe there is still room for a book by a single author, who can then express both the detail and the range of his experience. This approach is all the more valid when the subject is clearly defined, as is the case for the treatment of cleft lip and palate. This is a highly complex malformation. A lifetime of surgery barely suffices to cover all its facets. Years of apprenticeship and teamwork, close observation of innumerable findings and long-term follow-up through adulthood are prerequisites for a valid discussion. The fine points of technique, so essential to successful surgical results, cannot be given their due in short articles.

The present book answers my urge to transmit this body of knowledge. Pierre Petit, Department Head in my earlier years, should have written a work of his own, and many of the findings related here are drawn from his teaching. It is to Pierre Petit that we owe the past 30 years of what can be termed an original therapeutic experience.

As Isaac Newton put it in 1675:

If I have seen further it is by standing on the shoulders of giants.

One of the first precepts I learned during my residency was drilled into me by my unforgettable mentor, Robert Merle d'Aubigne. He forbade me to say 'I believe that...' or 'it seems to me...' when I presented oral or written descriptions of a clinical observation. Everything had to be clear-cut: an anatomical lesion is or is not.

Orthopedics is a field where such strict accuracy comes naturally, and I soon realized that this precept applies to surgery as a whole. This is a field of medicine where there are always anatomical disorders to correct.

Consequently, each chapter of the present book includes a study of anatomical pathology preceded by a background refresher on normal anatomy, which must be second nature to a surgeon. Correction of these disorders is the purpose of surgical repair, and always implies the same aim: to re-establish a state of anatomy which is as close to normal as is humanly possible. The operating technique used to attain this objective, however, may vary from one specialist to another.

The problem is not a simple one, and is not restricted to the correction of lesions that do not evolve as time goes by. When the growth process comes into play – and this is the case in our field – it is essential to understand how surgery may influence the development of the anatomy once it has been repaired.

What is more, the physio-pathological consequences of these lesions have not clearly been determined as yet. They are open to a wide range of interpretations. The individual evolution of the functional mechanisms involved, whether spontaneous changes or those resulting from initial surgery, remains to be clarified. We will attempt to provide a detailed analysis of these phenomena.

A whole chain of factors enters into the valid assessment of a therapeutic method:

- the extent of the disorders linked to the malformation itself, and of their effect on adjacent growth;
- the consequences of the surgical act (not only the iatrogenic effect, but the repercussions of a poor surgical technique, for instance);
- the importance of the age of the patient at the time of surgery;
- the timing of the different stages of the treatment; and
- the implications of associated malformations, etc.

In conclusion, it seems obvious that, like it or not, the therapeutic concept continues to include a certain element of individual consideration. It cannot be reduced to a mere technical question of lesions to be corrected as best they can.

Despite the principles of accuracy and thoroughness on which this study is based, we must admit that it is influenced by an initial body of beliefs, and that the factors involved cannot always be applied from one case to another, particularly those which depend on operating techniques, since surgeons all have their own techniques. This explains the infinitely broad range of therapeutic policies on how to treat cleft lip and palate, and no genuine consensus of opinion has been reached:

> Bold affirmations, biased criticism, baffling debate, gratuitous derision litter the field without regard for those arguments which, in order to convince, must first be recognized as plausible and therefore worthy to present their case (Changeux and Ricoeur, 1998).

The absence of a therapeutic consensus poses an inevitable dilemma for those families unfortunate enough to consult a series of different practitioners.

Let us remember that only the experience acquired from a vast number of operations over a period of several decades – the time necessary to provide objective detachment – can justify the publication and promotion of a given method. The method which we call early palate repair fulfills both of these requirements.

The following pages, therefore, recount our personal experience. It is not our intention to present an encyclopedia of all that has been said and done concerning this boundless subject.

Thanks to the presence of our mentor, Pierre Petit, during our early days at St Vincent de Paul Hospital, and to his encouragement during the later years, we have had the good fortune to share, since 1962, in an original experience. The innovations have been numerous in the techniques of lip and cleft palate repair, in the indications of primary treatment and in the timing of secondary surgery. Our purpose is to develop them in detail.

René Malek

Acknowledgments

I dedicate this book:

To Pierre Petit, who determined the course of my professional career. He had faith in me to treat clefts and taught me the surgical and spiritual rigour it requires. Through him I feel that, in my modest way, I have carried on the life's work of Victor Veau. May neither find anything to embarrass them in these pages.

To Raoul Tubiana, who meant a great deal more than a spiritual father to me. His constant presence and encouragement were essential from a material and intellectual standpoint. At the outset of my professional life, he instilled the incentives for hard work, which did not come naturally to me. He was my sole mentor in plastic surgery and enabled me to create the new title of Pediatric Plastic Surgeon in France. He faithfully sponsored and supported me in the circles of learned societies and granted me the honour of collaborating on his publications, in particular on his *Treatise on Surgery of the Hand*, which is monumental in the field. Without his steadfast encouragement, I would never have undertaken the present book.

To all my collaborators and friends who, over these many years, have helped me to make a few breakthroughs in this difficult domain.

The vital role played by the multidisciplinary team in the treatment of labio-palatine clefts is often stressed. It was essential for me.

I was fortunate enough to benefit from the teaching of Jean Psaume, without whom the experience we call 'Primary Palate' would never have taken place.

Hervé Martinez, who followed him in Orthodontics, has made fine work of a difficult succession.

Ms Mousset and Ms Trichet, our speech therapists, generously provided their precious assistance.

Patrice Oger is 'holding the fort' in cleft surgery. I trust he will find that these pages further clarify the ideas that he constantly stimulated throughout the years.

I owe a debt of gratitude to the anesthesiologists in our team, and in particular to Monique Dautheville and Jean-Claude Crabol, who helped me to make a success of so many operations with no setbacks or fatalities to mar the record.

My secretaries, Jeanne Cabaret-Lemoine, who was my assistant and helpmate throughout my surgical career in private practice, and Evelyne Menguy, during my hospital career, deserve an altogether special note of homage.

Lastly, my warm appreciation to Ms Peggy Castex, who translated this work into English.

Note on illustrations for complete clefts

Throughout this study, the line drawings used to illustrate the text conform to a conventional technique adopted in our Department.

In order to picture the incisions, flaps and sutures of each layer, the drawings show a projection of the lip which is sliced across its thickness and laid out: the vestibular surface is tangential to the plane of the alveolar rim and palate; the cutaneous surface continues the nostril sill and nose in the opposite direction.

This technique artificially lengthens the image of the nasal floor between the upper reference point for the lip and the bottom of the vestibule where it is continuous with the nasal layer of the palatal shelf.

The illustrations speak for themselves. They are far easier to understand than a written description of the elements they display (Fig. 1a, b, c). The sketches of unilateral clefts treated according to the 'classical' procedure appear in Fig. 2 and bilateral clefts appear in Fig. 3.

It is also important to be familiar with the technique for picturing the lip once the cutaneo-muscular incisions have been performed (Fig. 4a and 4b).

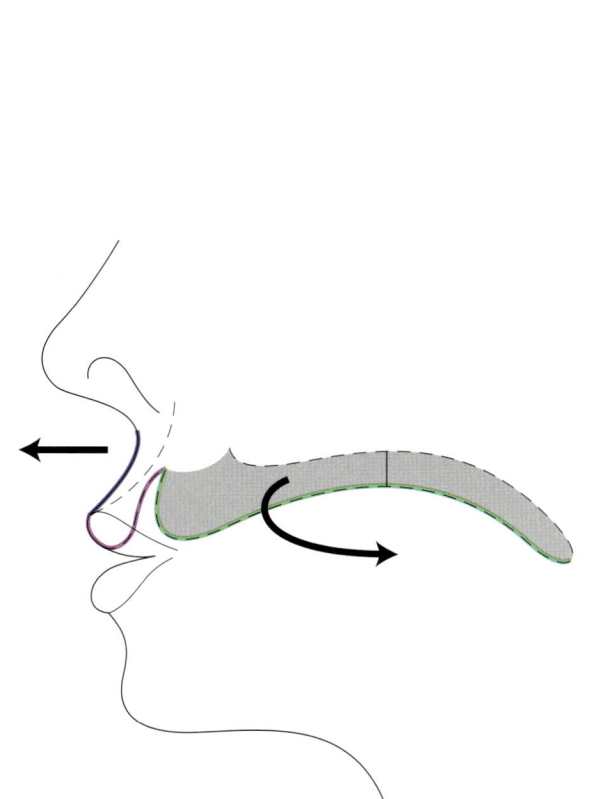

Fig. 1a

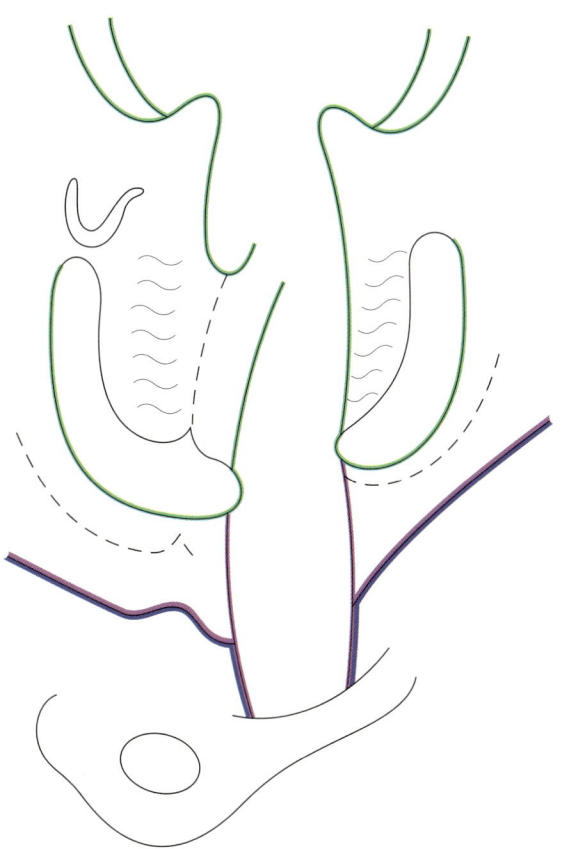

Fig. 1b

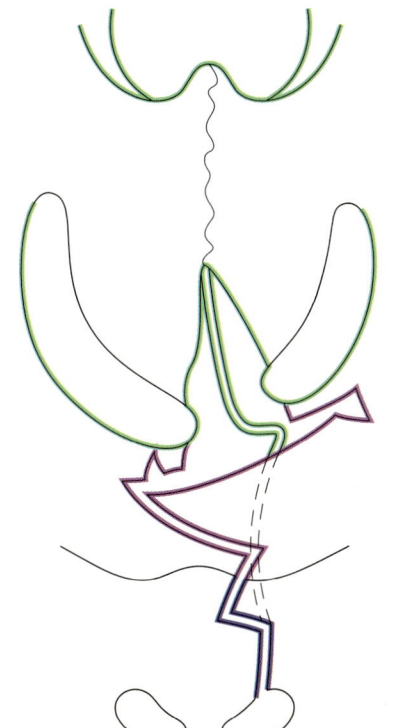

Fig. 1c

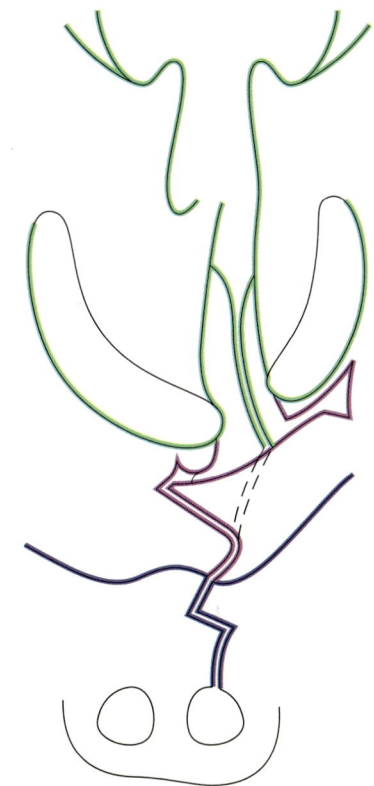

Fig. 2

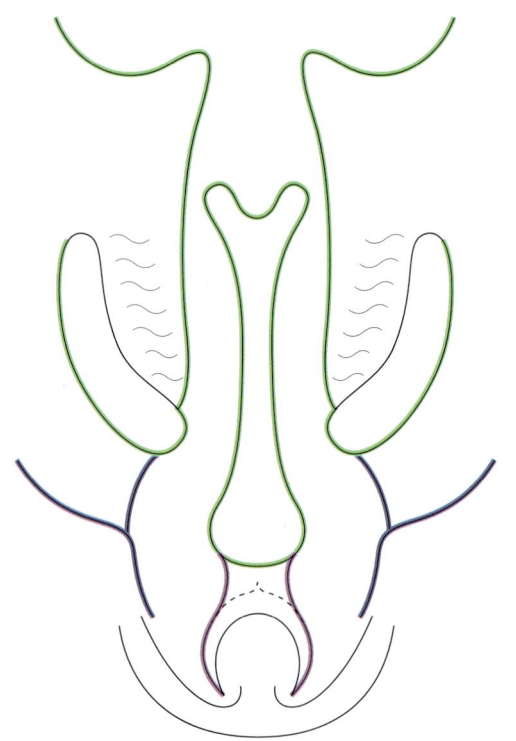

Fig. 3

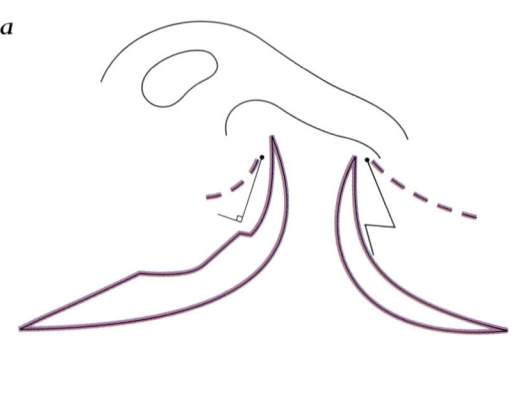

a

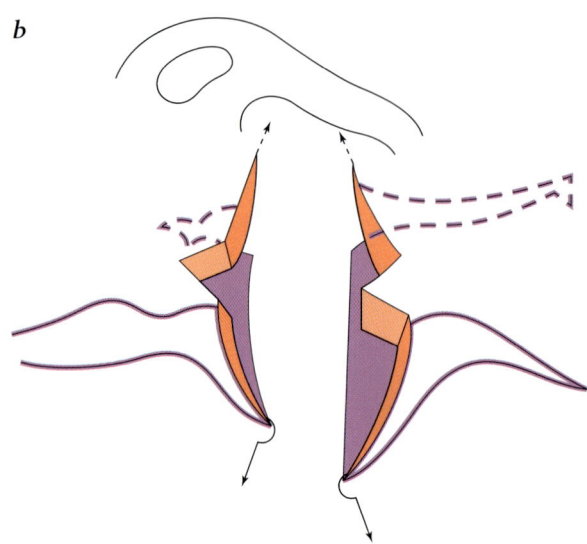

b

Fig. 4a and b
a. The incision.
b. The inferior triangular flap.

I GENERAL

1. Circumstances of the initial examination

THE ANTENATAL EXAMINATION

Due to improvements in ultrasound techniques and to its present routine use during the second trimester of pregnancy, a cleft lip/palate is often diagnosed before birth. Research in embryology has established that the fetus is completely formed after 2 months of gestation, and it is therefore possible to make a very early diagnosis of this anomaly. In most cases, however, the defect is not detected until some time between the fourth and sixth months, when ultrasound is generally first performed. It is at this point that the consulting surgeon in a cleft palate center first comes into contact with the prospective parents.

As soon as the diagnosis is made, often after a second examination that confirms the first, the ultrasound radiologist feels bound to inform the parents of his findings. However, the pros and cons of this practice bear discussion.

Detection of a cleft lip depends on a clear coronal view of the infant's face. This is often a problem, since it requires accurate orientation of the probe and may be also hindered by the position of the fetus. The cleft shows up as a gap in the labial muscle layer and may include a division of the nasal floor on one or both sides (Fig. 1.1). When a profile view is obtained, it may reveal a forward position of the premaxilla, which is particularly pronounced in bilabial clefts.

It is far more difficult to confirm the presence of a cleft palate, whether isolated or combined with a cleft of the lip and alveolus. Retrognathia with a slightly posterior position of the tongue may provide an indication. If the examiner is fortunate enough to

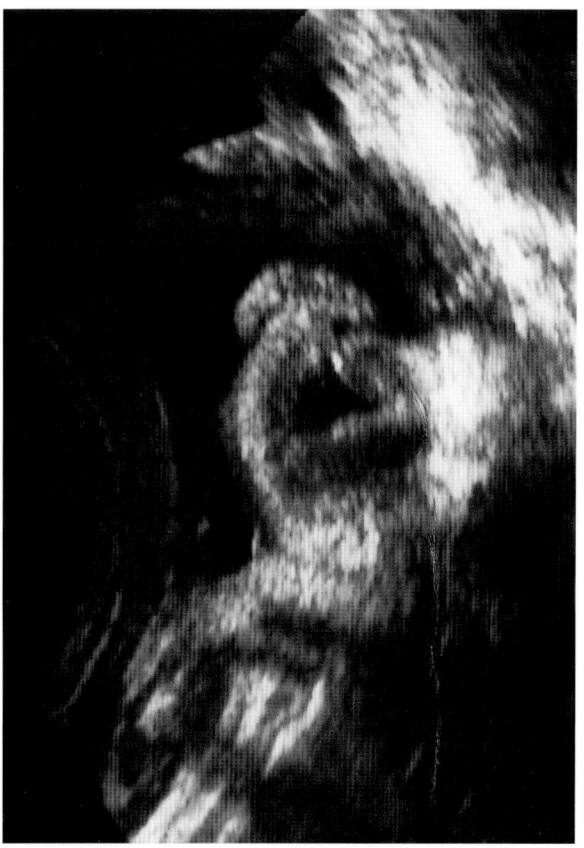

Fig. 1.1 *Left unilateral complete cleft discovered at ultrasound examination.*

observe the swallowing process, a telltale upward and backward movement of the tongue may be seen, which might suggest the existence of a cleft palate

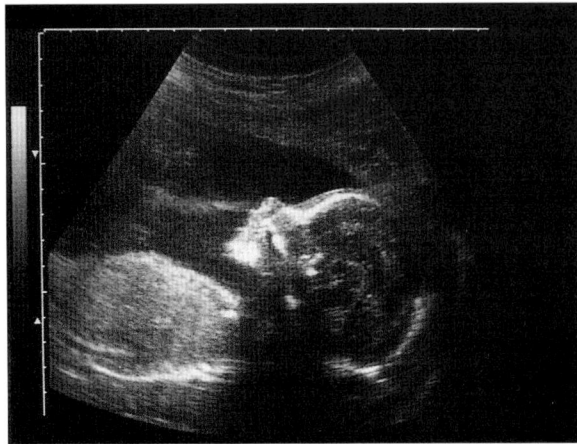

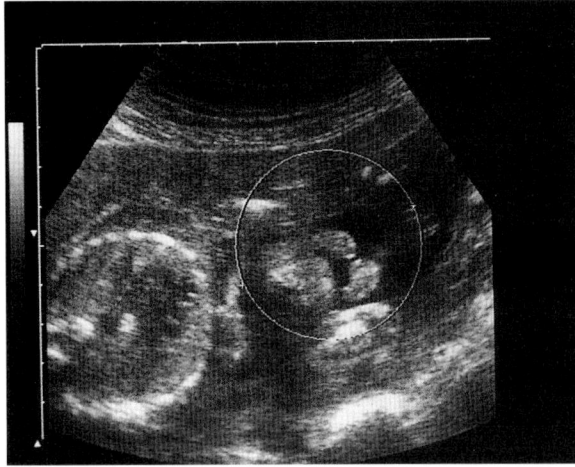

Fig. 1.2 Indirect signs can only indicate the suspicion of an associated cleft palate:
—retrognathia;
—displacement of the tongue backward.

(Fig. 1.2). In most cases, confirmation of this diagnosis is postponed until after birth; nonetheless, it is important to point out the consequences of such a malformation before the child is born.

Thus far, there is no treatment that can be applied *in utero* although a number of specialists are presently investigating the possibilities. Prenatal surgery would be doubly beneficial. The parents would never actually see the malformation, and would thus be spared major psychological distress and, above all, as a result of *in utero* experimentation on animals, many surgeons are convinced that scarring can eventually be reduced if not altogether eliminated. Still, for the time being this prospect lies in the distant future.

Parental reactions

Once the diagnosis has been communicated, the parents find themselves in a state of acute distress. Their anxiety is heightened by the information that further examinations (amniocentesis, for instance) are necessary to investigate the possibility of associated malformations. A certain number of parents may contemplate terminating the pregnancy. Since legalized voluntary abortion permits the elimination of normal embryos, they feel justified in rejecting an abnormal child. They have no clear idea of the difference between an embryo and a foetus. (Is this a valid distinction in the case of one and the same individual?) In many countries, present legislation does not authorize abortion at the stage of pregnancy that corresponds to the usual time of ultrasound diagnosis. Nevertheless, due to the ongoing debate on abortion ethics, there is no denying that a loophole does exist since grave psychological repercussions for the mother and/or child can be a criterion. Furthermore, legislation differs widely in neighboring countries so that, in actual fact, the abortion can simply be performed elsewhere. Although no statistics are available, a decision to abort can and regrettably does sometimes follow a prenatal diagnosis of cleft lip.

Even without resorting to such an extreme, parents are exposed to considerable psychological trauma on learning of the malformation. On the other hand, it is thought that an early diagnosis helps to prepare them for the birth to come. Above all, it is important to convince them of the relatively benign nature of the anomaly and then reassure them as to the beneficial effects of later treatment. Experienced teams have been trained to perform this task with praiseworthy efficiency. However, it must be granted that, before birth, the infant is not present in the flesh; nor have the parental feelings which alleviate the trauma of a malformation had time to take root. Once the newborn is on the scene, parental imagination no longer runs rampant.

Be that as it may, prenatal diagnosis is now routine. The question of when is the most opportune moment to inform the parents remains open to discussion, and depends on their state of mind. Theoretically, the information should not be communicated too early on in the pregnancy; a few weeks before birth allows for the aforementioned psychological preparation, which has widely acknowledged benefits. On the other hand, present legislation must be revised. In our day and age, a practitioner – the ultrasound radiologist in this instance – cannot withhold a diagnosis for any length of time without risking prosecution. Moreover, without such a diagnosis, additional examinations would no doubt be deemed superfluous.

To summarize these remarks on the prenatal diagnosis, a quotation from Cicero seems particularly apt:

Ne utile quidem est scire quid futurum sit. Miserum est emine nihil proficientem angi (It is not useful to know what is going to happen; it is quite wretched to be tormented without gaining anything from it).

THE EXAMINATION AT BIRTH

There is nothing urgent about the examination in the maternity ward. Nor is there the slightest need, as frequently occurs, for the child to be rushed to the hospital or cleft palate center complete with a motorcycle escort! Still, especially in cases where the family were not forewarned by a prenatal diagnosis, rapid examination of the infant is advisable in order to reassure the distressed parents, satisfy their questions and set up a program of treatment.

Obstetricians, midwives and the family physician share a key responsibility in the choice of the surgeon called in to examine the newborn. The initial operations are of major importance to these children's future (after all, no two surgeons are alike...); however, as yet there exists no foregone consensus on the treatment that might best guarantee a favorable outcome for these infants. The choice of surgeon is therefore essential, and it is disturbing to see that the decision can be determined by such factors as the distance between a given hospital and the parents' place of residence. It is equally distressing to find social security agencies pressuring parents to opt for the closest available center simply to reduce the costs of transportation.

The prime purpose of the examination is to identify the exact anatomo-clinical form of the cleft.

In complete forms, initial photographs are helpful in evaluating the width of the bony cleft and in documenting its spontaneous evolution towards transverse narrowing. The width of the palatal cleft and the size of the velar stumps are also noted. Photography is obviously difficult at this early age, and may arouse parental resentment if performed in the maternity ward. If need be, it can be postponed until a later examination. The detection of associated malformations is conducted in collaboration with the pediatrician. The investigation must be as thorough as possible. When new lesions crop up at each successive examination, the psychological impact can be disastrous.

Interviewing the parents

The interview with the parents must focus on events (whether medical or not) that may have occurred during the first 2 months of pregnancy. It is important to emphasize the accidental nature of the malformation, which can seldom be explained. This helps to relieve the parents of the guilt they inevitably feel. Hereditary forms are rare, and account for only 10–15% of cases.

Depending on the clinical form of the anomaly, a therapeutic program is set up. Despite their legitimate desire to see the problem solved as quickly as possible, the parents are usually willing to admit the necessary delays entailed in the series of operations. Their feeling of parental responsibility helps them to accept a certain period of waiting provided it is essential to the infant's welfare. In our practice, there is generally an initial interval of 3 months between birth and the first operation. In complete forms, a palatal plate is installed (known as a passive appliance since it is not intended to modify the bony segments). This maintains the width of the cleft and, on a psychological level, gives the parents peace of mind. The plate simplifies feeding since the infant can compress the teat of the baby bottle against it with his or her tongue.

Feeding instructions are extremely important. The parents must understand the sucking problems linked to bucco-nasal communication, if such is the case. The teat must be properly perforated, and feeding takes place in a vertical position to facilitate swallowing. It goes without saying that gavage is proscribed despite the advice of certain practitioners who are less famil-iar with this pathology. The advantages of the so-called spoon-bottle (teat replaced by a small spoon) must be clearly explained since normal bottle feeding is prohibited, at least temporarily, until after the series of operations (Fig. 1.3).

Finally, the long-term prognosis is broached. This is not the time to raise the prospect of secondary surgery or future follow-up, but rather an opportu-nity to convince the parents that their infant will be able to lead a normal life with a satisfactory facial appearance.

If conducted in this way, the initial examination should reassure the parents and guarantee a cooper-ative relationship with the surgical team. The surgeon must remain open to the many questions left hanging

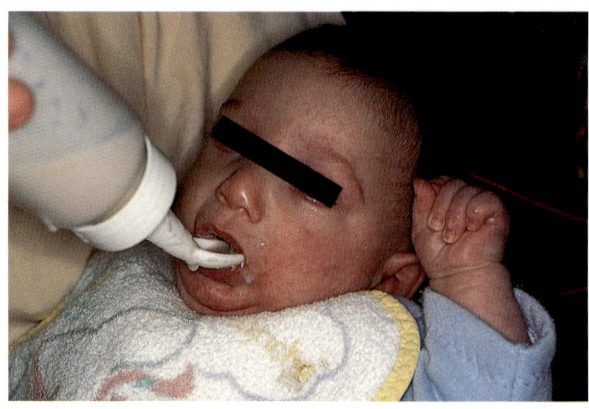

Fig. 1.3 *The spoon-bottle.*

during this key encounter, which is always fraught with emotion.

2. Embryology

INTRODUCTION

It is not the author's purpose to sum up the present state of embryological research, and nor do I intend to delve into what remains to be discovered. I would simply like to contribute to a clear understanding of the anatomo-clinical forms of cleft lip and palate, although we do not presume to furnish a full explanation of their original cause.

The 'classic' account of development, proposed by Dursy (1869) and His (1874), remains the most comprehensive, if not necessarily the most accurate. These authors contended that embryological mesenchymal processes migrate towards one another to form the facial structures at the fore end of the embryo. These processes are covered with ectoderm and, as they come together, their epithelial layers are brought into contact. At these points of apposition, the epithelium disintegrates so that fusion can occur between the mesenchymal masses.

This theory was heatedly contested before and after World War II. Veau (1936) subscribed to the theories of Hochstetter (1944), who held that, prior to the development of a cleft, there existed an original continuous layer of epithelium. Hochstetter believed that this original tissue was later colonized by the mesenchyme. A defect in the progression of the mesoderm and its associated blood supply was thought to be the factor responsible for the disintegration of the epithelial layer and, therefore, for the existence of a cleft. In this context, it is easy to explain the presence of residual bridges or bands of tissue between the two borders, which will subse-

quently be discussed. They were believed to correspond to subsisting portions of the original epithelial covering.

The next theory to develop suggested that the mesenchymal cells were produced by the neural crests. This did little to clarify the process, but did contribute the esoteric term of 'neurochristopathies' to designate errors in cell migration and development.

Modern techniques of exploring and visually observing embryonic growth tend to support the existence of initially developed and independent growth centers or processes which fuse together or, for some reason, accidentally fail to fuse (Hinrichsen, 1963).

THE NORMAL EMBRYOLOGY OF THE FACE

At the earliest stage of formation, there is a shallow depression in the cephalic extremity of the embryo. On its upper margin there appears a rounded prominence known as the frontal process and, on its lower, a bulge that corresponds to the primitive heart. In the floor of the depression lies a membrane composed of a double layer of epithelial tissue, which separates the surface of the embryo from the cavity of the primitive foregut. This two-layered membrane, known as the oral plate, gradually undergoes spontaneous rupture, no doubt due to the rapid outward growth of the elements developing around its margins. This primitive oral opening or mouth is called the

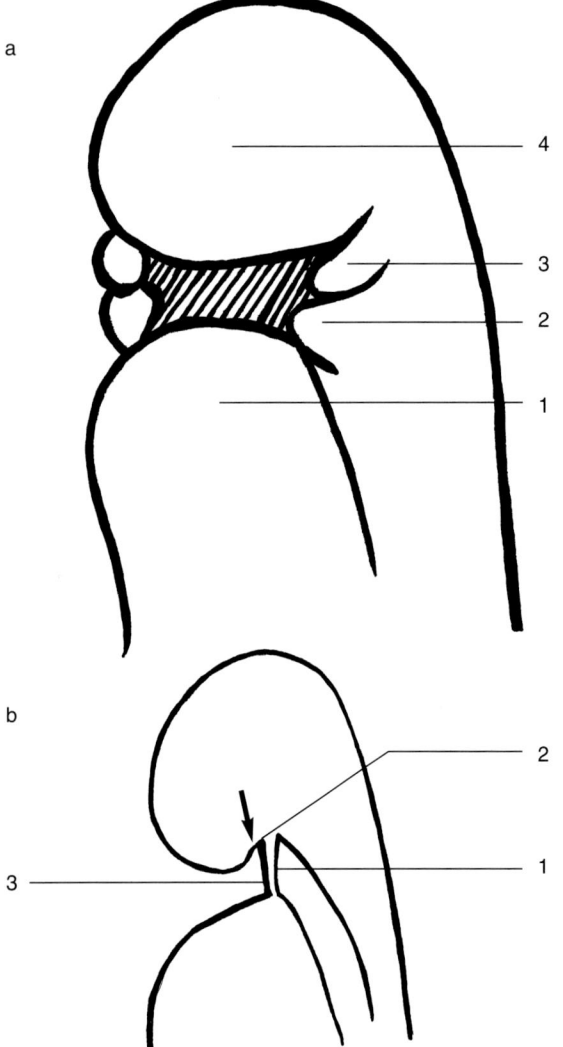

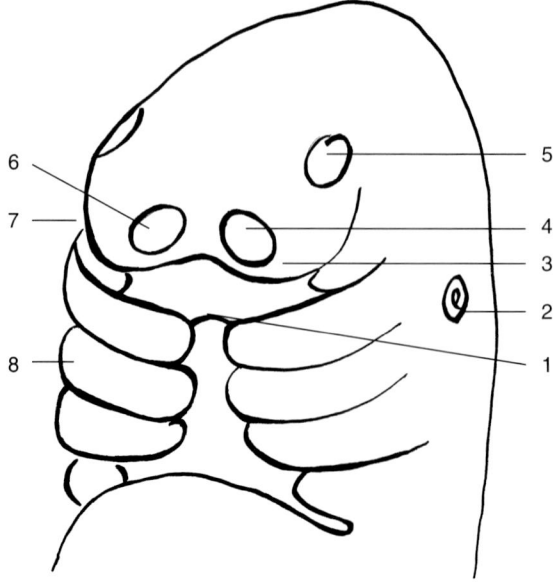

Fig. 2.2 *Development of the branchial arches. The first arch produces the maxillary and mandibular processes; the second is the hyoid arch.*

1. Endo-ectodermal function
2. Otic depression
3. Lateral nasal fold
4. Nasal placode
5. Lens placode
6. Olfactory pit
7. Naso lateral process
8. Hyoid arch

Fig. 2.1 *The primitive mouth or stomodeum: a. 3/4 view and bordering elements (frontal process, maxillary and mandibular processes, pericardiac bulge). b. Profile: The stomodeum closes the front end of the primitive foregut. The arrow marks the position of Rathke's pouch, which gives rise to the ectodermal portion of the pituitary gland.*

a
1. Pericardic bulge
2. Mandibular process
3. Maxillary process
4. Frontal process

b
1. Endoderm
2. Rathke's pocket
3. Ectoderm

stomodeum (Fig. 2.1a). The stomodeal depression rapidly deepens as the frontal process develops (Fig. 2.1b).

A number of thickenings or elevations can be distinguished on the ventral surface of the frontal process. These elevations curve together and merge on the midline to form a series of arches separated by deep grooves, which resemble fish gills (hence the term 'gill clefts' or, more accurately, branchial grooves) (Fig. 2.2). The branchial arches eventually close into a tube which forms, in order from top to bottom, the nasal fossae, the mouth and the pharynx. The rostral portion of the tube gives rise to the facial structures (primarily derived from the first or mandibular arch) and, behind the facial elements, the

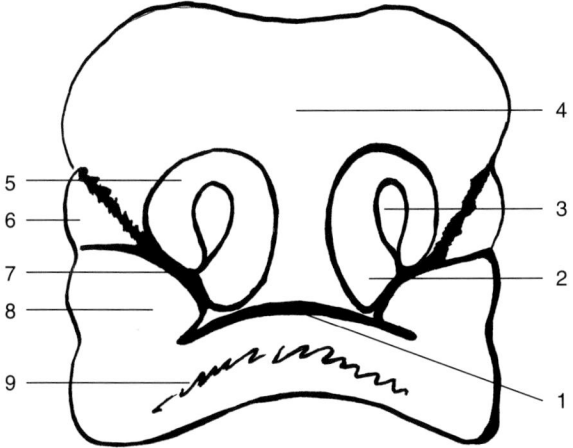

Fig. 2.3 *Development of the nasomedial and nasolateral processes around the olfactory orifices (nares).*

1. *Mouth cleft*
2. *Medial nasal process*
3. *Primitive anterior naris*
4. *Frontal nasal process*
5. *Lateral nasal fold*
6. *Eye*
7. *Medial nasal fold*
8. *Maxillary process*
9. *Mandibular process*

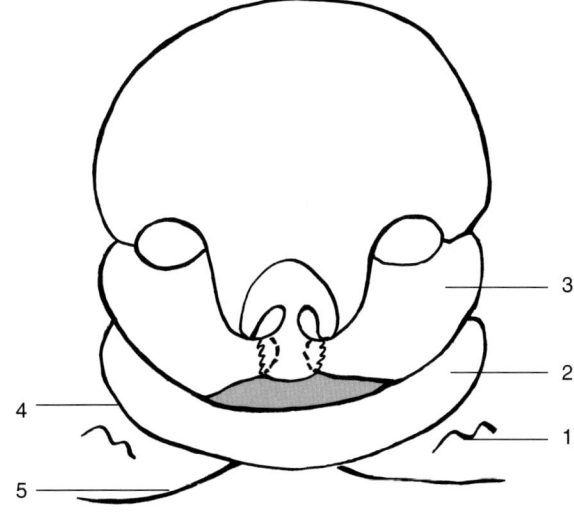

Fig. 2.4 *The face between the seventh and eighth weeks of gestation. The upper lip is derived from the superior maxillary processes and the nasomedial processess (which form the prolabium).*

1. *Beginning of the ear lobe*
2. *Mandibular process*
3. *Maxillary process*
4. *Hyomandibular cleft*
5. *Hyomandibular arch*

processes gradually cover the initial portion of the digestive tube to produce the anterior section of the neck. Thus, the true anterior orifice of the digestive tube (or oral opening) is displaced forward at a considerable distance from the original opening. The stomodeum eventually corresponds to the isthmus of fauces, or tonsillar isthmus, which separates the mouth from the oropharynx. The prime importance of this major functional center will be examined in a later section (Chapter 15).

On the twenty-fourth day of embryonic life, this primitive mouth opening is delimited by the frontal process above it, and by structures emerging from the first arch – i.e. below it the mandibular process, and laterally the two superior maxillary processes. The latter are the only paired primordia which do not fuse in their anterior portion, because they are separated by the nasomedial processes which originate in the frontal process. At the cephalic extremity of the embryo, more medial than the oculary placodes, two horse-shoe-shaped elevations develop, one on either side, which become the nostrils (or external nares). The outer portion of the nostrils represent the nasolateral processes, which merge with the upper portion of the superior maxillary processes to produce the nasal alae. The nasomedial process contributes to the formation of the nasal sill, and grows downward with its paired counterpart into the space between the superior maxillary processes (Fig. 2.3).

Towards the forty-eighth day, formation of the upper lip is completed through fusion of the two superior maxillary and the two nasomedial processes. The latter produce the medial portion of the upper lip, corresponding to the philtrum and the Cupid's bow, as well as the premaxilla. The maxillary and mandibular processes, which are initially separated, fuse together horizontally. Fusion stops at the corners of the lips (Fig. 2.4).

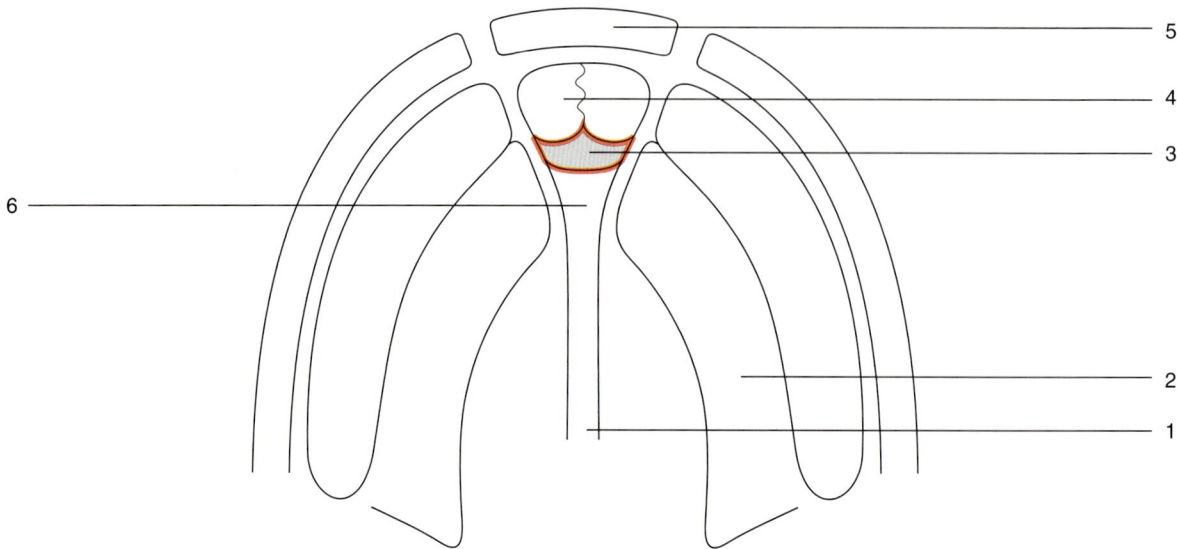

Fig. 2.5 *Intra-oral view. The philtrum of the upper lip, the premaxilla and primary palate (anterior palatine processes of the premaxillary bones) derived from the nasomedial processes. The lateral palatine processes of the upper maxilla give rise to the secondary palate.*

1. *Nasal septum*
2. *Palatal shelves*
3. *Primary palate (median palatine processes)*
4. *Premaxilla*
5. *Prolabium*
6. *Site of the anterior palatine foramen*

On a deeper level, the superior maxillary processes give rise to the jaws and alveolar ridge with the exception of its central portion, the premaxilla, which originates in the nasomedial process and carries the incisor teeth. The upper maxillary processes also produce palatine processes, from which shelf-like outgrowths advance towards the midline. These are the palatal shelves, which come to separate the oral cavity from the nasal fossae.

To its rear, the premaxilla emits a small anterior palatine process. Coupled with its counterpart from the opposite side into a double process, it forms a segment called the primary palate – as opposed to the secondary palate, which arises from the lateral palatine processes. At the junction of the three components of the palate lies the anterior palatine or incisive suture, which represents the center of this evolution. It will later figure in the study of clinical forms of the malformation. The line where the components of the palate fuse forms the shape of a 'Y'. Its branches embrace those elements that arise from the nasomedial process (Fig. 2.5). Once the paired branchial arches merge together on the midline, they constitute the anterior portion of the digestive tube, the mouth and the pharynx.

As a brief reminder, the different branchial arches undergo the following evolution:

• The first arch is subdivided into an upper portion, which corresponds to the superior maxillary process, and a lower mandibular portion. The point at which these two sections of the first arch cease to fuse determines the site of the oral opening. The body of the tongue develops within

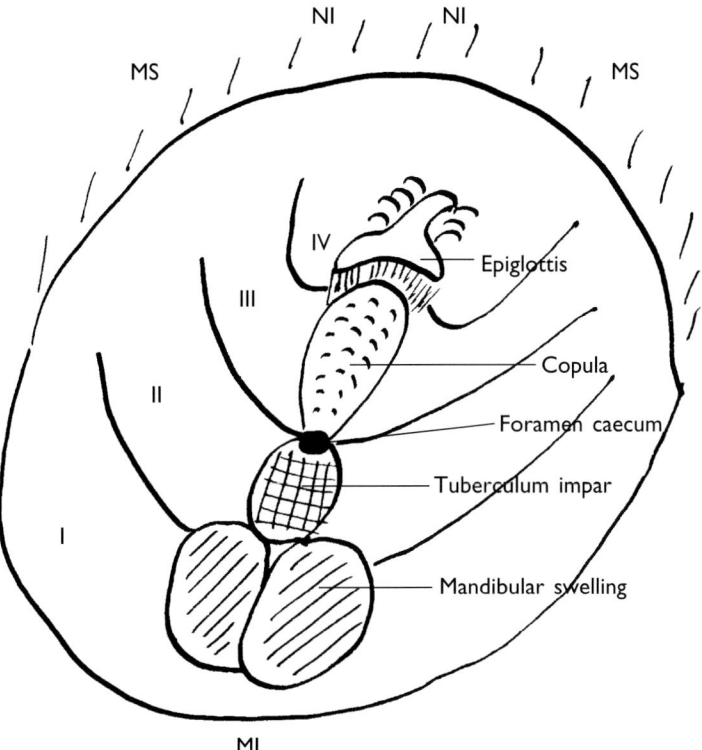

Fig. 2.6 *The primitive tongue in the floor of the oral cavity showing the lingual processes of the first arches, the tuber-culum impar of the second, and the copula of third and fourth arches. The primitive epiglottis is between the copula and the arytenoid processes. The foramen caecum is visible at the lingual V between the copula and tuberculum impar.*

the curve formed by the union of the paired mandibular arches.

• The second arch produces the superficial facial muscles, which can be said to envelop those structures that originate from the first arch. The tuberculum impar is a small medial component that contributes to the formation of the tongue.

• Arches three and four merge in a thick bulge, or copula, which produces the base of the tongue. The copula is separated from the tuberculum impar by a blind recess (foramen caecum), and from the underlying embryonic structure (arytenoid processes) by a zone that gives rise to the epiglottis (Fig. 2.6).

The airway, and particularly the larynx, originates as an evagination of the digestive tube, which develops forward and downward. It is initially situated between the epiglottis and the arytenoid processes.

Massive growth of the cephalic process and of those processes just described causes a right-angled flexion to appear between the first four arches and the underlying embryonic structures, which creates the neck. This cervico-cephalic angulation is located at the level of the hyoid bone and the epiglottis at the base of the fourth branchial arch.

From an embryological point of view, the tongue is composed of three elements:

1. The body and the tip arise from the lingual processes, which are derived from the mandibular portion of the first arch.
2. The tuberculum impar, which shares the same origin, is separated from the zone which is followed by the foramen cecum.
3. The copula, which forms the base of the tongue, is derived from the third and fourth arches. It is separated from the arytenoid processes by the

a

b

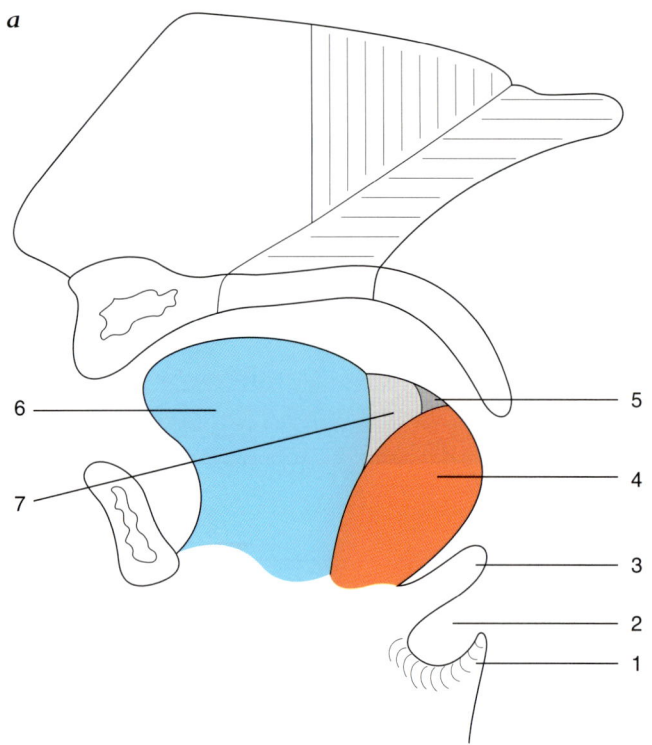

Fig. 2.7 *a Embryological components of the tongue.*
b Dorsal view of the tongue.

a

1.   *Arytenoid swelling*
2.   *Trachea*
3.   *Epiglottis*
4.   *Copula 3rd–4th arches*
5.   *Foramen caecum*
6.   *Mandibular swelling*
7.   *Tuberculum impar*

b

1.   *Vallecula*
2.   *Glosso epiglottic fold*
3.   *Sulcus terminalis*
4.   *Vallate papillae*
5.   *Foramen caecum*
6.   *Epiglottis*

epiglottis. Between these two elements, an evagination of the digestive tube produces the trachea and respiratory apparatus (Figs 2.7a and b).

The evolution of the embryo may seem highly complex. Its study, however, provides useful background information for a better understanding of how and why malformations of the facial structures occur; in particular, cleft lip and palate and the potential associated anomalies specific to them.

The figures that accompany this section do not presume to be models of precise detail, but they furnish what we hope are helpful illustrations of the material discussed.

PATHOLOGICAL EMBRYOLOGY

A basic background in normal embryology permits a better understanding of the pathological anatomy of clefts.

The site of the cleft

The site of the cleft theoretically corresponds to the lines along which the embryonic processes fuse together.

'Classic' authors establish a fundamental distinction between the primary and the secondary palates. As Victor Veau (1936) pointed out, these two zones undergo different embryonic evolutions. The primary palate corresponds to elements derived from the nasomedial processes, and which are located in front of the anterior palatine (incisive) suture. This term, therefore, includes structures such as the lip and alveolar ridge, which are not part of the palate in the strict sense. The secondary palate is derived solely from lateral palatine processes, and corresponds to the bony palatal shelves.

It is easy to understand why we are not fully satisfied with this rather hazy nomenclature. For most people, the palate represents the anatomical region that is encompassed by the alveolar ridges and lies strictly within their limits. It would therefore no doubt be less confusing to choose another set of terms for these two embryonic zones – for instance, superficial (alveolar ridge and lip) and deep (palate). The term 'primary palate' would be reserved for that small bony median palatal triangle which originates in the anterior palatine outgrowth of the nasomedial processes and is not derived from the palatal shelves of the superior maxillary process (Hamilton *et al.*, 1964) (Fig. 2.8).

- A cleft that occurs in the superficial zone is always lateral, and is situated on the line of fusion between the maxillary and nasomedial processes in front of the anterior palatine foramen. The parents are usually told that the cleft passes through the growth centre of the lateral incisor tooth to prepare them for potential bifidity or absence of the tooth, a frequent finding. This phenomenon is not easy to explain from an embryological point of view, since the four incisors are produced by the premaxilla (composed of the paired premaxillary bones). There is no trace of elements derived from the nasomedial processes on the lateral segments. Veau (1938) did refer to the fact that this question had aroused considerable debate, but concluded that it was not of any great significance. Be that as it may, there is almost always a 'pre-canine' tooth on the lesser segment (Fig. 2.9). If the premaxilla contains a lateral incisor, it is generally abnormal and is situated above the level of the central incisor. It tends to be undersized and decayed-

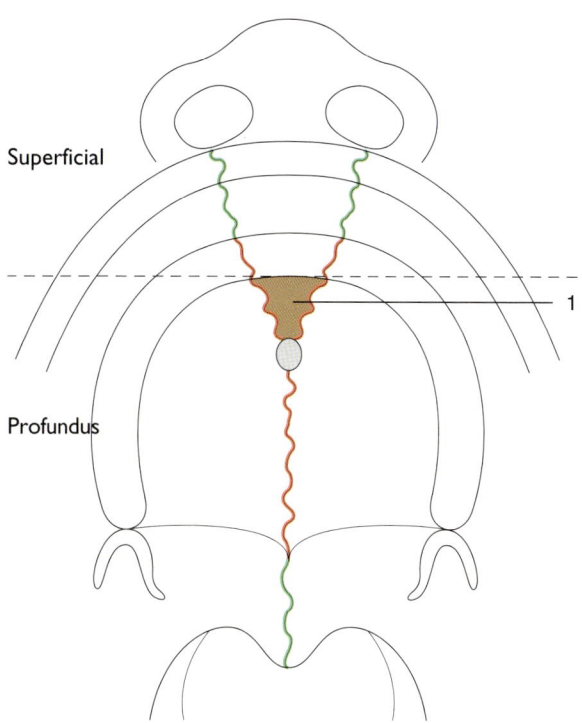

Fig. 2.8 *Fusion line of processes. The primary palate is between the branches of the 'Y' in front of the anterior palatine foramen (for classic authors).*

1.   *The true primary palate.*

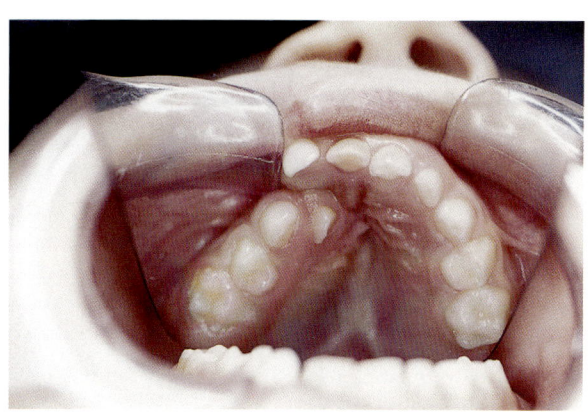

Fig. 2.9 *Split lateral incisor on the lesser segment.*

looking, often jutting out sideways. At times, it emerges high inside the cleft on the level of the nostril sill. It is usually removed in the course of lip surgery (Fig. 2.10).

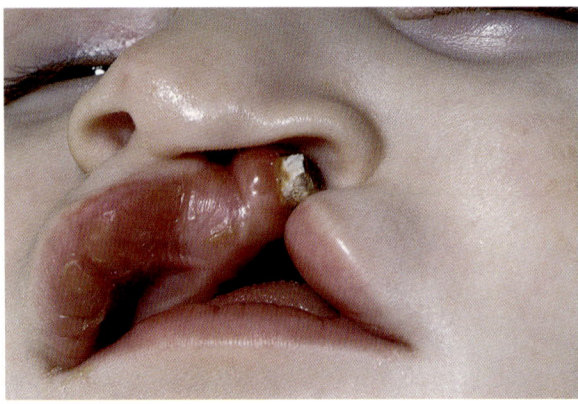

Fig. 2.10 *Abnormal tooth on the premaxilla (split lateral incisor or supernumerary tooth bud).*

- A deep cleft concerns the palate and, unlike the superficial cleft, it is always median. It follows the line of fusion where the lateral palatine processes should unite, and is located behind the anterior palatine suture, which separates the small retro-alveolar zone of the primary palate from the rest of the vault. The lower border of the vomer is attached to a palatal shelf to a greater or lesser degree, depending on whether the cleft is uni- or bilateral (Fig. 2.11). It is thought that the muscles of the soft palate develop before the palatal shelves have reached a significant size, which might explain their abnormal insertion along the margins of the cleft (Veau's fissural muscle).

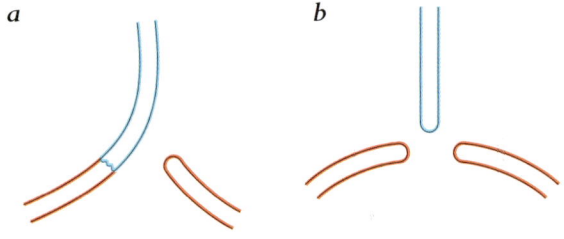

Fig. 2.11 *Palatal cleft: a. Unilateral cleft palate, where the lower border of the vomer is attached to one palatal shelf. b. Bilateral cleft palate, where the lower border of the vomer is free of any attachment.*

The size of the cleft

Whatever the original reasons for the failure of the embryonic processes to fuse (lack of intimate contact, secondary disintegration of epithelial tissue that has not been colonized by the highly vascularized mesenchyme), the initial dimensions of the cleft are never as wide as they eventually are at the time of birth. It seems that the space between the margins of the cleft is gradually widened by two main factors:

1. Distorted traction of the facial muscles due to the effect of the cleft, and the resultant abnormal insertions.
2. Lingual pressure exerted when the tongue intrudes between the bony elements, which are not fixed but mobile due to the gap in the superior maxillary processes (as is the case in complete clefts).

The parents can therefore be reassured that the size of the cleft does not indicate a corresponding loss of tissue. Consequently, it is possible to re-establish a virtually normal anatomical structure by using the tissues that already exist along the margins of the gap without resorting to a graft. There is, however, a variable degree of tissue hypoplasia, and this is obvious in the height deficit of the lip, for instance. This defect in development involves all three dimensions. Whatever their location, congenital malformations all share this characteristic.

Anatomical distinctions

From an anatomical standpoint, a distinction is made between the bone structure and the soft tissues.

The bone structure, when observed from below (i.e. the endobuccal view), presents two distinct sections: The alveolar ridge or dental arch, which encloses the second zone, the bony palatal vault. The alveolar ridge is composed of the two superior maxillary processes and the two intermaxillary bones, which form the premaxilla. The bony palatal vault consists of the palatine processes of the upper maxilla, which are separated from the intermaxillary segment by the anterior palatine foramen, and the palatal shelves of the palatine bones.

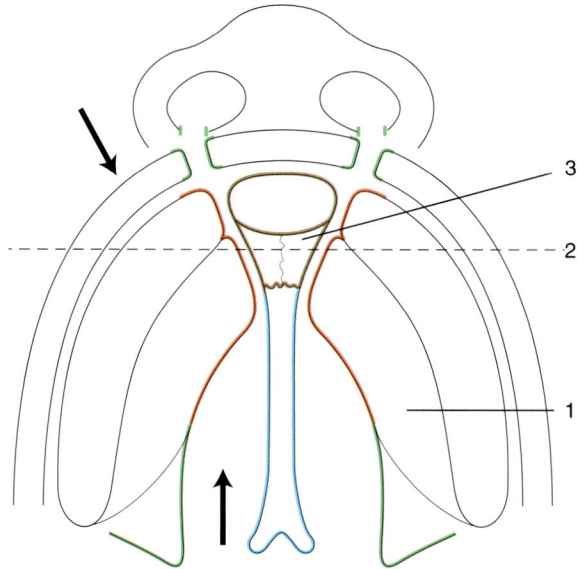

Fig. 2.12 Simple clefts involve soft tissue only (the lip, nostril sill and soft palate). A cleft is classified as complete if the bone tissue is affected (the alveolar ridge and palatal shelves). The severity of the cleft increases as it converges on the anterior palatine foramen: from the outer surface, for the lip and alveolar ridge, from front to back; from the uvula, for the soft and hard palate, from back to front.

1. Palatine process
2. Level of the anterior palatine foramen
3. Premaxilla and its palatine process

The soft tissues are also considered as two distinct sections. First, those anterior to the bone structure; the lips and the nostril sills in the extension of mucous membrane that covers the bony palatal vault on the nasal side. Labial mucosa is a continuation of the layer that covers the alveolar ridge and the palatal vault. Second, the soft palate behind the bony vault (Fig. 2.12).

A cleft that involves only the soft tissues is called a simple cleft, whereas a cleft that concerns both bony and soft tissue is known as a total or complete cleft. There is no perfect parallel between the disorders that affect each of these two elements, bone and soft tissue, and the anatomo-clinical form is determined solely on the basis of the absence or presence of lesions to the bone structure. Thus, even when the lip is only partially cleft, if the alveolar process is affected, the malformation is identified as a complete cleft.

The width of the cleft increases from the free border of the lip to the anterior palatine foramen (front to back) and, for the palate, from the uvula to the anterior palatine foramen (back to front). There are no forms of palatal cleft that begin within these two limits (uvula and anterior palatine foramen).

The distinction between simple and complete clefts permits the description of the different forms into which these two major categories are subdivided.

3. Classification and anatomo-clinical forms

All of these forms can be either unilateral or bilateral.

Initials are used to refer to the different types or forms: U = unilateral, B = bilateral, CP = cleft palate, S = simple, C = complete, L = lip, etc. The initials that correspond to the form described appear in parentheses.

We have not drawn up statistics of our own to illustrate the relative frequency of each form. To give a general idea, we have quoted the figures provided by Victor Veau on the basis of 1000 of the cases on which he performed surgery.

The clinical forms are illustrated by an inferior endobuccal view (Fig. 3.1).

Unilateral clefts

Simple cleft lip (SUCL)
Relative frequency: 27.3%.

The alveolar ridge is intact (Fig. 3.2). The cleft involves the height of the lip to some degree (Fig. 3.3a and b). The condition known as congenital scar of the

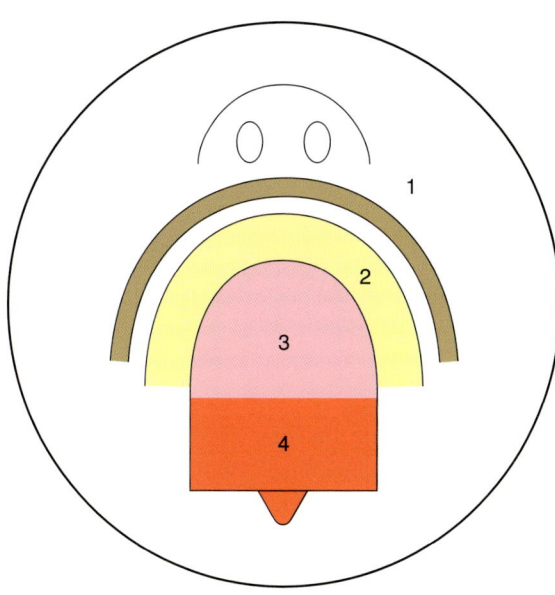

Fig. 3.1 *Diagram of structures potentially affected by a congenital cleft (seen from below).*

1. *Lip and nose*
2. *Alveolar ridge*
3. *Bony palate*
4. *Soft palate*

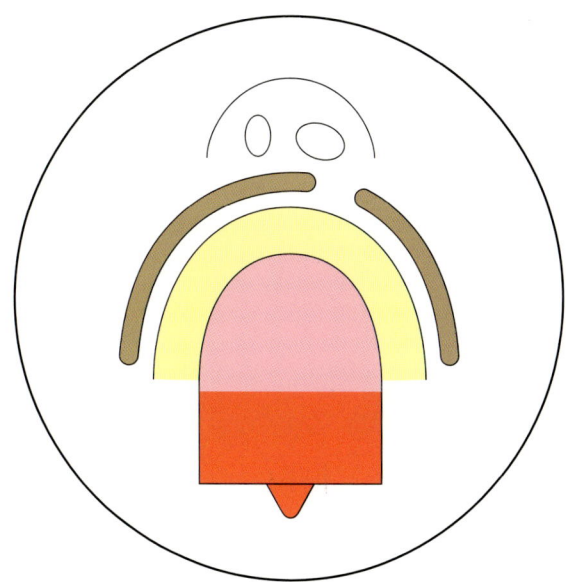

Fig. 3.2 *Simple unilateral cleft lip. Involvement of the lip and nostril sill varies.*

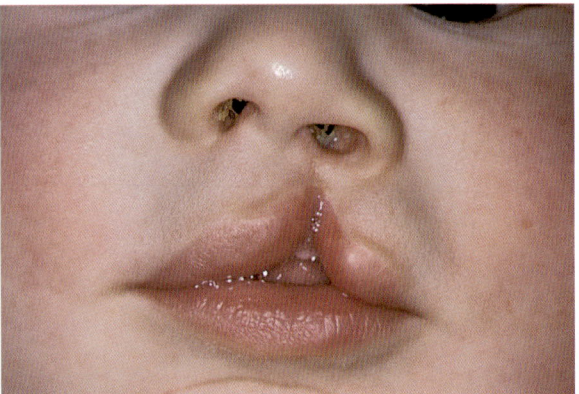

a

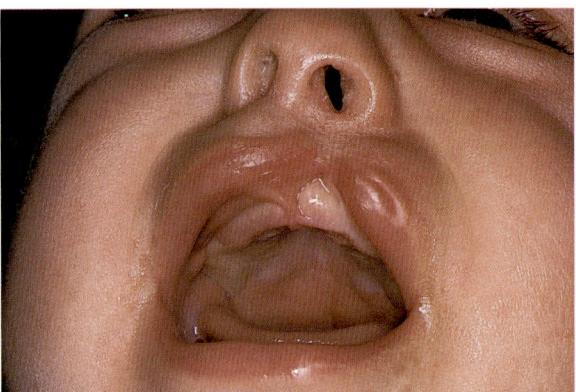

b

Fig. 3.3 *a and b Simple cleft: lip cleft three-quarters of the way, nostril deformity linked to the gap in the muscle fibers. The alveolar arch is intact.*

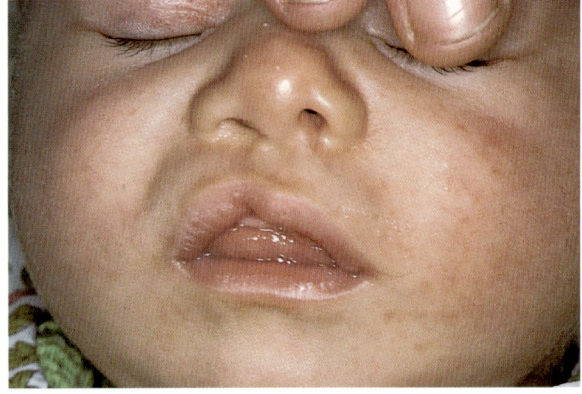

Fig. 3.4 *Congenital scar of the lip. There is no real cleft, but the furrow in the vermilion border and the nostril deformity are obvious.*

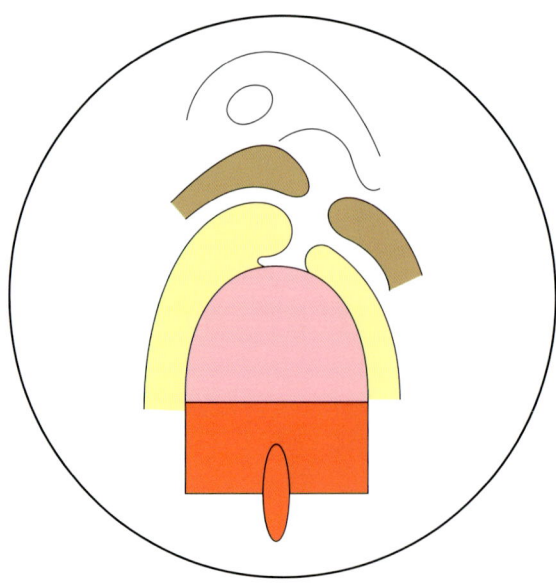

Fig. 3.5 *Complete cleft lip without cleft palate.*

lip appears merely as a furrow, which is more or less obvious on the free border of the lip (Fig. 3.4).

Complete cleft lip without cleft palate (CUCL without CP)

The lip and alveolar ridge are affected (Fig. 3.5). In the characteristic forms without a cleft palate, the cleft extends only as far as the anterior palatine foramen (Figs 3.6a and b).

There are less typical forms where the distinction between simple and complete is not clear-cut because the alveolar cleft appears only as a groove beneath a continuous layer of mucosa. It resembles a bridge with its posterior end abutting the bone (Fig. 3.7). In some cases, the clinical form cannot be identified until surgery is performed.

Simple cleft palate (SUCP)

Only the velum or soft palate is affected (Fig. 3.8a and b).

Complete cleft palate (CUCP)

Relative frequency: 0.53%.

Both the soft and the hard palate are divided. A complete palatal cleft is classified as unilateral if the

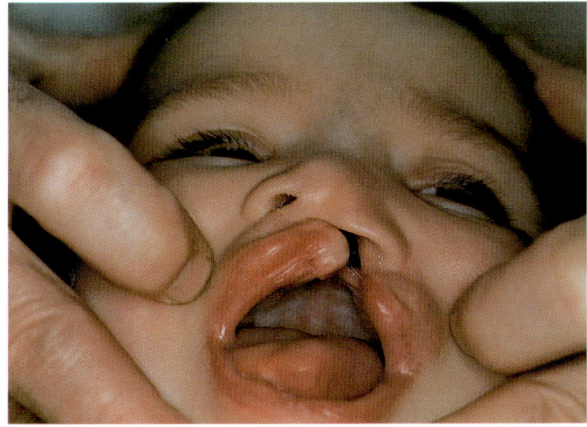

a

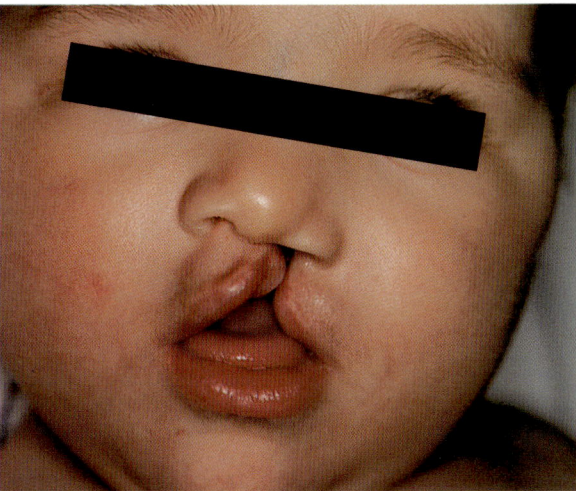

b

Fig. 3.6 *a and b Examples of complete unilateral cleft without cleft palate. Misalignment of the borders and nasal deformity are pronounced. Notice the anterior edge of the intact palatal shelf.*

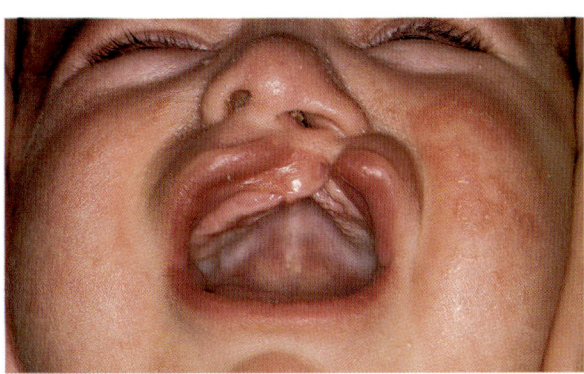

Fig. 3.7 *Complete unilateral cleft (complete division of bone structures), but a 'bridge' or band of soft tissue exists at the nostril sill.*

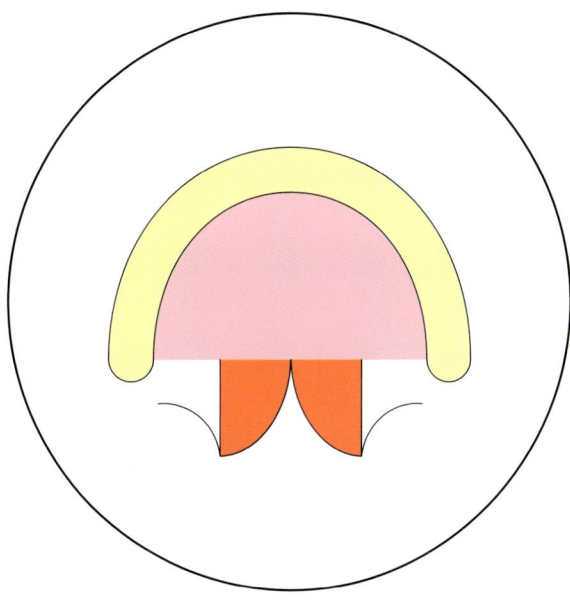

a

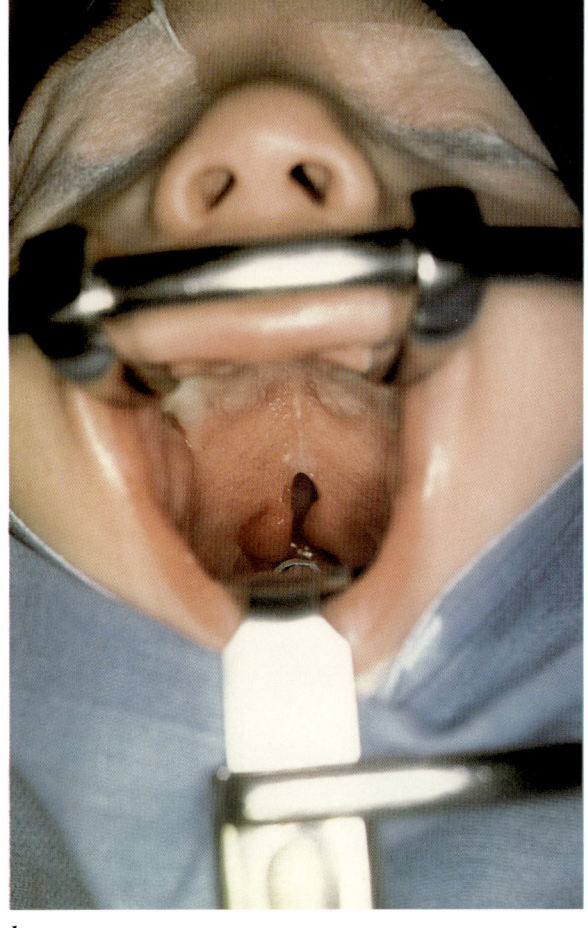

b

Fig. 3.8 *a and b Isolated simple cleft palate: strictly velar or posterior palatal cleft.*

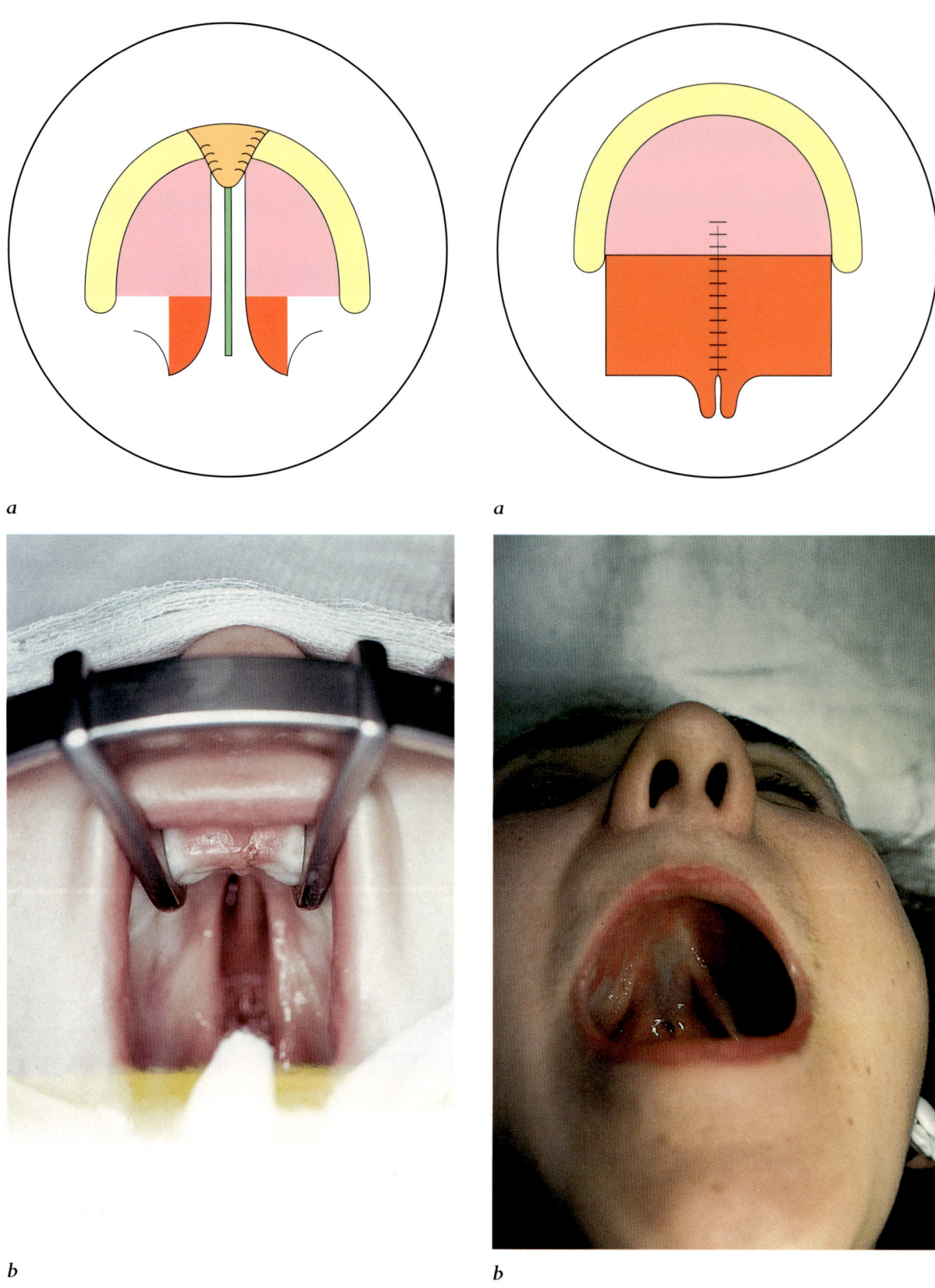

a

b

a

b

Fig. 3.9 *a and b Complete cleft palate involving the bone structure of the vault. The lower free border of the vomer is visible.*

Fig. 3.10 *a and b Submucous cleft. Virtually the entire bony vault is affected.*

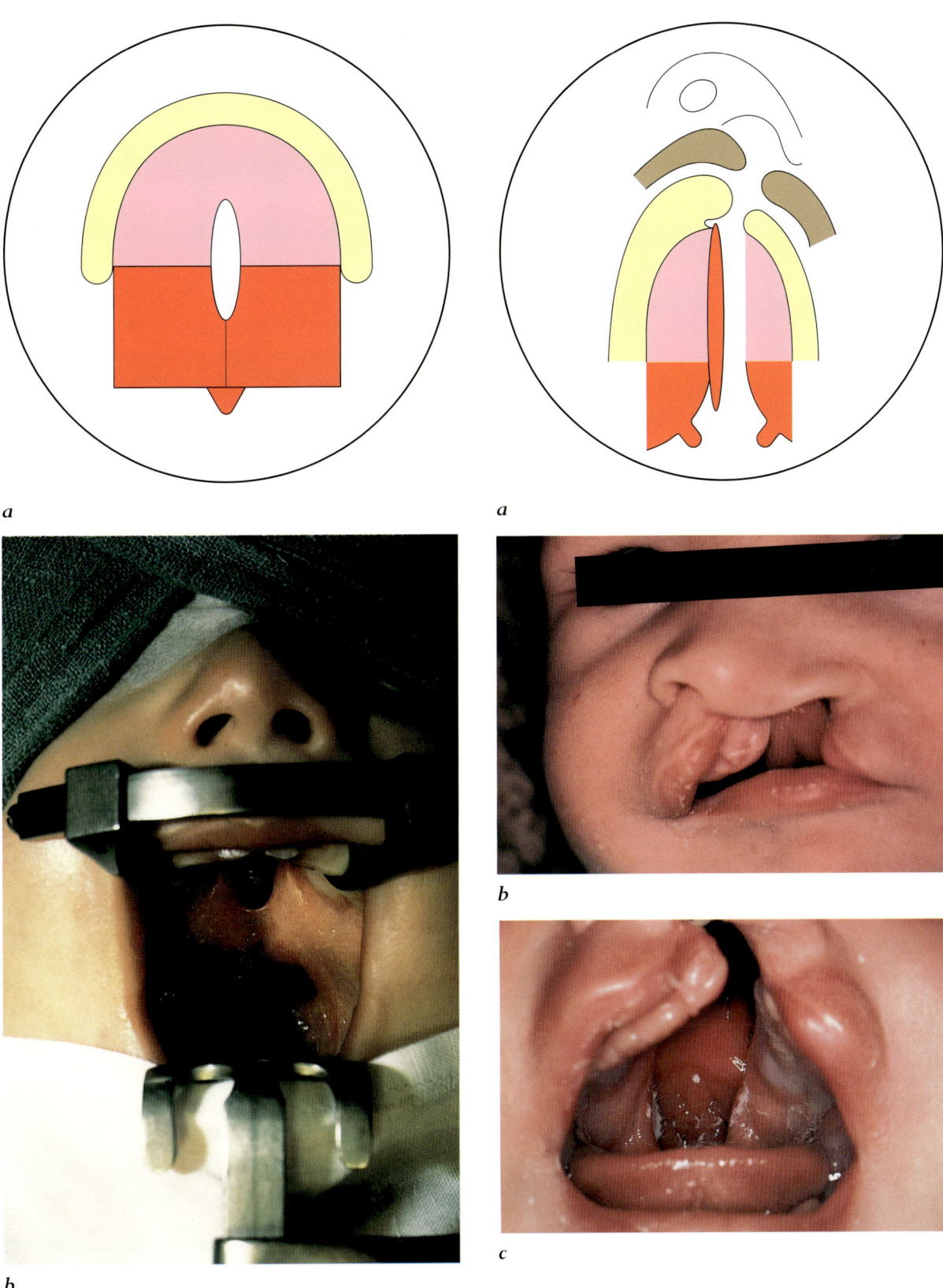

a

a

b

b

c

Fig. 3.11 *a and b Only traumatic rupture could be responsible for the absence of the mucosal layer in this submucosal cleft.*

Fig. 3.12 *a, b and c Complete labio-maxillo-palatal cleft affecting the lip, alveolar ridge, hard and soft palates. The postero-superior wall of the pharynx is visible when the mouth is opened.*

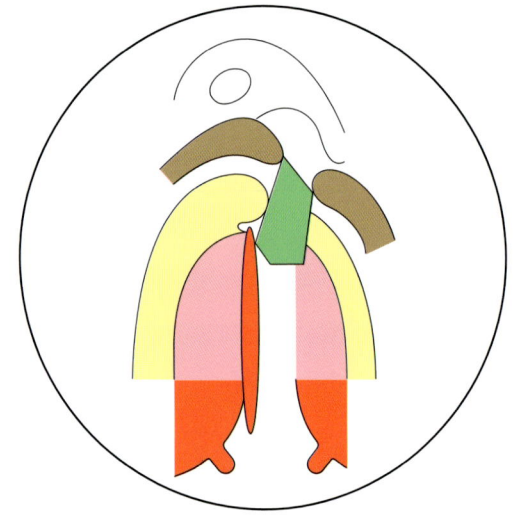

a

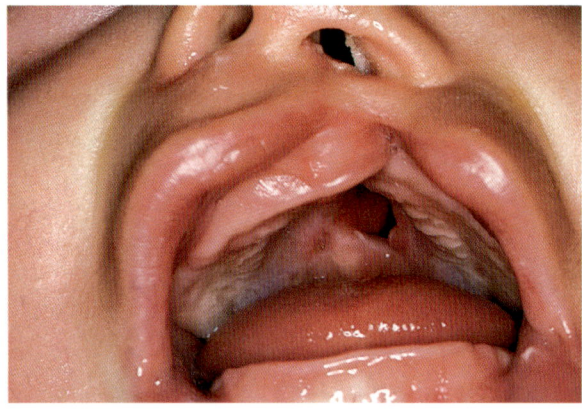

b

vomer is attached to one of the palatal shelves. When the vomer is totally separated from the palatal shelves, its lower free border can be detected between them. The cleft is then classified as bilateral, although it remains median (Fig. 3.9a and b).

In the category of isolated palatal clefts, there is a reasonably uncommon form known as the submucous cleft.

The cleft appears to affect only the uvula and a portion of the soft palate. In reality, it extends forward through the rest of the velum and into the hard palate, at times as far as the anterior palatine foramen. It is masked by a double layer of oral and nasal mucosa (Fig. 3.10a and b). It seems logical to assume that a secondary rupture in some portion of the continuous layer of these mucosae is responsible for the rare forms where a palate is non-cleft or only moderately so towards the back of the mouth is perforated in front of an apparently normal zone (Fig. 3.11a and b).

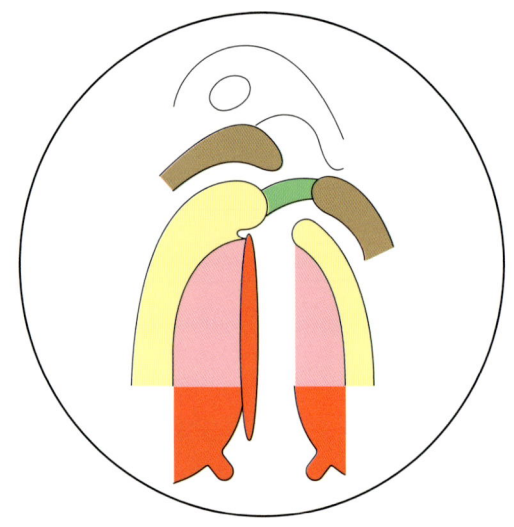

c

Fig. 3.13 *a, b and c Complete cleft with a mucocutaneous band. These bands are generally located between the alveolar borders, and are often very frail.*

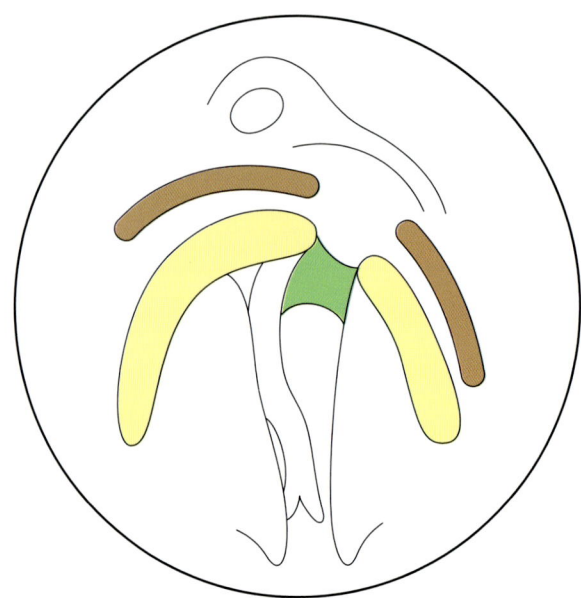

Fig. 3.14 *Mucocutaneous bands can be broad and composed strictly of soft tissue.*

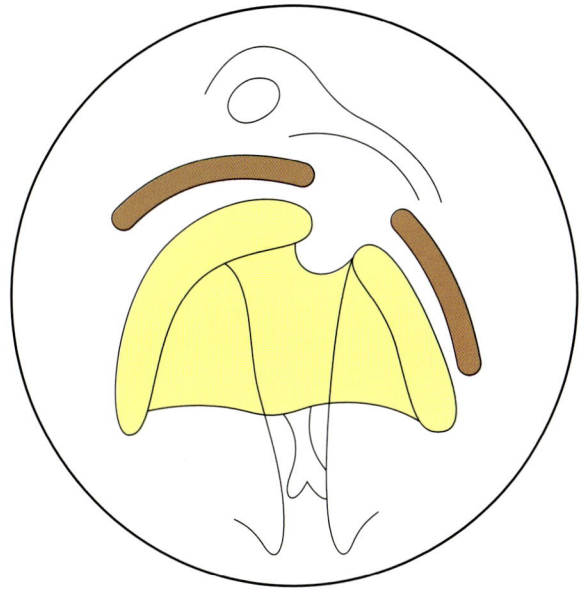

Fig. 3.15 *A rare form of lesion combining a labio-maxillary and a posterior palatal cleft. The hard palate is intact.*

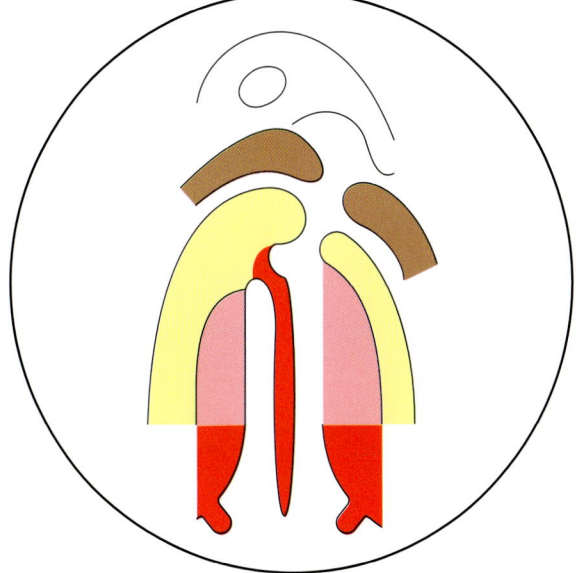

Fig. 3.16 *Unilateral labio-maxillo-palatal form with bilateral palatal cleft.*

Complete labio-alveolo-palatal cleft (CUCL + CP)

Relative frequency: 47.6% (Fig. 3.12a, b and c). Labial and palatal clefts can also be combined. The most common form is a combination of complete cleft lip and cleft palate, which is known as a complete labio-alveolo-palatal cleft. Although the palatal cleft is always median, rotation of the vomer may cause it to appear lateral.

In these forms, bands of soft tissue (see Chapter 6, page 46) may exist in the inter-alveolar area (Figs 3.13a, b and c). Depending on their size, there may be some doubt as to precisely which anatomo-clinical form is involved. Bridges of bone tissue also exist in forms that combine complete labio-maxillary clefts and palatal clefts that do not affect the entire hard palate (CBCL + CP + bridge) (Figs 3.14, 3.15 and 3.16).

Bilateral clefts

Bilateral forms represent about 25% of the total defects. They may be symmetrical, when the lesions are identical on both sides, or asymmetrical if the lesions on either side are different.

A distinction is made between simple and complete forms. Simple forms (SBCL) may occur with or without a palatal cleft (CP) (Fig. 3.17a and b). At times, the form appears as a congenital scar of the lip (Fig. 3.18). Complete bilateral forms (CBCL) may occur with or without a cleft palate and/or band (Figs 3.19a and b, 3.20a, b and c, 3.21).

A complete asymmetrical cleft usually involves a cleft palate (CBCL left, S right, for instance + CP) (Fig. 3.22a, b and c).

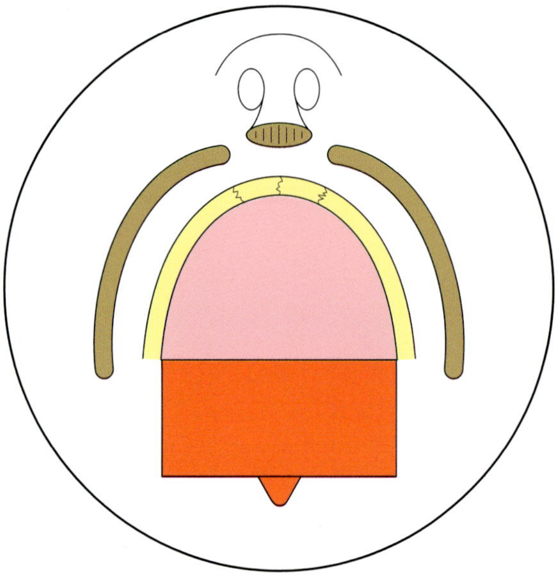

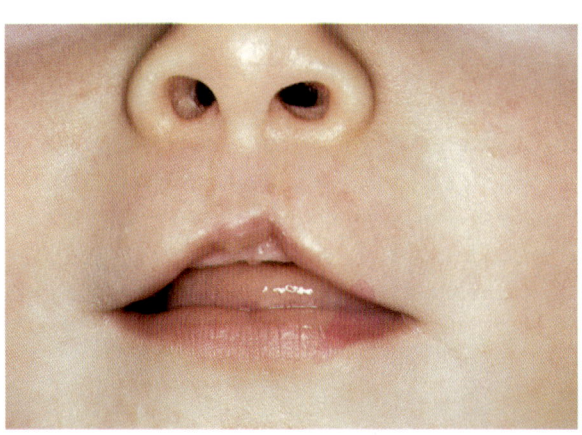

a

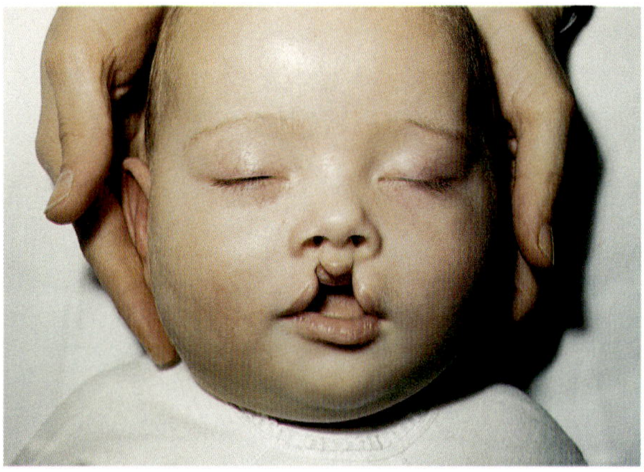

b

Fig. 3.17 *a and b Symmetrical simple bilateral cleft.*

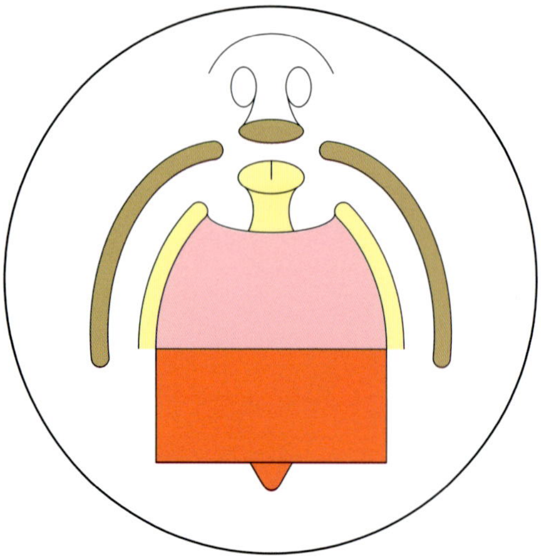

Fig. 3.18 *Simple bilateral form of congenital scar of the lip.*

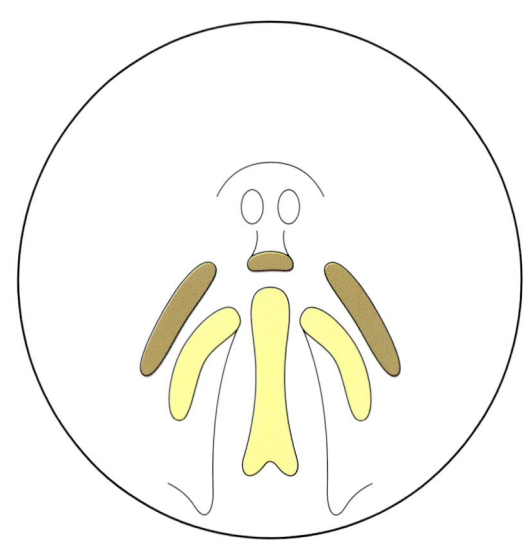

a

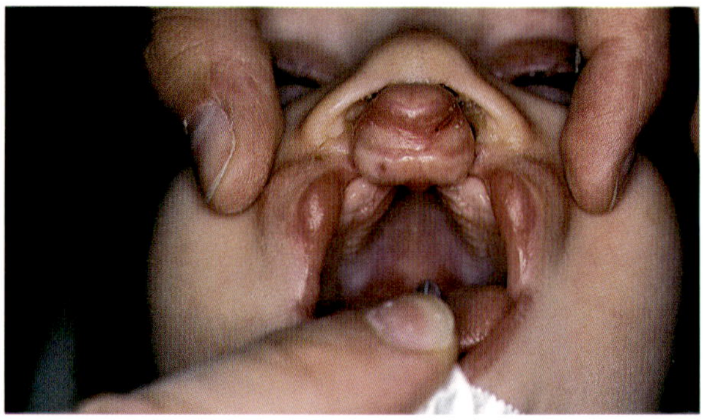

b

Fig. 3.19 *a and b Complete bilateral form without palatal cleft.*

Fig. 3.20 *Symmetrical complete bilateral form with palatal cleft.*

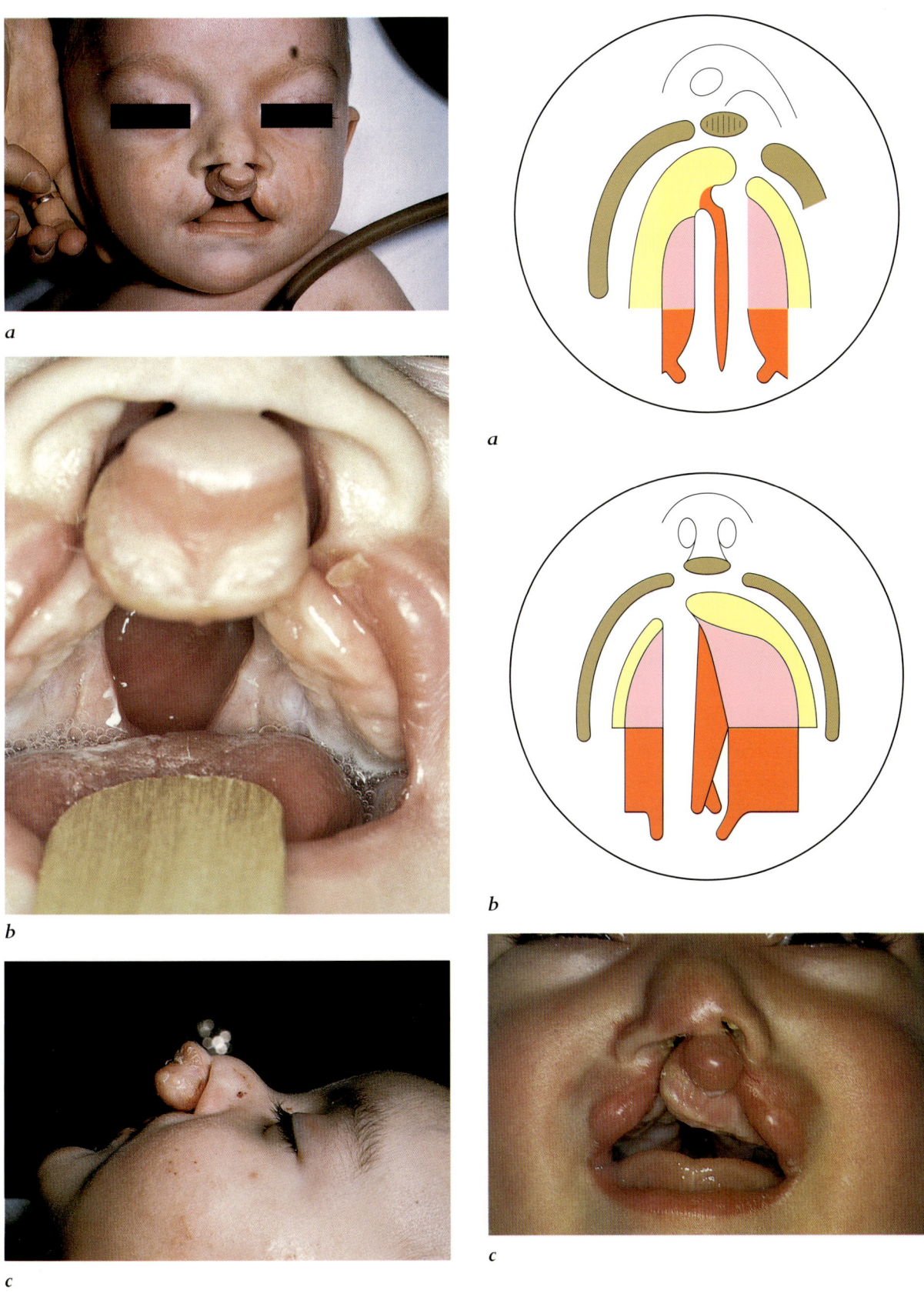

a

b

c

a

b

c

Fig. 3.21 *a, b and c Different angles of complete bilateral cleft.*

Fig. 3.22 *a, b and c Asymmetrical bilateral clefts: a, b. complete on one side, simple on other; c. complete on both sides with unilateral bridge.*

4. The lesions and their consequences

INTRODUCTION

The congenital cleft is a gap which may involve the lip, the upper maxilla and the palate, either independently or in combined forms (Fig. 4.1). The anatomical and physiological consequences increase in proportion to whether one, two or all three areas are affected. As soon as the cleft appears during the early stages of embryonic development, both anatomy and function are modified.

THE CLEFT LIP

The cleft in the lip interrupts the continuity of the superficial facial muscle layer.

The orbicularis of the lips is only one component of this muscle layer; however, all the facial muscles are nonetheless continuous with it. Due to its malformation, these muscles all lose their insertions in the midline; in other words onto the anterior nasal spine of the upper maxilla. This can occur on one or on both sides, depending on whether the cleft is uni- or bilateral. Consequently, the muscle bundles develop abnormal orientations and insertions, and their action is significantly altered.

The orbicularis oris, which normally functions as a sphincter, exerts an uncustomary divergent action as its two portions, which are divided by the cleft,

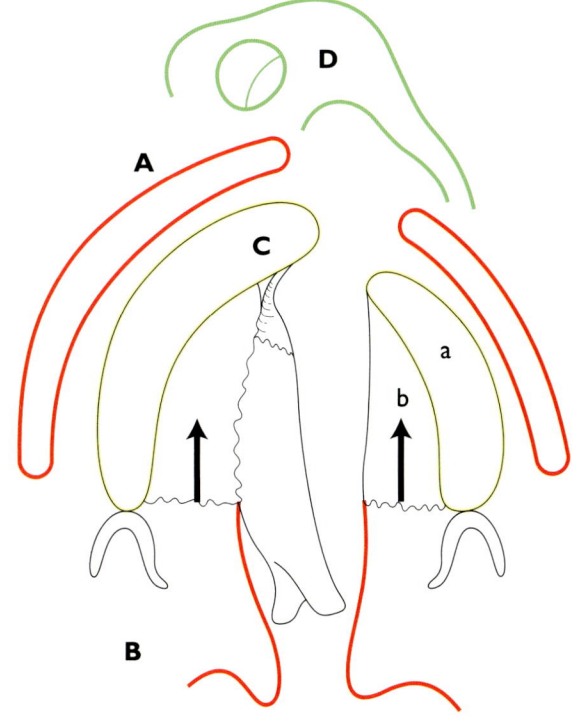

Fig. 4.1

The anatomical regions affected by complete cleft lip and palate:

A. The lip

B. The velum

C. The maxilla and its two components a. the alveolar ridge and b. the palatal vault, or palatine shelves. These may be deformed and/or displaced

D. The nose

tend to pull away from one another. This anomalous muscle action leads to deformities of the bones and cartilages, even in simple forms. Its effects are particularly obvious on the septal structures and alar cartilages.

Muscle pressure exerted on the underlying bone structure is affected as well. Since facial bone growth follows the resorption/deposition principle described by Enlow (1975) (see Chapter 16), changes in muscle pressure can hinder growth and contribute to deformity.

THE CLEFT PALATE

The cleft in the palate disrupts normal muscular continuity in the roof of the oral cavity. Here, too, the velar muscles lose their insertions in the midline. The fibers are oriented differently and develop abnormal insertions. The transverse continuity of the soft palate is disrupted.

The widening of the nasopharynx might find a simple explanation in the action of intact antagonistic muscles, yet no such antagonists exist when the velum is cleft. The explanation, as we shall see, lies elsewhere.

The palatal cleft has a major impact on physiology. Its functional consequences are of the utmost importance, according to Veau. The palate represents the upper wall of the oral cavity, and is the anatomical element that serves to separate the respiratory from the digestive passages. With a cleft palate, the digestive function is seriously impaired. The velum no longer seals off the airway during swallowing, and closure can only be obtained by contact between the base of the tongue and the anterior aspect of the superior pharyngeal constrictor, which advances to meet it.

To ensure an airtight seal, the base of the tongue broadens to exert pressure along the side walls. The tongue rises higher than usual during elevation of the aero-digestive bract, which represents the first phase of deglutition. The tongue presses against the velar stumps, which cannot fulfill their function, and causes them to rotate outwards on either side (Chapter 10). This is not an incidence of lingual dystopia, as some have interpreted it, but an intermittent disorder of the swallowing process, which is clearly displayed on videofluoroscopy. In our opinion, this pressure of the tongue upward and towards the back of the oral

cavity is responsible for enlarging the pharynx and, more particularly, for causing the pterygoid processes to spread apart, the telltale sign of this enlargement.

The palatal cleft also leads to respiratory problems. Breathing tends to become oral, primarily because tongue pressure deforms the palatal shelves and vomer, thus reducing the height of the choanas.

The opening and closing mechanism of the eustachian tube is impaired by the cleft and by changes in nasopharyngeal air pressure.

Finally, the permanent passage of air in the nasal fossae impedes phonation even in the first stages of development, which occur at a surprisingly early age.

DIVISION OF THE MAXILLA

The division of the maxilla in complete forms adds its own specific problems to the lesions and disorders listed above.

Modified muscle action tends to cause displacement of the bony segments, which have become mobile due to the cleft. Their attachments to the rest of the skull are extremely fragile. A combination of factors must be taken into account; dysfunction of the orbicularis oris and of the superficial facial muscles, compounded by modified tongue action. The tongue may intrude into the posterior velar cleft, and often into the gap in the bony vault as well. There may be considerable bone displacement, with subsequent alteration of the child's facial appearance.

Displacement due to abnormal muscle action produces bone and cartilage deformities specific to the type of cleft involved, uni- or bilateral. In unilateral forms, for instance, major septal deformity is common.

For the sake of clarity, given the complexity of these notions, the following order of presentation has been adopted for this book. Granted, it may seem somewhat arbitrary.

1. Lesions of the lip, which concentrates on the simple form.
2. Lesions of the palate, with the main focus on the isolated cleft palate.
3. Complete forms (labio-maxillo-palatal), involving the most complex problems of repair and the most controversial methods of treatment.

II THE LIP AND THE NOSE

5. Normal anatomy

The purpose of cleft lip repair is, of course, to obtain a result that is as close to normal as possible. This supposes a precise understanding of those criteria that define normality. The upper lip, however, involves a multitude of features that are not usually considered in the traditional medical curriculum. We therefore intend to present a detailed study of the outer aspect of the upper lip, including a certain amount of histological data.

Two factors are involved in determining the characteristics of the normal lip: the age of the subject and the facial expression. There is a dynamic aspect to the lip, which is specific to each individual.

MACROSCOPIC ASPECTS

The upper lip is defined as follows:

- Laterally, by two vertical lines drawn at the extreme corners of the lips and by the naso-labial folds. Thus, the lip is continuous with the cheek and the lower lip.
- Above, superficially, by a horizontal line drawn under the lower portion of the nose. This, moving from the outside in, corresponds to the sub-alar furrow and then, in the midline, to the transverse groove of the columella. These two anatomical features are often inconspicuous if not invisible, in which case the upper lip appears to be continuous with the nostril sill and the lower surface of the columella. At a deeper level, the limit lies at the bottom of the vestibular sulcus, where the

mucous membrane of the lip continues the gingival mucosa.
- Below, by the upper half of the oral aperture, which the upper lip encloses.

The lip is of variable thickness, and presents two surfaces, superficial and deep. The superficial (or outer) surface is itself subdivided into two parts: the cutaneous or white lip, and the mucous membrane or vermilion. The transition between these two zones is represented by the mucocutaneous ridge, or white roll, which extends from one corner of the mouth to the other. It is characterized by the V-shaped indentation it forms in the midline, which is called the Cupid's bow.

The cutaneous lip

The cutaneous portion of the lip presents a series of elevations and depressions above the white roll (Fig. 5.1).

Immediately above the line there is an unnamed ridge of variable size, which also involves the upper portion of the Cupid's bow. Directly above the Cupid's bow, the upper lip forms a vertical groove-shaped depression called the philtrum. This is bordered by two rounded vertical elevations of variable prominence, known as the philtral ridges. The latter tend to converge towards the midpoint of the transverse columellar groove if it exists or, if not, towards the centre of the base of the columella. On either side, the zone between the philtral ridge and the ipsilateral transverse columellar groove forms a

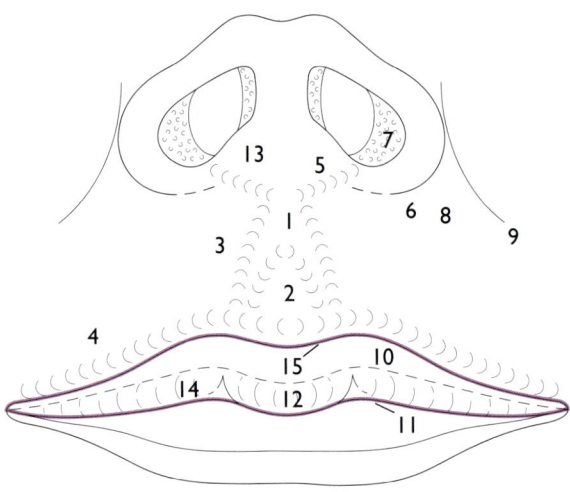

a

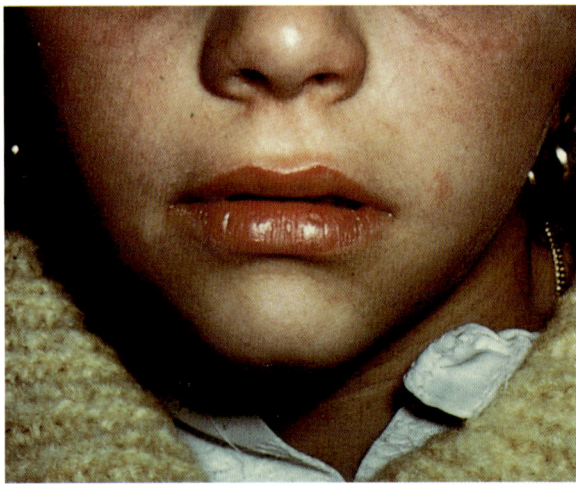

b

Fig. 5.1 *Macroscopic aspect of the normal lip.*

1.　*Philtrum*
2.　*Philtral dimple*
3.　*Philtral ridges*
4.　*Unnamed crest above the mucocutaneous ridge*
5.　*Transverse groove of the columella*
6.　*Sub-alar furrow*
7.　*Stippled skin in the vestibulum of the nares*
8.　*Nasogenial triangle*
9.　*Nasogenial fold*
10.　*Matt zone of the vermilion*
11.　*Moist zone of the vermilion with vertical striations*
12.　*Tubercle of the upper lip*
13.　*Columellar base lifted by mesial crura*
14.　*Vertical creases of the vermilion*
15.　*Cupid's bow*

triangle. Its apex, oriented inwards towards the midline, projects forward compared with the rest of the lip. This triangular portion of variable size is therefore set on a slant from back to front and from outside in, which contrasts with the overall plane of the upper lip (Fig. 5.2). As it nears the Cupid's bow, the philtral depression deepens into the philtral dimple.

At times, a whitish scar-like line runs vertically down the centre of the philtrum. In all probability, it is a trace of the fusion line between the nasomedial processes (see Chapter 2).

The vermilion

The visible portion of the vermilion is, in fact, subdivided into two superposed zones which are not

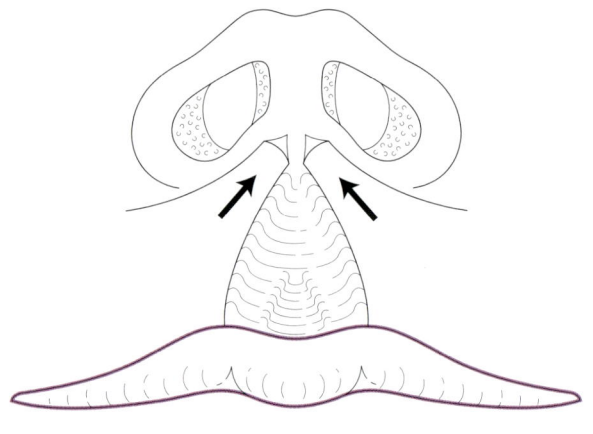

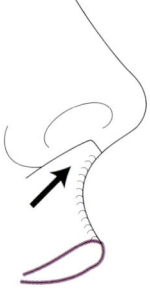

Fig. 5.2 *The triangular portion of the lip under the columella is set on a slant back to front and from outside in contrasting with the general plane of the upper lip.*

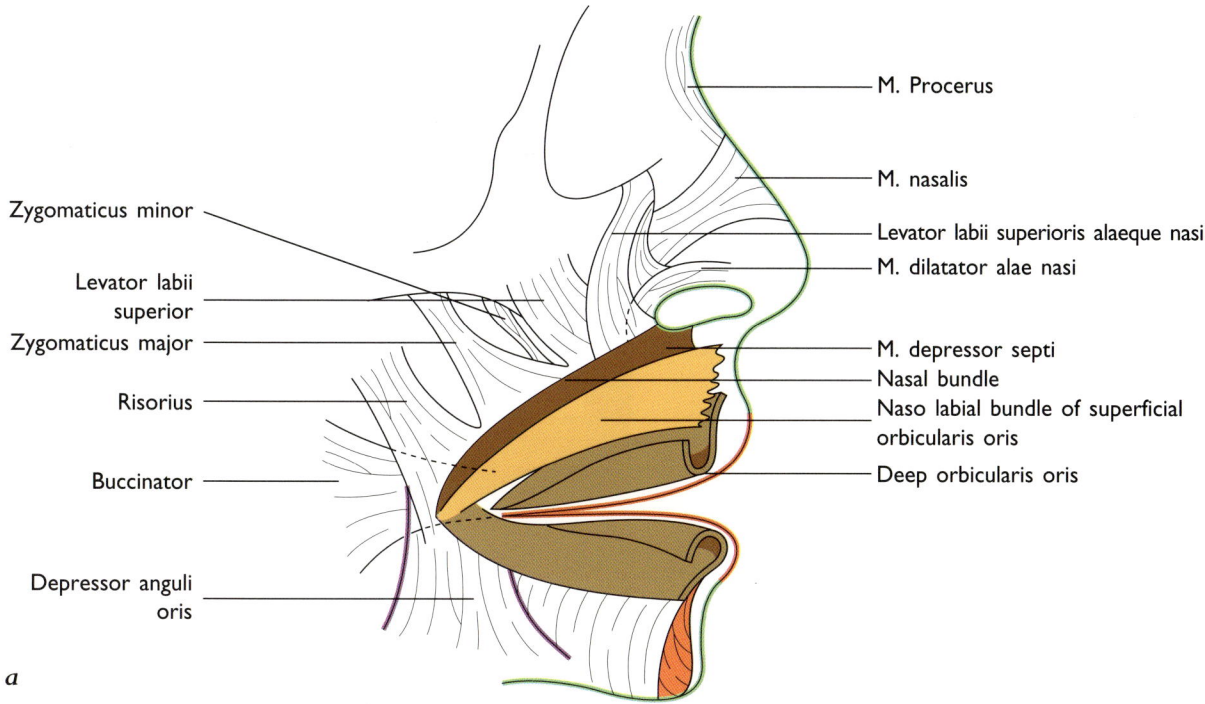

Zygomaticus minor

Levator labii superior

Zygomaticus major

Risorius

Buccinator

Depressor anguli oris

a

M. Procerus

M. nasalis

Levator labii superioris alaeque nasi

M. dilatator alae nasi

M. depressor septi

Nasal bundle

Naso labial bundle of superficial orbicularis oris

Deep orbicularis oris

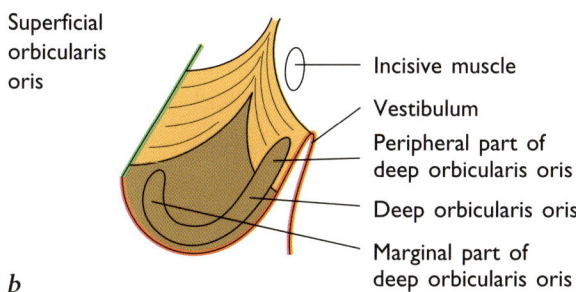

Superficial orbicularis oris

b

Incisive muscle

Vestibulum

Peripheral part of deep orbicularis oris

Deep orbicularis oris

Marginal part of deep orbicularis oris

Fig. 5.3 *Orbicularis oris muscle fibers (according to Nicolau, 1983). a. In a profile view, the two parts of the orbicularis: the outer bundle and the inner bundle. All facial muscles are tightly connected with it and are thus anchored to the anterior nasal spine. b. Cross-section of different parts of the outer bundle; both deep and superficial fibers are visible, as is the arrangement of the inner bundle.*

clearly delimited. The upper zone is a pinkish red and, since it is not generally moist, it appears matt. The lower zone is a richer, translucent red. Its moist aspect resembles that of the mucosa with which it is continuous.

Among black infants, there is a much clearer distinction between the coloration of these two zones; brownish above and red below.

The entire visible portion of the vermilion, both zones included, presents tiny vertical striations. Two of these are more clearly defined, and correspond to what are called the vertical creases of the vermilion. They are situated in line with the peaks of the Cupid's bow.

The free border of the upper lip which defines the oral aperture follows the contour of the mucocutaneous ridge or white roll.

Below the Cupid's bow, the vermilion forms a protrusion in the midline called the tubercle of the upper lip. Its centre, like that of the cutaneous lip, is marked by a vertical ridge (Fig. 5.1). On either side, the free border follows a moderately convex curve (as opposed to the concavity of the white line) as far as the corners of the lips, where it passes in front of the lower lip.

The inner surface of the upper lip is covered with red mucosa marked by the protruding labial salivary glands that lie beneath it. As stated earlier, it is continuous with the gingival mucosa at the deepest part of the vestibular sulcus.

In the midline, the upper lip is attached to the gum by a fold of mucous membrane known as the frenum of the upper lip. It is broader on the lip than on the gum side. In certain cases, it may appear short and hypertrophic. At times, it is continuous with the retro-alveolar mucosa, and this may create a gap between the middle incisors. Additional lateral frena may also be present, particularly in certain malformations such as cleft lip or oro-facial-digital syndrome (OFD).

THE STRUCTURE OF THE LIP

The orbicularis oris

The lip is composed essentially of muscle tissue. The major muscle of the upper lip is the orbicularis oris. Its fibers extend from the commissures to the midline, where they meet their contralaterals.

The fibers of the orbicularis oris are customarily described as two units: an outer or superficial group, and an inner or deep group. These fibers are arranged in a circular pattern around the oral aperture (Fig. 5.3a).

The outer or superficial bundle

This is itself subdivided into two types of fibers:

1. Extrinsic fibers are rightly affixed to the skin, thus including the orbicularis among the superficial skin muscles (it is thought to determine the expressions of the lip). After crossing the midline, the fibers from either side become densely interwoven in the central portion of the upper lip where they form both the philtral ridges and the depression of the philtrum (Fig. 5.4). The upper fibers of the bundle insert into the anterior nasal spine of the upper maxilla and into the lower end of the nasal septum, forming the septo-maxillary ligament (Latham and Deaton, 1976). This is the true major midline insertion of the entire facial muscle layer, since a large number of its fibers interlace laterally with the orbicularis oris.

2. Intrinsic or deep fibers separate into two bundles:
   a. the incisive labii superioris, which inserts into the periosteum of the incisor region;
   b. the incisive labii inferioris, which inserts into the mucosa.

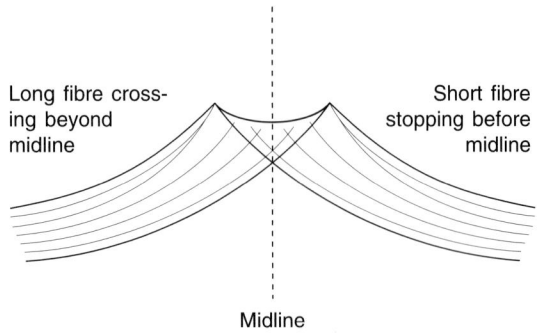

Long fibre crossing beyond midline

Short fibre stopping before midline

Midline

Fig. 5.4 *Composition of the philtrum (according to Nicolau, 1983). The fibers of the extrinsic part of the superficial bundle interweave at the midline; only the deeper long fibers cross the midline to create the furrow and the ridges.*

The outer or superficial bundle makes up approximately three-quarters of the height of the upper lip.

The inner or deep bundle

This is arranged on the lower half of the upper lip, and is partially covered by the superficial muscle fibers. It forms a true sphincteric loop near the free border of the lip. On a deep level, its fibers are thought to be laterally continuous with those of the buccinator.

Just outside the corners of the lip, the inner muscles concentrate into two layers between which are interlaced the fibers of the orbicularis of the lower lip. Thus they are arranged so as to form a scissor-like closing mechanism, which seals the commissures.

In the lower portion of this deep group, the horizontal fibers curl in upon themselves, thus causing eversion of the vermilion near the white roll (Fig. 5.3b).

On the outer contour at the corners of the mouth, the orbicularis oris, as has been stated, is intimately attached to other superficial facial muscles of the upper lip (Fig. 5.5). These also influence skin movements:

- the nasalis;
- the superficial and deep levators of the alar wing and lip;

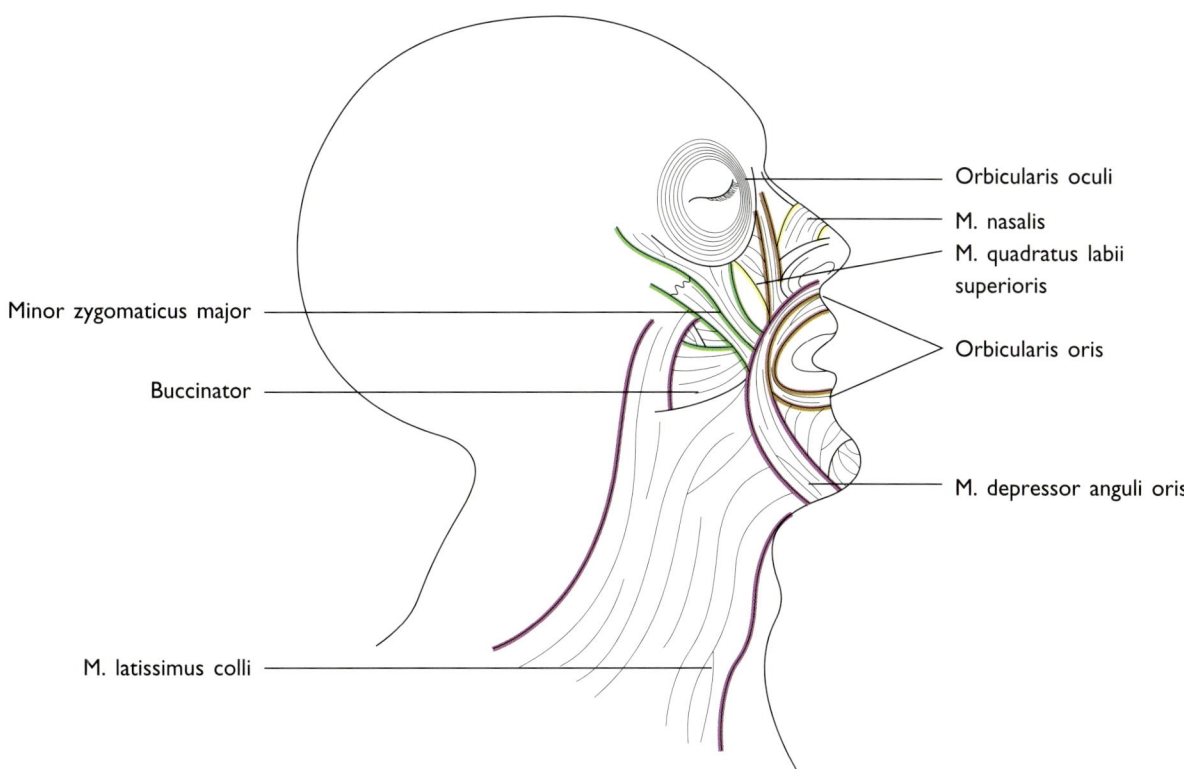

Orbicularis oculi

M. nasalis

M. quadratus labii superioris

Orbicularis oris

Minor zygomaticus major

Buccinator

M. depressor anguli oris

M. latissimus colli

Fig. 5.5 *The facial muscles (according to Rouviere 1943).*

- the levator anguli oris or caninus;
- the risorious;
- the zygomaticus major and minor;
- the platysma; and
- the deep-lying buccinator.

THE BLOOD AND NERVE SUPPLY

The arterial vessels of the upper lip originate in the superior labial artery, a branch of the facial artery, near the corners of the lips. The right and left labial arteries anastomose in the midline of the upper lip. The midline anastomosis gives off a vertical ascending branch, the subseptal artery, which extends as far as the tip of the nose.

Each superior labial artery produces numerous smaller vertical arteries, which in turn anastomose laterally to irrigate the highly vascularized zone of the entire upper lip. These labial arteries course between the layers of muscle and mucosa near the free border of the upper lip.

Additional vessels that arise from other facial arteries contribute to the vascularization, particularly towards the lateral limits of the lips.

The motor nerve supply is provided by the facial nerve and, more specifically, by the superior branches, which arise from the parotid plexus. The terminal nerve ends lie deep beneath the muscle fibers described above.

The sensory nerve supply is furnished by the descending branch of the buccal nerve, which originates in the temporo-buccal nerve, itself an offshoot of the anterior terminal stem of the trigeminal nerve.

THE NORMAL NOSE

This section is included here to provide a helpful reminder of the characteristics of the normal nose. To understand abnormal development, a thorough knowledge of the relevant anatomical structures and of the terms used to refer to them is required.

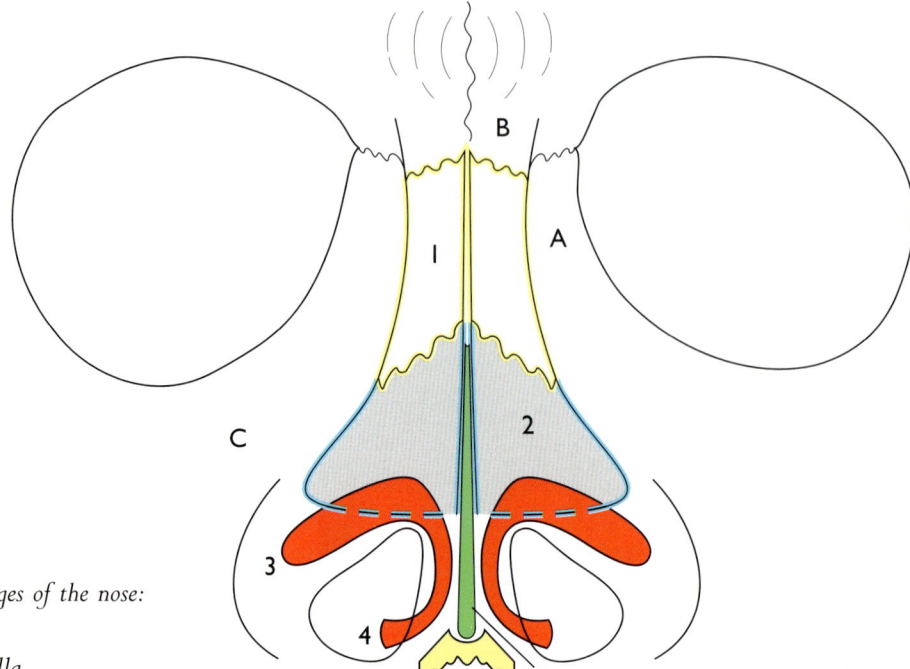

Fig. 5.6 *Bones and cartilages of the nose:*

A. Maxillary Process

B. Frontal bone and glabella

C. Nasal components:

    1. Nasal bones

    2. Lateral cartilage

    3. Lateral crus of alar cartilage

    4. Medial crus and its protrusion into the nostril

    5. Nasal septum

    6. Anterior nasal spine of maxilla

The nose is a protruding structure composed of both a bony and a cartilaginous skeleton. Its elements are arranged in symmetrical pairs.

The external protrusion of the nasal bones is completed by the frontal processes of the maxilla, connected above with the frontal bone, which is characterized by the transverse projection of the glabella. This area corresponds to the base of the nose (Fig. 5.6).

The nasal cartilages comprise:

* The triangular (lateral or upper lateral) cartilages. These are connected to the lower border of the nasal bones, and extend the nasal structure downward.
* The alar cartilages. These form a partial circle connecting the anterior nasal spine to the piriform aperture. The U-shaped cartilages are composed of two segments: an external segment or lateral crus, which overlaps the lower border of the lateral cartilage to which it is attached by dense connective tissue, and an inner segment or medial crus, which joins its contralateral to form the lower mobile portion of the cartilaginous nasal structure. The base of this segment forms a ridge inside the nostril, since it is elevated by the nasal spine that supports it (Fig. 5.6).
* The septal cartilage or nasal septum. This is formed of very sturdy cartilaginous tissue (Fig. 5.7). Quadrilateral in shape, it is connected by its antero-superior border to the nasal bones and triangular cartilages. Its postero-inferior border fits into the groove of the vomerian bone to which it is attached, and its postero-superior corner is connected to the perpendicular plate of the ethmoid bone. Lastly, its antero-inferior border slips between the medial crura of the alar cartilages and helps support the tip of the nose. Jacobson's

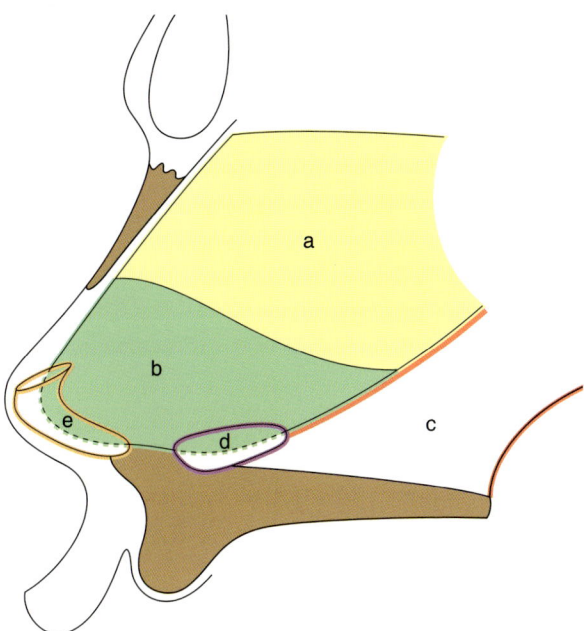

Fig. 5.7 *Components of septum:*

a.   *lamina perpendicularis of ethmoid*

b.   *septal cartilage*

c.   *vomer*

d.   *Jacobson's cartilage*

e.   *Medial crus of alar cartilage*

cartilages correspond to two small lamellae of cartilage, which enclose the lower portion of the septum on the level of the vomer and the posterior section of the anterior nasal spine. The septum separates the two nasal fossae. A more detailed description of the lateral surfaces characterized by the ridge of the nasal conchae appears elsewhere.

The tip of the nose is therefore the protuberance created by the domes of the alar cartilages and supported by the nasal septum. The medial crura form the columella while the lateral crura support the wings of the nose, which are attached to the cheek at their outer base. The lower borders of the triangular cartilages form the plica nasi inside the nose. The nasal vestibule is located between this fold and the superficial external base of the nose.

The nares are therefore enclosed from below, by the nostril sill (described earlier in this chapter); on the inner side, by the columella; and on the outer side and front, by the wings of the nose and its external base. These openings are normally symmetrical, and have a larger antero-posterior axis.

Figure 5.8 shows the nasal muscles.

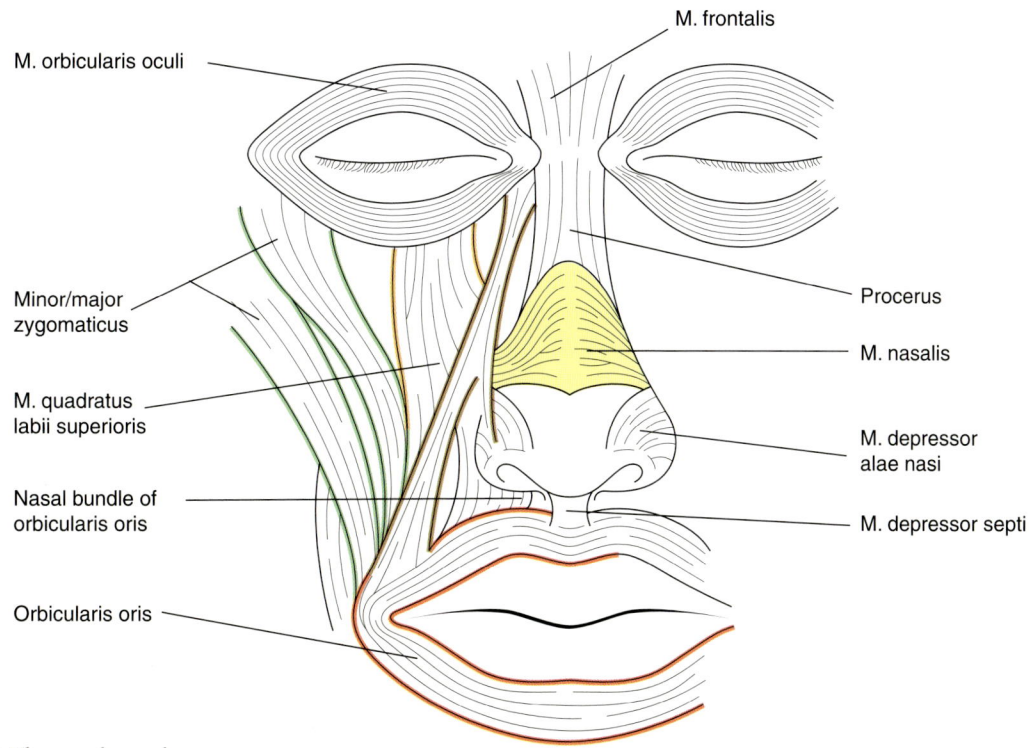

Fig. 5.8 *The nasal muscles.*

6. Pathological anatomy

The upper lip is a highly complex anatomical region, and its structure is profoundly altered by the existence of a congenital cleft.

What immediately strikes the eye in these cases is the fact that, on each side of the cleft as far as the divided nostril sill, it is possible to identify the structures of a normal lip. In other words, the cutaneous and mucosal portions are both present and are perfectly continuous with the rest of the lip (Fig. 6.1a). What is more, at the apex of the cleft on either side, the lip is anchored to the underlying bone structure by the mucous membrane and the periosteum. A detailed analysis will be devoted to this point of attachment, which corresponds to the junction between those elements that make up the lip and those that pertain to the nasal floor (Fig. 6.1b).

Unilateral and bilateral forms of cleft lip each require a separate study.

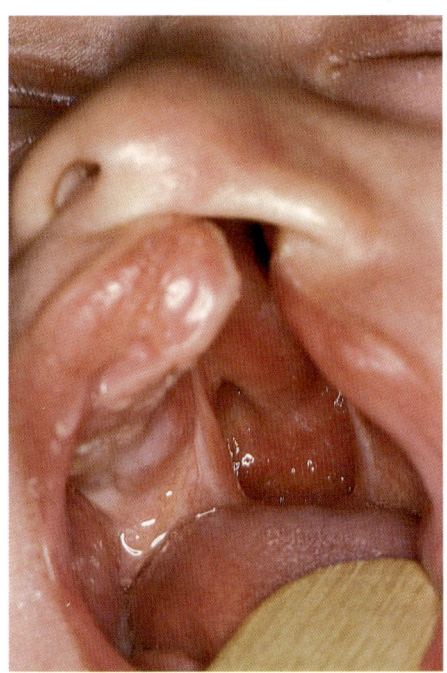

a

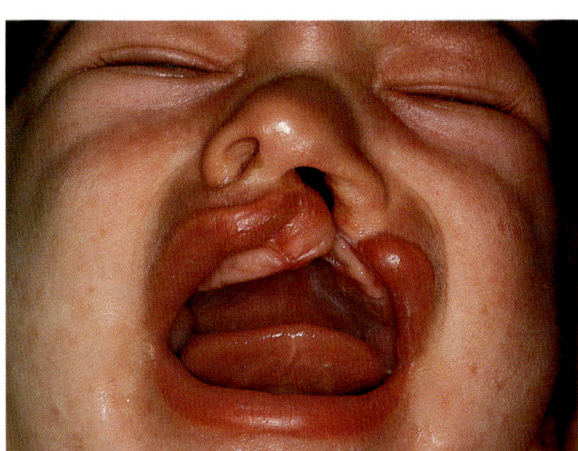

b

Fig. 6.1 *Lip lesions in a unilateral cleft: a. The cutaneous and mucosal portions of lip continue as far as the nostril sill. b. Due to the cleft, the upper portion of the labial structures is anchored to the periosteum of the greater and lesser segments.*

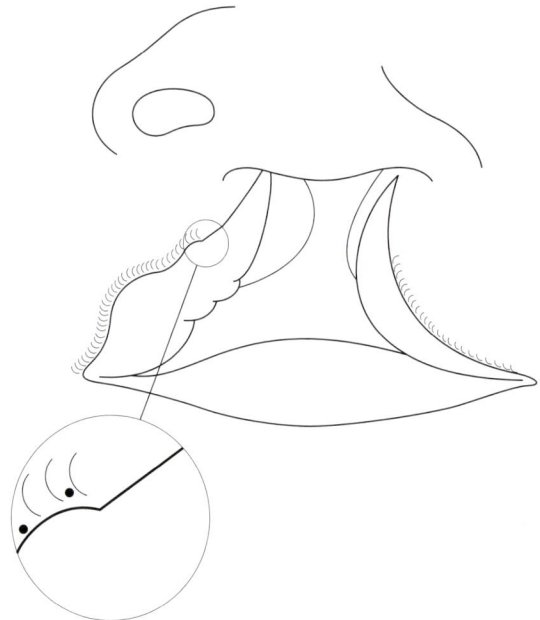

Fig. 6.2 *The notch in the skin–vermilion line on the inner border.*

THE UNILATERAL CLEFT LIP

Form involving the entire height of the lip

This is the most characteristic form of unilateral cleft lip, and has the following features.

The inner border

1. The mucocutaneous ridge or white roll consistently presents a Cupid's bow, which is more or less clearly outlined. A notch that indents the cutaneous integument in the direction of the vermilion marks the junction between this ridge and the line of transition from skin to mucosa on the border of the cleft. This factor is very important when the reference points are marked (Fig. 6.2).

2. The philtral ridge on the cleft side is usually ill-defined, if not absent. The philtrum is therefore difficult to define. The philtral dimple, which forms a hollow just above the Cupid's bow, remains however far more conspicuous (Fig. 6.3).

3. Abnormal vertical shortness of the lip compared with its height on the normal side is obvious on the margins of the cleft. Nevertheless, it must be kept in mind that hypoplasia of the structures involved begins before the inferior reference point that serves to measure lip height.

4. There is noticeable thinning of the vermilion, which starts before the peak of the Cupid's bow.

5. The distinction between the two zones of vermilion, dry and moist, continues for a short distance on the lower portion of the borders of the cleft beyond the reference points.

6. The frenum of the vermilion is often hypertrophied, and the base of its implantation on the lip seems abnormally wide.

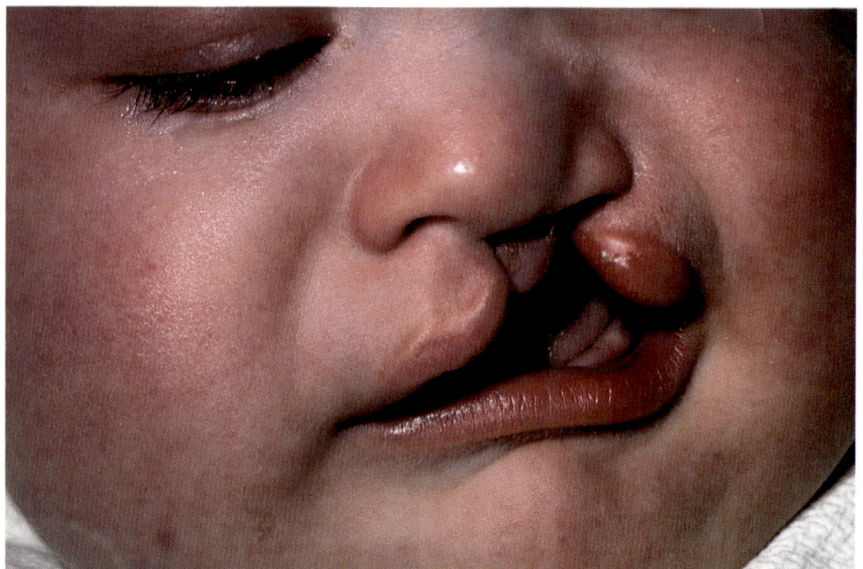

Fig. 6.3 *The philtral dimple is clearly visible above the Cupid's bow on the inner border.*

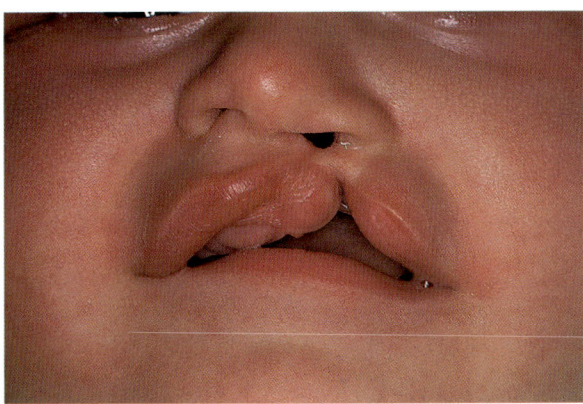

a

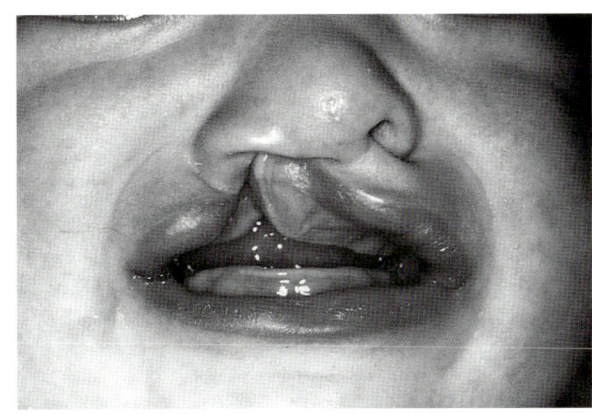

b

Fig. 6.4 *Lesions of the outer border: a. The end of the ridge above the skin–vermilion line. Note the separation between the dry and moist zones. b. Everted alar wing with the crease in the upper part of the border with the sub-alar furrow.*

7. The depth of the vestibular sulcus can only be evaluated on the non-cleft side.

Victor Veau (1938) contended that the mucosa on the inner border of the cleft was abnormal, and readily subject to desquamation and crusting. Since he considered it 'sterile', he advised that it be removed and replaced with the more healthy mucosa from the outer border. In our practice, we have always retained the inner mucosa and have never encountered any long-term ill effects.

The outer border

1. The ridge that normally runs above the white roll becomes blurred in the vicinity of the cleft. This helps in positioning the lower reference point. Unlike the inner border, the outer side does not present a step in the dividing line (Fig. 6.4a).
2. The cutaneous portion of the lip is often convex in both vertical and horizontal directions. The underlying muscles, which have lost their medial insertions, tend to draw up into a ball of fibers. In its upper portion and along the cleft, the aspect of the outer cutaneous border differs from that of the skin around it. This area seems to be defined below by a furrow, which continues the existing crease between the outer base of the ala and the cheek (Fig. 6.4b). We are not referring here to the naso-labial crease, which is a different entity. In reality, this portion of skin pertains to the nose

and corresponds to a part of the vestibule that is normally inside the nares but is drawn outward, in this instance, by eversion of the alar base. This eversion is linked to contraction of the facial muscles, which have lost their medial insertion, while the deep-lying soft tissue remains anchored to the periosteum. A true torque effect is thus produced.

3. On the external border, the vestibule of the lip is normal; however, the presence of one or several abnormal mucosal frena is not uncommon (Fig. 6.5).

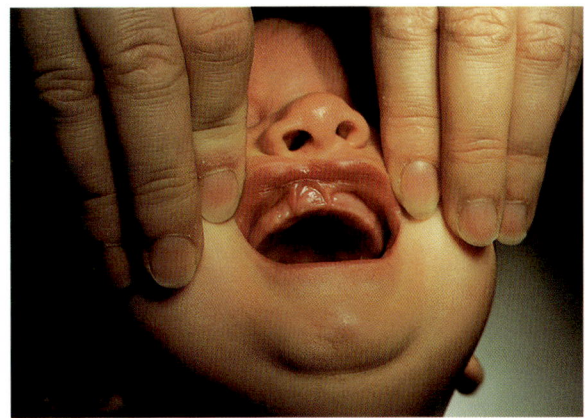

Fig. 6.5 *Supernumerary lateral frenum.*

4. Palpation of the lip between the thumb and forefinger reveals muscle thickening on the outside, which gradually thins as it nears the cleft.

5. The dividing line between the dry and moist zones of the vermilion extends inward beyond the reference point and therefore beyond the end of the horizontal ridge. It meets the transitional line between skin and mucosa on the lower portion of the cleft. In other words, the mucosa bordering the cleft is, for the most part, moist.

6. Vertical shortness of the outer border varies in degree. Generally, when there is no bridge, the height of the inner and outer borders is the same. However, this is not always the case. The outer border often looks longer, but this visual impression must be confirmed or otherwise by using calipers to verify the actual height of the cleft. It is always advisable to double-check that no error has been made in siting the reference points or in evaluating the width of the outer border. The distance between the lower reference point and the corner of the lip on the cleft side should be identical to that between the corner of the lip and the peak of the Cupid's bow on the intact side. Thus, the width of the cleft itself in no way indicates a corresponding tissue deficit in a transverse direction.

   However, local tissue shortfall can be considerable in certain cases. For instance, in what are termed hypoplastic forms, there is an obvious deficit than can be checked objectively by measuring the width of the lateral stump to confirm that there has been no miscalculation. In these cases, the entire border shows a three-dimensional lack of development.

7. Finally, congenital clefts consistently present a deformity that has received little mention. When the infant is observed from the front, it is obvious that the labial and nasal structures on the outer margin are lower than their counterparts on the inner side (Fig. 6.6). Granted, the inner margin is raised by the premaxilla and therefore seems to have 'ascended'. Nonetheless, the outer border is clearly lower than it should be. The commissure on the cleft side follows this general movement, and is below its normal level as well.

This latter phenomenon is again related to the loss of midline insertions for the facial muscles, and to the

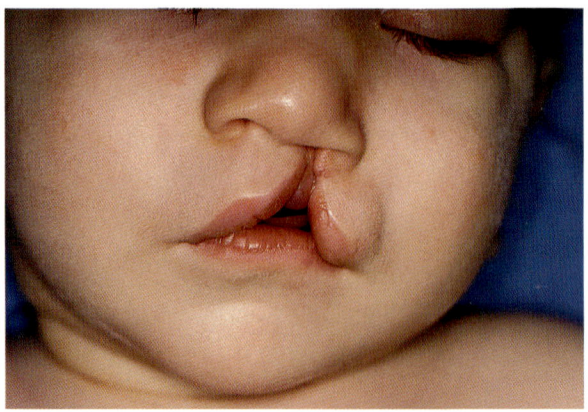

Fig. 6.6 *Lateral ptosis involving the nose, outer margin and corner of the lips.*

downward traction exerted at the oral aperture. Delaire's sketch of the peri-orofacial muscle rings clearly illustrates this mechanism (Fig. 6.7). Although the bilabial ring is divided by the congenital cleft, the upper nasolabial ring around the bridge of the nose remains intact, as do the muscle unions of the lower lip and neck. The facial muscle layer draws back the

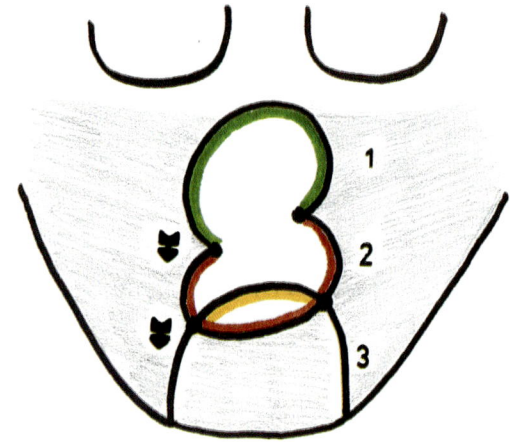

Fig. 6.7 *Delaire's (1983) illustration:*
1. *Muscle ring around the nose.*
2. *Split ring of the superior orbicularis. The dominant action of the inferior muscles when mouth is opened explains the deformity.*
3. *Lower ring around the chin and neck.*

soft tissues covering the lesser segment (effect of the buccinator), and pulls the corners of the lips down due to the dominant action of the lower muscles. Furthermore, the muscle mass brings abnormal pressure to bear on the anterior end of the lesser segment, which deforms it into an inverted J-shape and distorts the upper maxilla into an oblique oval (see Chapter 17).

The deep structures of the lip

These are also altered by the cleft.

The terminal insertions of muscle fibers at the cleft have not yet been accurately identified. Fara (1966) described the fibers as running up the cleft towards the nostril sill. Other specialists speak of direct insertions into the margins of the cleft for the lower fibers of the orbicularis, while the upper fibers are thought to rise towards the nasal spine on the non-cleft side (Fig. 6.8) (De May *et al.*, 1989).

These factors have a significant effect on the results of lip repair. The orientation of the muscle fibers conditions the dynamic as well as the static results obtained by the repair, as will be seen a little later on.

The blood vessels, and in particular the terminal branches of the orbicular artery, rise along the borders of the cleft. It is essential to sever this vascular bundle which, in a sense, 'locks' the height of the cleft as it is, whereas the aim of the cutaneo-muscular repair is an attempt precisely to lengthen its abnormal shortness.

These vessels are multiple and lie parallel to one another below the mucosa, and it is often necessary to venture some distance from the cleft in order to locate them. They are then severed and hemostasis is performed.

Simple forms

A distinction should be made between partial clefts and 'masked' forms, which cannot really be classified as clefts since there is no visible gap.

In masked forms (forme fruste), a scar-like line usually runs along the outer slope of the philtral ridge, which itself is not always clearly visible. This is often referred to rather irreverently in French as 'the Good Lord's scar', as if to imply that God has not done a proper job... (Fig. 6.9). The white roll is

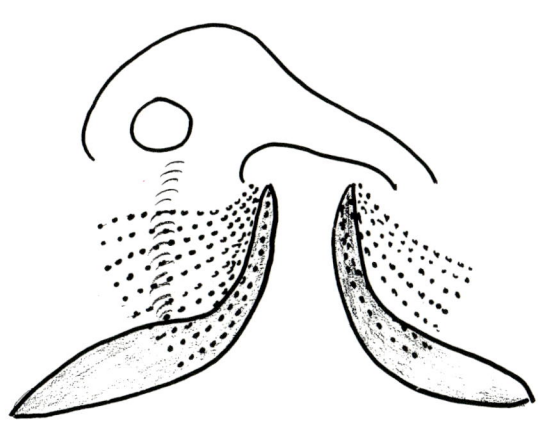

Fig. 6.8 *Orientation of the muscle fibers towards the upper part of the cleft concerns only a portion of the orbicularis.*

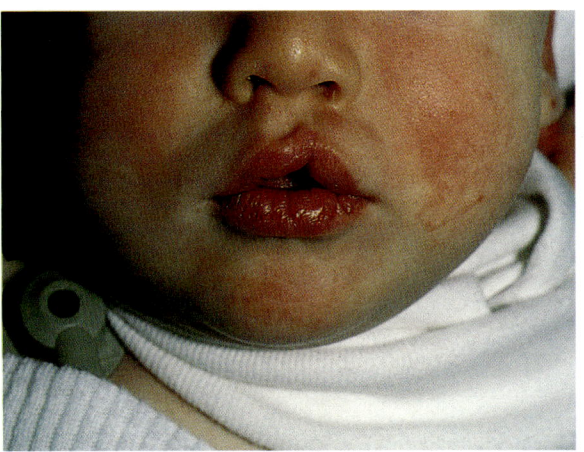

Fig. 6.9 *Congenital scar of the lip. Note the ball of orbicularis fibers on the outer margin. Despite the absence of a cleft, the muscles have lost their midline insertions.*

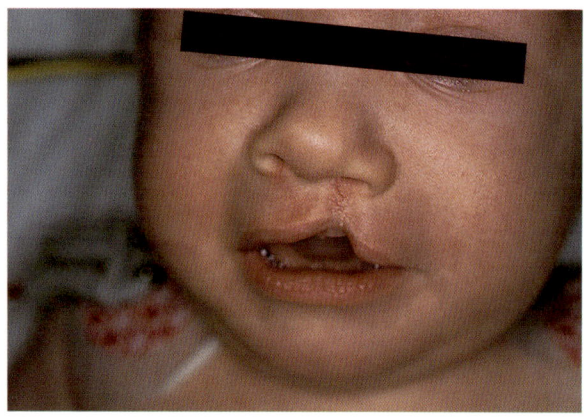

Fig. 6.10 *The angiomatous appearance often observed in the upper part of the lip.*

always more or less clearly notched, and the Cupid's bow is situated high on the inner border, which is a sure sign of deficient lip height. Neither the nostril sill nor the nares are symmetrical with their counterparts on the normal side, and angiomatous skin is often observed in the upper part of the lip (Fig. 6.10).

It is extremely important that the parents understand the full implications of these anomalies. Even these apparently benign forms indicate defective muscle insertions, which require surgical repair of the entire height of the lip. The muscular defect is evident in facial expressions. It can also be verified by palpating the lip between thumb and forefinger, which reveals an obvious difference in the thickness of tissue along the 'scar' line.

There is no urgency in the repair of masked forms, and therefore no reason to rush the surgical procedure. It is up to the parents to choose a suitable date. This leaves them time to get used to the idea of a scar along the entire height of the lip, especially if an over-optimistic picture was presented at the time of their infant's birth.

The same holds true for simple clefts, which stop at various levels on the lip yet all require repair of the entire labial structure.

Anomalies of the nose

These are considered further in a later section.

It has become customary to say that there are no malformations of the nose in unilateral clefts; the nasal structures are said to be simply deformed due to skeletal anomalies and abnormal muscle traction. The major role of the various muscles in the etiology of deformities must be stressed here. In actual fact, this is definitely not the case, and there is always a certain degree of malformation involved. This is obvious not only at the nostril sill, where the lip and the nose are continuous, but also at the base of the columella and the outer wing of the nose.

THE BILATERAL CLEFT LIP

These lip anomalies are altogether different.

In those forms that affect the entire height of the lip, whether simple or complete (and therefore involving bone structures), the medial portion of the lip known as the prolabium presents very specific characteristics (Fig. 6.11).

The medial portion of the lip

1. The mucocutaneous ridge or white roll is rounded, and the angular peaks and dip of a

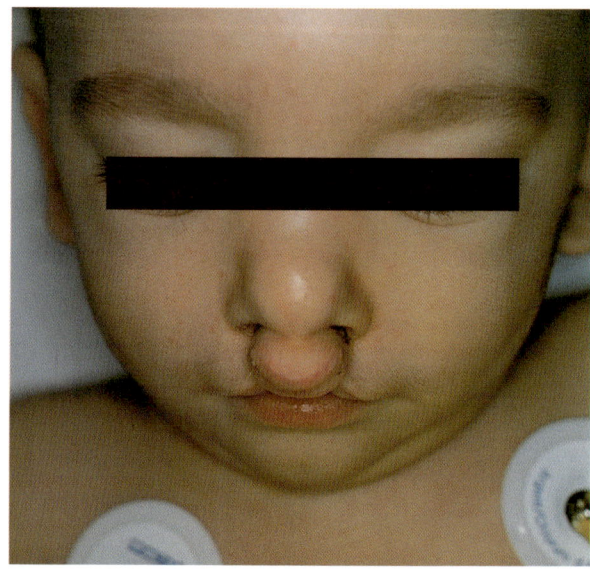

Fig. 6.11 *Typical prolabium in a symmetrical bilateral cleft.*

typical Cupid's bow are generally absent. The ridge extends into the dividing line between the skin and mucosa at the cleft, with no visible notch or indentation to serve as a guide for the reference points.

2. The cutaneous portion often presents a convex surface, shaped like a lens. There is no trace of a philtral ridge or depression. The prolabium is continuous with the base of the columella, which is abnormally short and widened in its lower section. It is elevated by the premaxilla, which tends to project forward. This causes a transverse crease to appear at the labio-columellar junction (Fig. 6.12).

3. The prolabium is usually devoid of properly developed muscle fibers. This is not always the case, particularly if a mucocutaneous band exists or if the cleft does not involve the entire height of the lip. It is likely that the mesenchyme was somehow prevented from penetrating this portion of the lip (as stated by Veau (1938), who used Fleishmann's hypothesis as the basis of his theory). As a result, after lip repair the orbicularis will have medial insertions in connective tissue that contains very scarce muscle fibers. The question is whether or not this zone is likely to grow and produce healthy, functioning muscle fibers after early repair. There is no valid histological data to support an affirmative answer. However, day-to-day clinical experience clearly demonstrates that the prolabium plays a major part in the development of the medial portion of the upper lip. For example, whenever surgery was performed based on the Abbe-Estlander procedure, we found that this portion of the lip contained a layer of well-developed muscle fibers. Without presuming to offer a clinching scientific argument, we have nonetheless come to the conclusion that the prolabium must always be retained, and that flaps from the lateral muscle segments should not be introduced beneath it to reconstruct the sphincteric loop of the orbicularis.

4. The mucosal zone (vermilion and borders of the cleft) is underdeveloped and often coated with desquamative scabs. The vestibule is either absent or is merely suggested by the existence of a furrow, which is frequently ulcerated in its deepest part (Fig. 6.13).

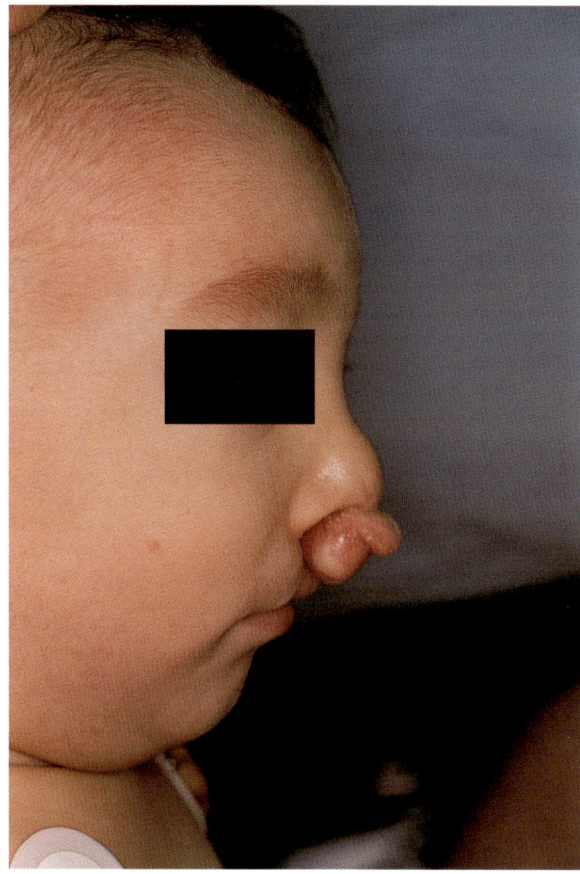

Fig. 6.12 *Forward projection of the prolabium angled out from the columella.*

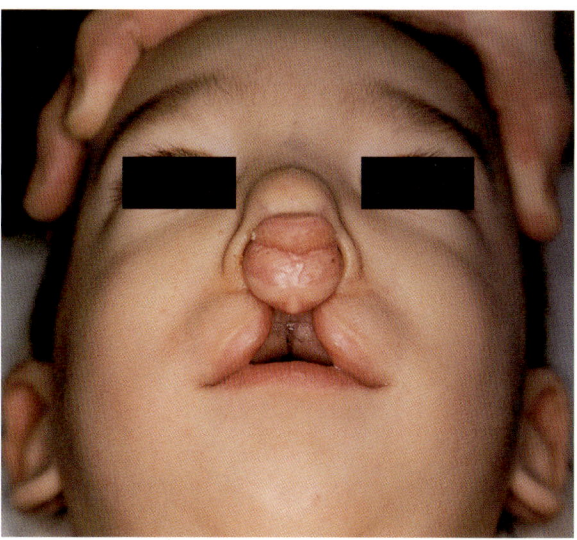

Fig. 6.13 *The shallow vestibule is often simply suggested by an ulcerated furrow.*

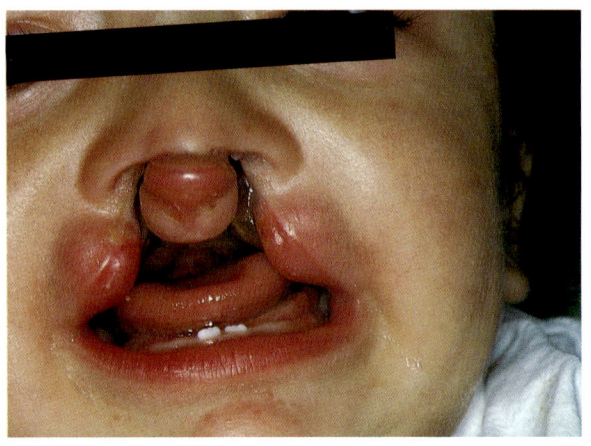

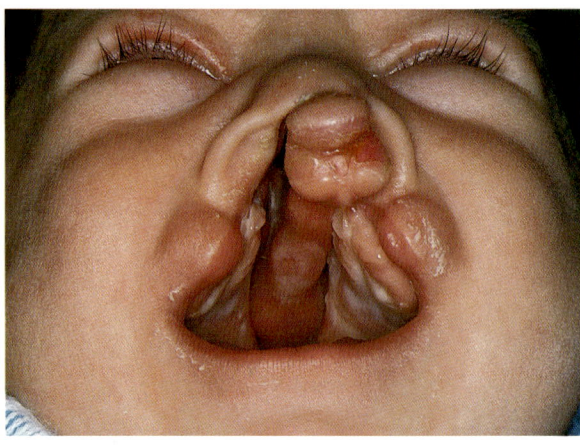

a   b

Fig. 6.14 *The outer portions of the lip seem to dangle well behind the premaxilla.*

5. Although there is no normal side to provide a basis for comparison, the shortfall in the vertical height of the lip is very conspicuous. This height deficiency may seem more moderate along the outer borders, which seem to dangle because they are relatively longer, particularly when mucocutaneous bands exist (Fig. 6.14a and b). It seem logical to assume that the (putative) height of the prolabium should be equal to that measured on a vertical line from the outer alar base. This measurement serves to determine the dimensions of the cleft repair.

The lateral portions of the lip

These present the same characteristics as those described for unilateral clefts. However, the relative deficit in transverse length may seem more striking.

We have also seen that the outer borders may be asymmetrical, particularly when mucocutaneous bands are present (Fig. 6 .15).

MUCOCUTANEOUS BANDS

In a certain number of cases, the borders of the cleft are united by a bridge of soft tissue known as a mucocutaneous band or cutaneous bridge (Veau calculated the ratio at 10%; statistics from Brazil suggest 19.6% (Silva Filho *et al.*, 1994)).

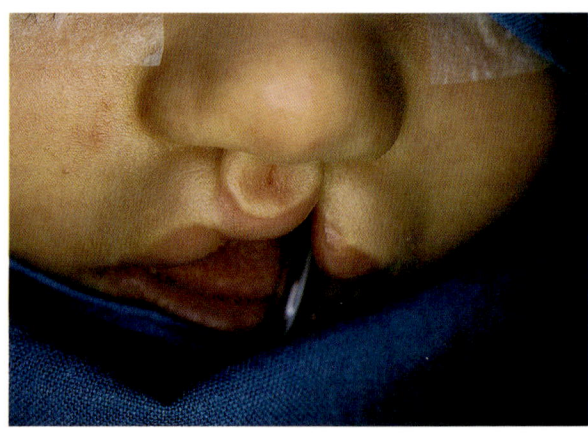

Fig. 6.15 *Unusual aspect of the mucosa in an asymmetrical bilateral form.*

Embryologists have proposed various explanations for the existence of these bands. The majority hold with a theory of incomplete disintegration of the epithelial covering due to abnormal migration of the mesoderm. These bands vary in size, but are always sited at the upper portion of the premaxilla on the inner border and at the junction between the lip and the nose on the upper part of the outer border.

These bands have no influence on the prognosis or on whether the cleft will be easy to treat or not. With respect to the position of the divided maxillary segments, although it is true that sizeable bands may limit the spread between the borders of the cleft, this may not prove to be an advantage in the long term. Conversely, bands cannot prevent the segments from collapsing. Therefore only unusually broad bands can be expected to have any positive effect from an orthopedic standpoint.

On the other hand, in the case of nostril repair, Veau (1938) remarked that the surgical procedure was simplified by the presence of a band (owing both to the lesser width of the cleft and to the more normal curve of the pre-existing nostril rim). The need for secondary nasal repair and the difficulties this involves, however, remain unchanged.

In these circumstances, the arguments put forward by certain specialists to justify the lip-adhesion procedure can be disregarded. These authors contend that surgical construction of a band or adhesion of soft tissue encourages better development of the bone structures and improves the results of nostril repair. On the contrary, the lip adhesion technique, as will be explained, presents serious drawbacks.

Depending on their size, the bands are covered by various types of integument. They may be exclusively cutaneous, or exclusively mucosal. At times, when they are of considerable breadth, they are both cutaneous and mucosal with a dividing line that continues the mucocutaneous line of the lip (Fig. 6.16).

By definition, a band is entirely encompassed by either skin or mucosa. Nevertheless, in simple forms where the cleft does not involve the entire height of the lip, the upper non-cleft portion can be assimilated to a band. Although continuous, it is composed solely of skin and mucosa. There is a gap in the underlying muscle layer, which is both palpable and visible to the naked eye. This zone requires resection during cheiloplasty (Fig. 6.17).

One rare form of band is attached to the cutaneous portion of the outer border at the narinary vestibule, and extends into the mucosa behind the alveolar ridge. This variant is known as Simonart's band, although no publications are available by an author of this name (Gibson, 1977; Gibson and Gustav, 1977) (Fig. 6.18).

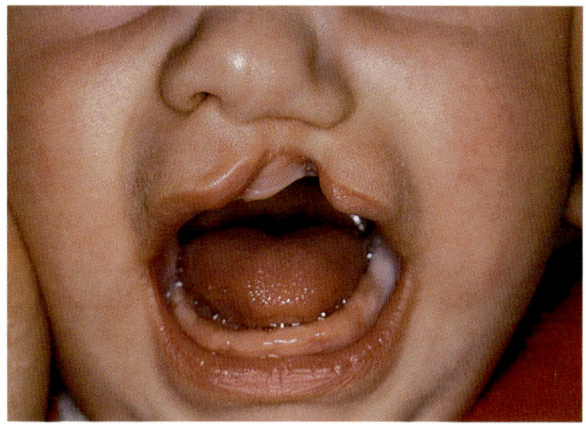

Fig. 6.16 *Band of cutaneous and mucosal tissue in complete cleft.*

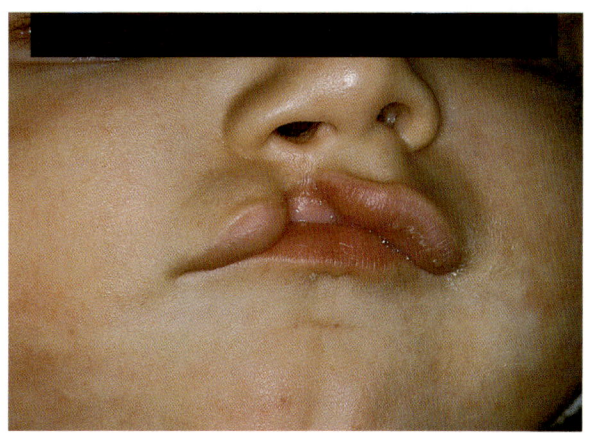

Fig. 6.17 *In simple forms, the band does not contain a muscle layer.*

In order to re-align the unequal height of the two borders and safely obtain the two planes (nasal and buccal) needed for repair, it is usually necessary to sever the bridges. In most cases, hemostasis must be performed on a blood vessel which runs through the centre of the bridge.

In particularly narrow clefts, or those where the bone segments are only moderately out of line, the band may complicate the procedure; for instance, it sometimes happens that the division between the superficial and deep planes that the scalpel should follow in incising the nasal floor no longer forms a

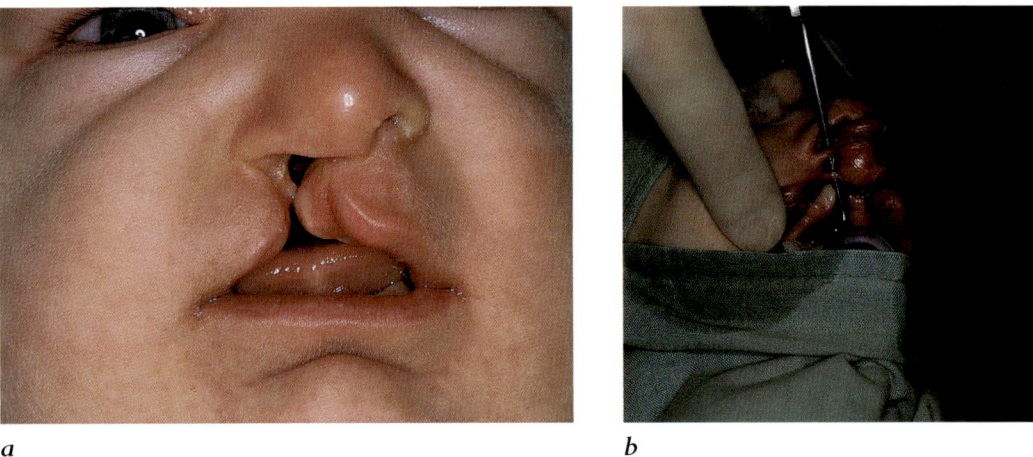

a   *b*

Fig. 6.18 *Simonart's band with an unusual case of a narrow double band.*

straight line. In this case, it is difficult to make the adjustments needed so that the two borders that are to be sutured together are of equal length.

NASAL DEFORMITIES IN SIMPLE CLEFTS

It is generally thought that the nose is deformed rather than malformed in congenital clefts. This is not altogether true if the following factors are taken into account:

1. The nostril sill that corresponds to the junction between lip and nose is affected in the majority of cases.
2. Like the other facial muscles, those that surround the nostrils have abnormal insertions. Therefore from the earliest period of fetal development, during the formation of facial structures, the action of these muscles is greatly altered.
3. Furthermore, local and regional malformative hypoplasia is a constant finding, and this automatically affects these nasal structures.

Simple unilateral cleft lip

In simple unilateral cleft lip, the major lesion concerns the gap in the orbicularis of the upper lip.

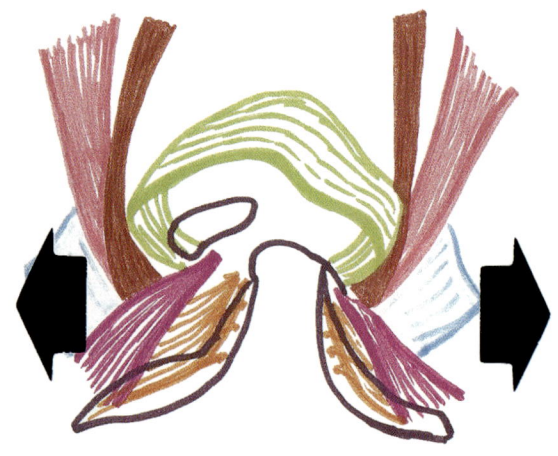

Fig. 6.19 *Muscle division creates opposing forces exerted on nasal structures.*

It follows that the muscle group affected develops a totally new and abnormal action. Instead of fulfilling a sphincteric function, the two portions of muscle separated by the gap tend to pull in opposite directions. One exerts traction on the outer alar base; the other on the base of the columella (Fig. 6.19). This divergent traction causes deformity of the tip of the nose and of the nostrils, which can be more or less pronounced but tends to conform to a certain type (Fig. 6.20):

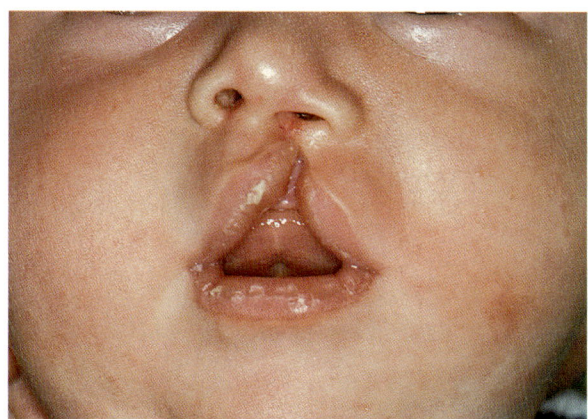

Fig. 6.20 *Nasal deformities in simple clefts are similar to those encountered in total forms.*

- Flattening and widening of the nostril aperture on the cleft side;
- The columella is slanted towards the affected side;
- The lower border of the septum is visible in the orifice of the normal nostril;
- The alar base is slightly everted, revealing the cutaneous zone of the vestibule, and is lower than its counterpart on the opposite side;
- The anterior nasal spine may be displaced towards the normal side;
- The free border of the nostril is somewhat lower than it should be; and
- The tip of the nose is slightly asymmetrical.

These deformities are minor versions of those encountered in complete forms, which are compounded by misalignment of the bony borders (see Chapter 18).

In simple forms, most of these deformities (with the exception of those involving the septal cartilage and the anterior nasal spine) can return to normal once the nostril sill is corrected and proper facial muscle insertions are restored.

Simple bilateral cleft lip

In symmetrical forms of simple bilateral cleft lip, the nose is not deviated. Its tip, however, is moderately

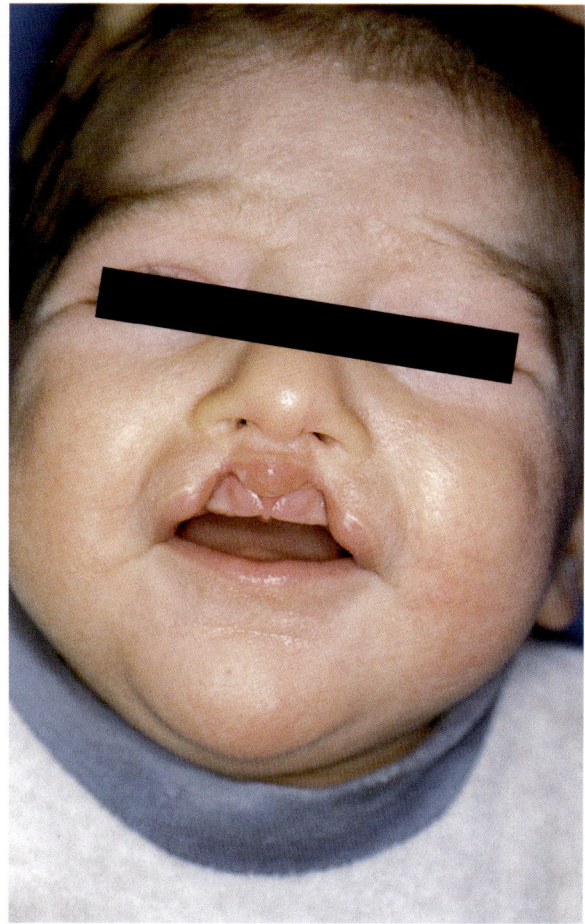

Fig. 6.21 *Medial hypoplasia of the columella and the prolabium in a bilateral simple form.*

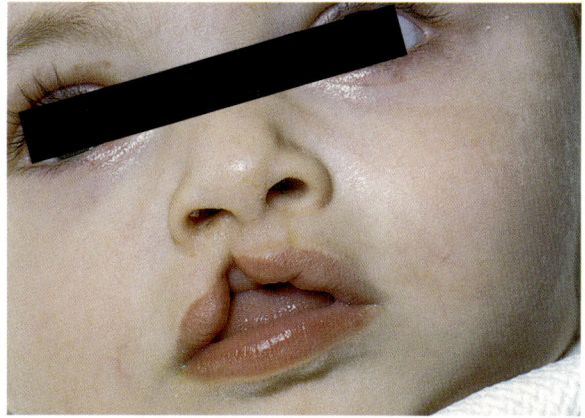

Fig. 6.22 *In asymmetrical forms, the nose more or less resembles the unilateral forms.*

flattened and widened. The columella seems too short, and its junction with the prolabium is not clearly marked. The septal cartilage is often underdeveloped, which is a sign of more severe regional hypoplasia than might ordinarily be expected in what is thought to be a relatively mild anatomo-clinical form (Fig. 6.21).

In asymmetrical forms, the imbalance of muscle forces produces nasal deformities resembling those of unilateral forms (Fig. 6.22).

7. Primary treatment

HISTORICAL LANDMARKS

The true men of progress are those who start with a deep respect for the past

(Ernest Renan)

A look at history is always enlightening. It bears witness to the continuity of human concerns and teaches a lesson in humility.

It has become commonplace to say that all there is to write has already been written. Conversely, today's beliefs will be erased tomorrow by other opinions and techniques. The dogged search for truth is ingrained in human nature, despite the knowledge that it will never be attained.

Works on labio-palatal clefts hark back to time immemorial, and a few landmark dates may help to explain the origins of our own therapeutic method. The data for the following list is drawn from an article published in *Cleft lip and palate* (Rogers, 1971).

The first cleft lip operation is thought to have been performed in the year 390 AD.

The Flemish surgeon Jehan Yperman (1295–1351) was the first to describe cleft lip repair. In 1510, Ambroise Paré coined the French term *bec-de-lièvre*, or hare-lip. Gaspare Tagliacozzi (1545–1599) called the cleft lip surgeon an 'artist' (Tagliacozzi, 1597).

In the seventeenth century, Hendrick von Roonhuyse (1674) recommended that infants be operated on at the age of 3–4 months.

The eighteenth century was the age of a generation of eminent cleft surgeons, notably in France. André Myrrhen inaugurated the use of a technique for lengthening the soft palate in the early eighteenth century (Myrrhen, 1721), and Levret emphasized the importance of oral and palatal sphincters (Levret, 1772). Eustache described his operation for suturing the split velum in 1783 (Dorance, 1933) and Desault introduced the use of a pre-operative retaining device in 1791 and advocated primary closure of the soft palate before cheiloplasty (Desault, 1798).

In the nineteenth century, true palatal surgery was initiated by Roux (1819), von Graefe (1817 and 1820) and Warren, in America, in 1820 (Warren 1828, 1867). Towards the mid-nineteenth century, the modern era of labial surgery was ushered in by Malgaigne in 1843 (Malgaigne 1861) and Mirault (1844), who is hailed as the forefather of flap techniques. Collis was the first to describe a double lip plasty (Collis, 1868) and, in 1884, Hagedorn introduced a flap procedure which was later adopted by Le Mesurier.

In the 1930s, no doubt thanks to the development of improved anesthesia, modern cleft surgery reached maturity. In France it is traditionally thought that Victor Veau was the pioneer of modern techniques. He is known for his fine descriptions of cleft lesions and his method of suturing homologous tissue layers.

GENERAL ASPECTS OF SURGERY

Anesthesia

Surgery is always performed under general anesthesia.

The pre-operative physical is extremely important in that it helps to prepare for potential difficulties related to associated malformations (such as the contraindication to local vasoconstrictors in the case of cardiac malformations). It gives a picture of the patient's general state of health and, thanks to complementary tests, furnishes data on the hemoglobin count, which is often low in very young infants. The examination also offers a good opportunity to appraise the family environment, since parental cooperation is essential for proper post-operative care.

It should be repeated on the eve of the operation, bearing in mind how frequently surgery has to be postponed due to infections in infants.

The anesthetic is generally administered through an endotracheal tube; using a mask is hardly feasible for operations involving the mouth area. Intubation also helps to prevent liquids or blood from seeping into the trachea. Theoretically, the endotracheal tube could be replaced by a 'laryngeal mask', which does not pass into the glottis and therefore precludes the risk of post-operative glottal edema, but the diameter of the tube of the mask itself can make its use a hindrance. Endotracheal intubation, which came into common use after World War II, has vastly improved the conditions for cleft surgery.

Except in a very few specific cases, the tube is inserted orally and is securely taped in the very center of the lower lip. This position permits the use of mouth-gags in palatal surgery, and does not present an obstacle to symmetrical lip repair. The use of 'preformed' tubes that are flexed to fit over the lower lip also represents a significant improvement. They avoid miscalculations in the length of the tube inserted into the trachea (and the risk of intubating only the right bronchus), and leave no protruding structures to interfere with the movements of the surgeon or assistant.

The endotracheal tube used for young infants is not equipped with an inflatable gas-bag. Pharyngeal packs are not necessary since the position of the tiny patient, with head extended, avoids the passage of fluids (antiseptic, saline solution, blood, etc.) into the larynx or trachea. As an extra precaution, a simple gauze can be placed in the oropharynx. If this is the case, it must be easy to retrieve, and a length of heavy suture material clipped to the drapes at some distance from the mouth area makes sure of this. It will not then be forgotten once the operation is over; such a mishap will result in serious ventilation problems.

The tube rests on the dorsal surface of the tongue, and holds it down in a central position.

Modern anesthesiology equipment greatly simplifies the anesthetist's task of monitoring these small patients throughout the procedure. A constant check can be kept on ventilation, blood–gas ratios and cardiovascular activity.

A flexible catheter is set up in a vein of the infant's hand or foot, for injections and per-operative drips.

In this type of surgery, blood transfusions are rarely needed thanks to the temporary hemostasis obtained by infiltration of an epinephrine solution.

Positioning the patient

The infant is installed at one end of the table, with the head resting on an adjustable support or, better still, on a plastic ring that holds the skull in a stable position. A rolled sheet or towel is placed beneath the shoulders to keep the neck extended (Fig. 7.1).

It is customary for the surgeon to stand at the head of the table, with the chief assistant on the right and the anesthesiologist to the surgeon's left. From this position, the surgeon will be better able to visualize facial symmetry and to judge the results of lip plasty, and will have free access to both sides of the bucco-pharyngeal cavity.

A tray is installed crosswise above the infant's chest. This gives the anesthesiologist more room to check the endotracheal tube and reach the child's thorax or limbs (where a vein or veins have been prepared).

The infant's eyes are taped shut with sterile strips. It is advisable to put a drop of vaseline oil or ophthalmic liquid in each eye beforehand to protect the corneas against irritation from blood or antiseptics.

To avoid skin and mucosal reactions, the favored antiseptic is a colorless, diluted solution of quaternary ammonium. After this solution has been applied, the lip is cleansed with alcohol to bring the surface tension up to normal; otherwise, the ink used to mark the reference points and trace the design of the repair might run.

Infiltration

The tissues of the operative site are usually infiltrated, both to facilitate mucoperiosteal undermining and to

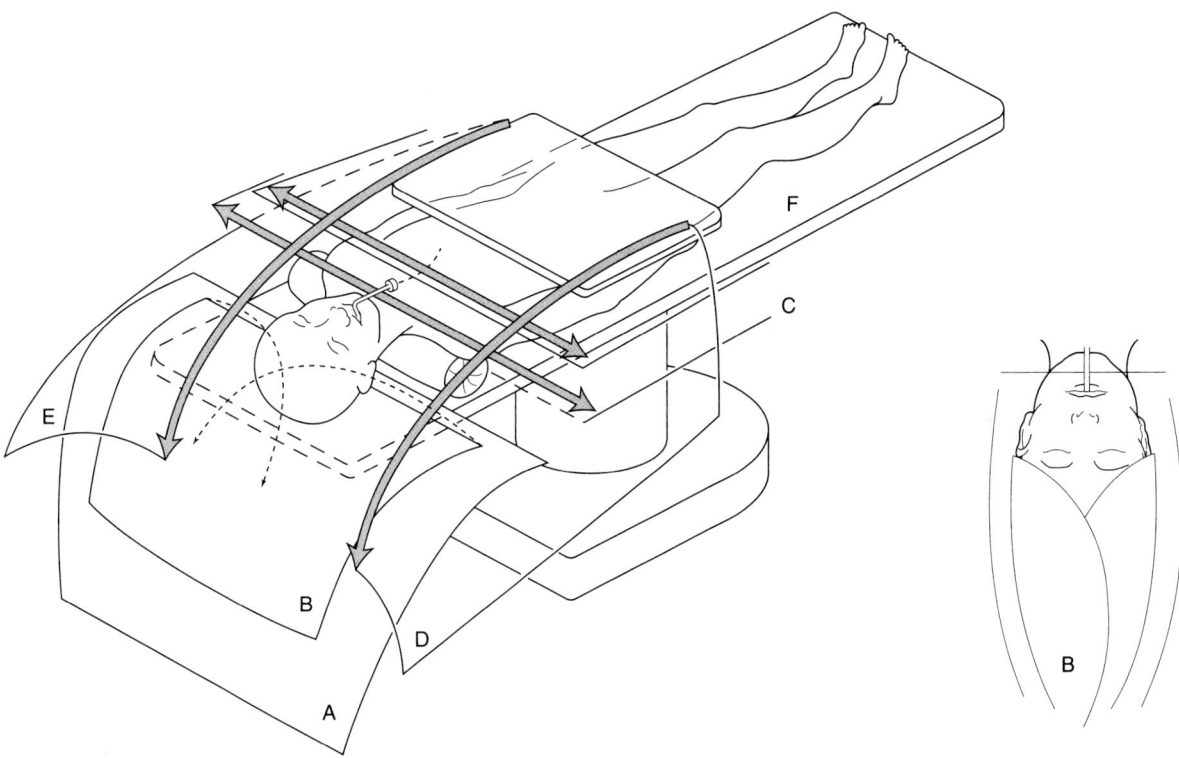

Fig. 7.1 *Installing the patient on the operating table. The head is positioned with the neck hyperextended (the table is fitted with an adjustable head-rest and a rolled towel is placed under the infant's shoulders). The drapes are arranged in the routine manner: A and B beneath the head, with B folded over across the child's forehead; C is on the tray set above the thorax, and is attached to the endotracheal tube under the child's chin; D and E are spread across the head-rest; F is also spread over the tray. Thus, the anesthesiologist has convenient access to the respiratory and cardiac regions and to the upper limbs, where venous catheters are in place.*

reduce bleeding thanks to the temporary hemostatic effect of a vasoconstrictor. A solution of Buvipacaine hydrochlorate (Marcaine) or of Novocaine containing a small dose of epinephrine (0.25%) is used. A special syringe with a very fine needle permits trouble-free infiltration under high pressure.

Both labial borders are infiltrated, as is the surface of the deeper bony elements. In the inter-alveolar and palatal region, the bevelled tip of the needle must be oriented so as to elevate the densely connected mucosa and periosteum. This will reduce the risk of tearing during the undermining procedure, which should be performed with a Veau elevator. To avoid

tissue damage during suturing, the needle should take a good bite of the periosteum, which is the only element sturdy enough to resist the tension inevitably exerted on the borders.

Preventive hemostasis greatly simplifies the procedure.

In certain cases – for example, an infant with associated cardiac malformations – the anesthesiologist usually asks the surgeon not to use epinephrine, which may cause episodes of hypertension or tachycardia. Nonetheless, the operative site must be infiltrated (with a simple saline solution if need be) to obtain the desired elevation of mucoperiosteal tissue.

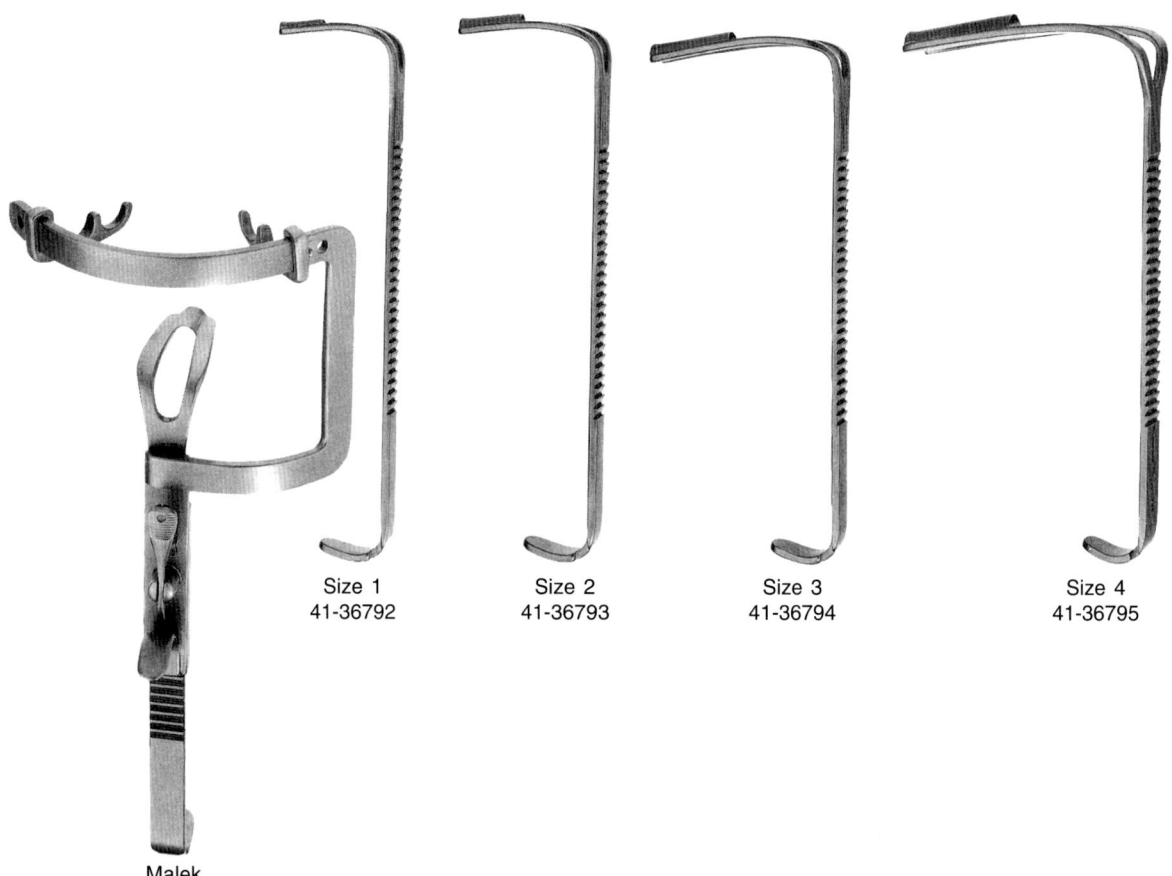

Size 1
41-36792

Size 2
41-36793

Size 3
41-36794

Size 4
41-36795

Malek

Fig. 7.2 *The Malek mouth-gag. The dimensions are specifically adapted to the mouths of infants, and do not collapse the endotracheal tube (D. Leibinger GmbH).*

Post-operative care

Barring special cases, a drip is no longer needed since fluids can be administered to the infant shortly after surgery.

Stiff cylinders are customarily used as elbow restraints on the upper limbs. These are easily constructed from sturdy cardboard, and prevent the infant from sucking his or her fingers or touching the wounds.

Feeding is quickly resumed post-operatively. To minimize sucking efforts and avoid contact between the fresh wounds and a teat, normal baby bottles are proscribed. This policy has been contested but, true to the old saying 'An ounce of prevention is worth a pound of cure', we stand by it. Even very small infants rapidly adjust to spoon feeding.

Although many pediatricians disagree, we also routinely prescribe antibiotics, particularly during wintertime.

Lateral rather than ventral decubitus is recommended, to avoid any rubbing against the labial sutures.

Lastly, the lip wounds require no local care. Any tape strips that come unstuck should be removed, but it is better to leave them alone during the period of edema, which lasts for about 48 hours.

The infant can be discharged on the fourth day after surgery. The stitches are removed on the sixth or seventh day.

SURGICAL EQUIPMENT

The surgical equipment should be specifically adapted to this type of operation (Fig. 7.2). The same kit can be used either for cheiloplasty or for palatal surgery, and includes:

- Angulated dissecting forceps (Adson type) with teeth and very fine jaws
- A second dissecting forceps, fine gauge and sharp-toothed for grabbing the tongue
- Six Halsted hemostatic clips (or mosquito hemostats), fine gauge and flat-edged
- Set of four drape clamps
- Set of four flat clamps (Terrier or Péan type)
- Two scalpel holders with interchangeable #11, 12, and 15 blades
- Pair of Metzenbaum scissors
- Pair of fine, curved, pointed scissors with spatulated blades
- Pair of blunt scissors with spatulated blades
- Pair of large Mayo scissors
- Two Gillies plasty skinhooks
- Veau elevator
- Blunt Trelat hook with right-angle bend
- Narrow blunt spatula
- Small suction tip with no lateral opening at end
- Set of four cups of different sizes with easy to identify colors for:
  Cleansing solution of quaternary ammonium (low concentration)
  Solution for local infiltration
  Saline solution
  Ink
- Pen-holder
- Small dividers
- Pre-printed card showing 120° and 150° angles with a common apex and side
- Veau toothed-rack mouth-gag.

In separate packaging (due to the size of the instrument or to the type of sterilization):

- A high-pressure syringe for local infiltration to dissociate tissues like the periosteum, complete with sets of fine needles and long needles
- A Malek mouth-gag (variation on the Dingman–Gillies version) featuring a choice of blade sizes (notably a very small caliber for early velar surgery) and a groove, which avoids compression of the endotracheal tube against the mandibular rim during palatal surgery (Fig. 7.3)
- One or several fine caliber Reverdin needles with a mobile eye (known in France as Petit needles),

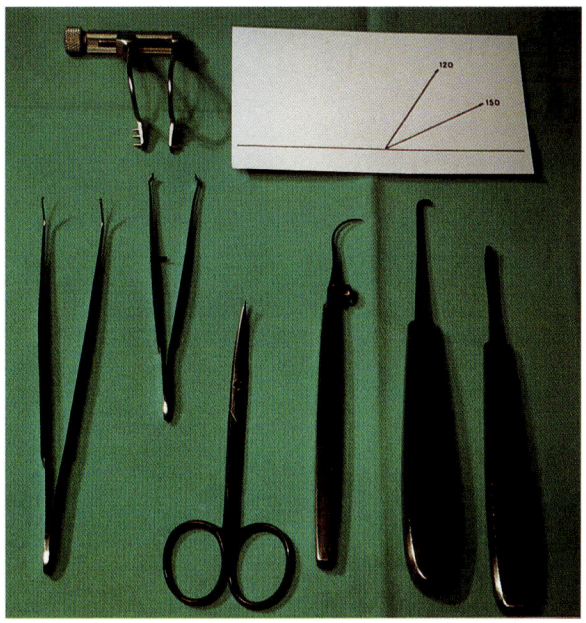

Fig. 7.3 *Specific instruments required for cleft lip/palate surgery. From left to right:*

- *Angulated Adson forceps*
- *Adjustable Veau mouth-gag (used in cleft lip surgery)*
- *Small, curved, sharp-pointed scissors*
- *'Aiguille de Petit', a variation on the Reverdin needle with a mobile eye, which is useful in cleft palate surgery (suture of nasal layer)*
- *Trelat's blunt hook — used for dissection and fracturing the hamulus*
- *Veau's elevator*
- *At the top: a sterile card on which 120° and 150° angles are pre-printed.*

indispensable for closure of the nasal layer of the vault.

Medium rather than small gauzes are used, to avoid the risk of leaving one behind. If a swatch of gauze is inserted into the pharynx to seal off the tracheal vestibule, it should be attached to a length of heavy suture material which is then clamped to an outer drape for easy identification and retrieval.

Suture materials should include the following:

- For palatal surgery: absorbable sutures, 4/0 and 5/0 as a rule, though sometimes 3/0 and 2/0 in older children
- For labial surgery: very fine, non-absorbable 6/0 nylon or equivalent, plus absorbable material for suturing the mucosa.

Bipolar coagulation and suction apparatus is indispensable.

Finally, dressings of adhesive tape are widely used at the end of surgery. They limit lip movement, provide temporary protection of the sutures from nasal secretions, and help combat post-operative edema.

Unlike many surgeons, we never use bandages within the mouth (vaselined dressings sutured over a roll of gauze).

MODERN PRINCIPLES OF LIP REPAIR

The major evolutions in cleft lip repair are relatively recent.

At first, surgeons sought, naturally enough, simply to close the gap by suturing the freshened borders together in a straight line. Since no adequate suture material was available at the time, their main problem was to keep the sutures from tearing apart while maintaining apposition of the raw tissues and, at the same time, relieving the tension produced by closure of the cleft.

Later, to correct the obvious shortening of the upper lip, surgeons began to curve their denuding incisions.

In 1848, Mirault from Angers suggested a technique that elevated a flap from the outer border and inserted it between the lips of an incision on the inner side of the cleft. This procedure was limited to the vermilion.

In Paris, Jalaguier (1910) used similar methods of repair of the white or cutaneous lip, thus heralding our modern techniques. His pupil, Victor Veau, however, returned to the technique of vertical straight-line incisions, no doubt to reduce excessive scarring. To compensate for the height deficit, this procedure required considerable resection along the

width of the two borders, which tended to produce a tight upper lip.

During the 1950s and 1960s flap techniques were resurrected, and have since come to be the most widely used methods of repair.

In 1945, Le Mesurier of Toronto devised a quadrilateral flap procedure (Le Mesurier 1949), which represented a modified version of the technique originally described by Hagedorn in 1892.

In 1952, Tennison introduced a triangular flap method which, for the first time, preserved the Cupid's bow. A wire stencil was used to outline its contours.

In 1955, Millard (1958) presented another version based on a lateral triangular flap.

These well-known techniques will be reviewed later, comparing their relative merits with those of our method.

In the past few decades, a general consensus has been reached concerning the criteria of satisfactory lip repair.

Unilateral clefts

1. The width of the lip must be preserved. As a rule, it seems clear that the horizontal width of the upper lip is not reduced in labial clefts. This is not totally true, of course, since most surgeons have come across hypoplastic clefts where the stump or stumps show three-dimensional lack of development. It is most important that tissues from the existing width are never sacrificed to gain better vertical height.
2. The natural Cupid's bow, which is always present on the inner border, must be preserved in its entirety.
3. The height of the lip on the cleft side and its symmetry with the normal side must be the surgeon's constant concern. To increase lip height, a flap procedure based on the principle of a Z-plasty is the only valid solution. Exact symmetry must be calculated with mathematical precision.
4. To ensure that the flaps retain their original dimensions and hold up under the strain to which they are subjected when the borders are drawn together, it is essential to use relatively thick cutaneo-muscular flaps. Subcutaneous undermining of the lip muscles is therefore to be avoided.

Since labial muscles are in fact skin muscles, their intimate connection with the surrounding tegument must be preserved.

5. The results of lip repair should be equally satisfactory from both a static and a dynamic point of view. The orientation of the muscle fibers depends on the outlines of the incision, since the cutaneomuscular flaps that are used must undergo a certain degree of rotation. The incision must therefore take into account the final direction of the muscle fibers, which are to be re-inserted into the bone and periosteum as naturally as possible. These factors dictate the appearance of the lip during muscle contraction (facial expressions).

6. The lip is naturally continuous with the nostril floor, which must be reconstructed when cheiloplasty is performed. Simple 'drawing the curtain' closure of the lip, which leaves the cleft open behind it, produces disastrous static and dynamic results despite being justified by some specialists as sparing those structures adjacent to bone and particularly to the periosteum in order to avoid osteo-dental disorders. Secondary repair of the ensuing defects requires complete surgical reconstruction of the lip.

7. In complete forms, labial repair should have as few repercussions as possible on the position and growth of the maxillary segments. Extensive undermining and minimal resection can help reduce subsequent tension.

It is advisable not to intervene in the first few months after birth, during which time the bone structures are particularly pliable and are therefore easily affected by the pressures around them. This influences the choice of techniques and, to an even greater extent, that of the date at which labial surgery is to be performed. Neonatal repair should be proscribed.

Bilateral clefts

1. As above, the entire width of the lip, and in particular that portion of white roll on the prolabium corresponding to the Cupid's bow, must be preserved. As a rule, the Cupid's bow is virtually non-existent in bilateral clefts.

2. As is the case with unilateral clefts, 'drawing the curtain' closures should be ruled out.

3. Lip closure in bilateral clefts must always be performed in two stages. In complete clefts, where undermining involves the premaxillary segment and the adjacent vomer, if enough tissue is to be dissected to close the inter-alveolar region, the primary palate and the bony palatal vault simultaneously, there are serious risks involved in closing both sides of the cleft in a single operation. Such extensive denuding might jeopardize the vascular supply to the bone structures. However, some surgeons continue to advocate simultaneous closure of both sides on the grounds that it makes symmetry more easy to obtain.

   In addition to the vascular risk to the bone structures, this procedure presents other drawbacks. It increases the transverse tension, which is detrimental to a satisfactory scar line and even more so to the proper position and growth of the bony segments. It also creates the danger of insufficient blood supply to the lower and medial portion of the lip. If the surgeon has chosen a flap procedure, whatever the specific technique, the incision on the inner border (needed for the insertion of the flap raised from the outer border) inevitably cuts across the prolabium. When both sides undergo surgery in a single operation, the two incisions (and the dissection of the mucosa that accompanies them) isolate part of the prolabium. Deprived of its blood supply, this portion is condemned to necrosis. Lip closure must therefore always be performed in two stages, separated by an interval of about 2 months, to ensure satisfactory vascularization of the first cicatricial zone.

4. The labio-columellar junction must be left intact in bilateral clefts. As already stated, an abnormally short columella is one of the hallmarks of these forms. However, any attempt to lengthen it during cheiloplasty automatically leads to surgery on both sides during the same operation, an unacceptable procedure. Since it is difficult to include correction of the short columella in either phase of the two-stage cheiloplasty, it seems advisable to postpone this until later.

5. Correcting a height deficit of the upper lip calls for a flap procedure involving its lower portion. If the surgical aim is simply vertically to lengthen

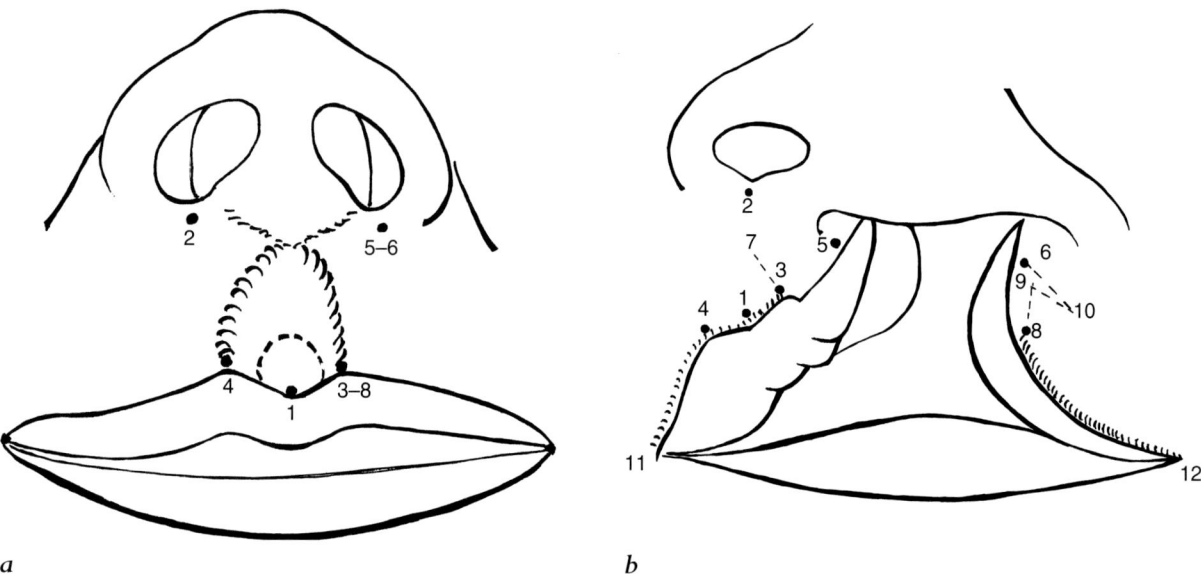

a   *b*

Fig. 7.4 *The numeral system generally accepted for a unilateral cleft corrected with an inferior triangular flap of the Tennison type:*

a.   Numbers on a normal lip.

b.   Numeral system used for unilateral clefts. Numerals 8, 9 and 10 designate the triangle to be inserted into the incision on the inner border indicated by 3 and 7.

the lip, it is better to avoid the upper or high plasties, which concern flaps elevated from the upper portion of the lip (see Malek's inverted triangle or Millard's procedures). These necessarily cut into the labio-columellar junction. Scar formation at this level is often highly visible, and may preclude secondary repair based on one of many techniques (local flap or Brauer plasty, Abbe-Estlander or the Millard forked flap method).

6. The height, which serves as a reference in bilateral clefts, is calculated by measuring the vertical segment from the mucocutaneous ridge to the outer alar base.

7. The labial vestibule is virtually non-existent in bilateral clefts, and must be constructed from scratch by advancing outer mucosal tissue during the two-stage plasty.

8. The absence of muscle tissue in the prolabium should not be corrected by suturing well-developed fibers from the outer borders together at all costs. This procedure tends to create an excessively tight upper lip.

REFERENCE POINTS

Numbering the reference points

Assigning a number to each reference point is not an easy task. In international literature, a consensus seems to have been reached. According to Tennison (1952), the numbers to be used range from 1 to 12 (Fig. 7.4). It can be difficult to retain this system, and a simpler method is proposed (Fig. 7.5). After points 1, 2 and 3 have been placed for the Cupid's bow, it seems only logical to continue clockwise to mark the nostril sill on either side. The reference points corresponding to the outer borders will be the same, distinguished by an asterisk (2' and 5'). The points for the corners of the lips will always be numbered 6 for the left side and 7 for the right.

Plotting the reference points

Plotting the reference points represents an essential step in the operation. Measurements are taken that enable the surgeon to calculate the precise dimensions of the plasty needed to obtain satisfactory lip

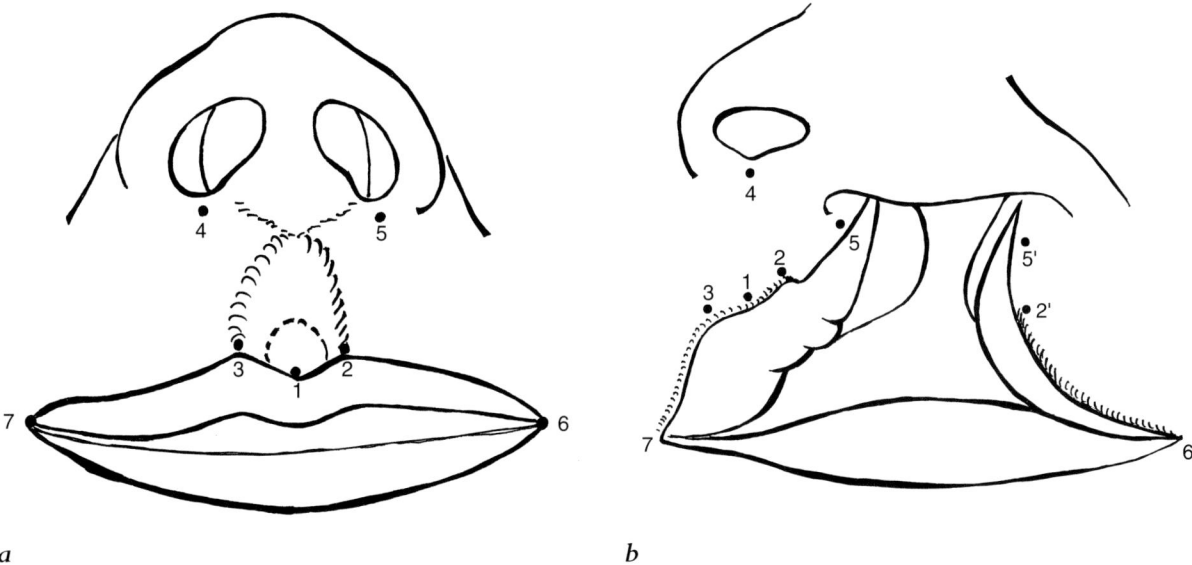

a

b

Fig. 7.5 *Alternative system, suitable for bilateral clefts as well as unilateral:*
a. *On a normal lip.*
b. *On a cleft lip. The reference points on the outer border equating to those for the Cupid's bow and nostril sill on the inner border(s) are distinguished by asterisks.*

height. If errors develop, these can seriously jeopardize the end results. The present chapter should therefore be read with close attention.

The height of the normal lip must be calculated. This is relatively simple in unilateral clefts, but more difficult for bilateral forms.

If a triangular flap plasty is programmed, it is important to establish the height of the cleft.

For both measurements, the precise position of the Cupid's bow must be determined. It is easy to detect on the inner border of a unilateral cleft. In bilateral forms, it corresponds to that portion of the mucocutaneous ridge belonging to the prolabium, which must be preserved to create the replica of a Cupid's bow.

The Cupid's bow

Unilateral clefts

In unilateral forms, it is not always easy to locate the exact site of those three points that correspond to the Cupid's bow. In certain cases, this feature is not clearly visible on the mucocutaneous ridge.

The inferior angle (or 'valley') of the bow is reasonably simple to find; by pinching the lip transversely, the lower angle of the V-shaped valley is accentuated. This marks the midpoint.

On the normal side, a concave curve is usually visible on the lower portion of the philtral ridge. Since there is no sharp angle to serve as a guide, the point that corresponds to the lateral limit or superior peak of the bow can only be surmised (Fig. 7.6). On the cleft side there is often a notch in the mucocutaneous ridge, which marks the beginning of the lower portion of the cleft. Here, it is always the cutaneous zone that encroaches on the vermilion to form a step. The lateral point or peak of the bow can be located quite accurately at this site.

Thus, with experience, the location of the opposite peak of the bow can be determined by marking off two small segments, which are symmetrically positioned on either side of the midpoint. A caliper can be used to check that the two segments of the bow are of equal length. It is important to preserve as much tissue as possible on the inner side of the stepped notch that indents the white roll on

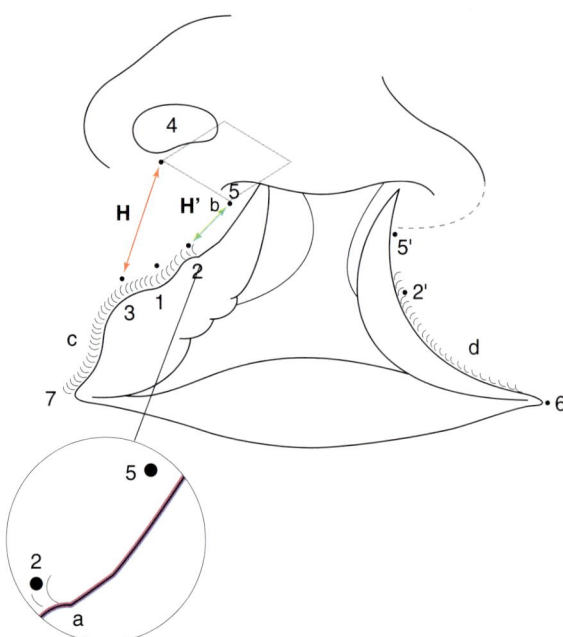

Fig. 7.6 *Reference points placed according to our numerical system. Diagram shows:*

a. *Step in skin–vermilion line on the inner border at the lower end of cleft (insert).*

b. *Line extending the contour of the medial crus of the alar cartilage, which helps to locate reference point 5 for the nostril sill. Segment 4–5 forms a tangent with the lower edge of the columella.*

c. *Cross-hatched zone in upper portion of outer border, corresponding to the skin of the nostril vestibule. Point 5′ must not be placed too high.*

d. *Distances c and d are generally equal, which helps to locate point 2′.*

the cleft side. The same holds true for the curved portion of white roll on the normal side.

Bilateral clefts

In bilateral clefts, the prolabium rarely presents a bow 'valley' with a clear-cut lower angle. This future midpoint of the replicated Cupid's bow can be located by referring to the frenum of the upper lip. It is determined by continuing the line of the frenum until it meets the mucocutaneous ridge (Fig. 7.7).

The choice of the two lateral points remains arbitrary. Enough of the white roll on the prolabium must be retained so that the triangular flaps, which are always located near the free border of the lip in bilateral clefts, do not overlap. This would seriously compromise the results and present a risk to the vascular supply of the lower portion of the prolabium.

It is true that, in most cases, the width of the prolabium will spread considerably once repair has been effected on both sides. However, rather than have the outcome compromised from the start, it is always better to work with a broad prolabium, which can furnish additional flap material for secondary repair if necessary. It is a characteristic of cleft surgery that the situation can easily be improved by removing excess tissue, whereas adding tissue where it is lacking is a far more difficult proposition.

The nostril sill

Next, the reference points for the nostril sill are located on the normal side and on the inner border of the cleft.

Unilateral clefts

In unilateral clefts, plotting is relatively easy on the normal side. The appearance of the sill varies from one individual to another. There is frequently a sub-narinary crease, on which the reference point for the lower pole of the nostril should be indicated. If there is no crease, it is possible to draw a line in ink that continues the curved contour of the outer alar base. The reference point is marked on this line at the centre of the nostril sill. Another way to determine this point is by exerting traction with a Gillies skinhook placed in the ala near the tip of the nose. This causes the structures of the base and lower border of the medial crus of the alar cartilage to protrude. Here, too, a line is drawn in ink, which continues the ideal curve of the protruding structures. The reference point for the sill is marked at the lower pole of the nostril opening.

On the inner border of the cleft, traction with the skinhook is the only maneuver that can locate the point corresponding to the nostril sill. It is in a considerably lower position than its counterpart.

The line formed by joining these two reference points for the nostril sills is normally tangential to the lower plane of the columella.

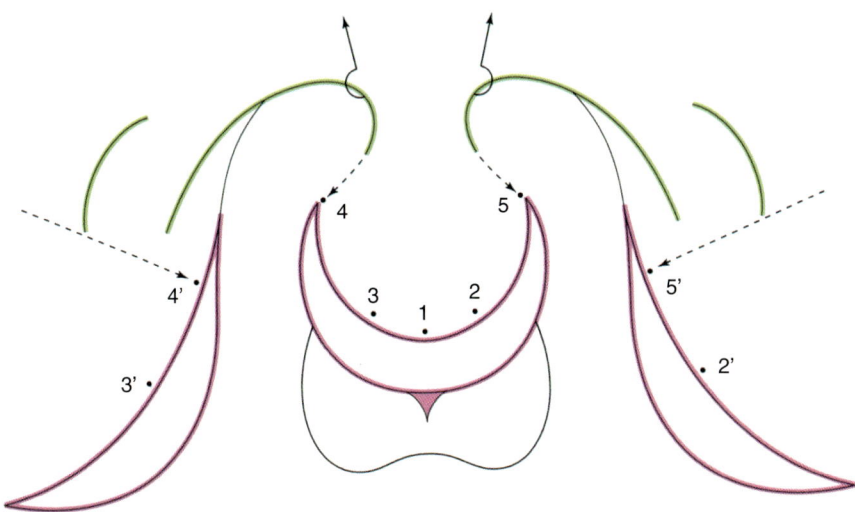

Fig. 7.7 *Placement of the reference points in symmetrical bilateral clefts. Point 1 is directly above the furrow in the premaxilla, on a line with the medial frenum of the prolabium. The reference height for measurement is the height of the lip measured from the outer alar base.*

Bilateral clefts

In bilateral clefts, the traction maneuver is also used to site the points that mark the inner border on either side.

The outer border of the lip

Unilateral clefts

The reference point equating to the lateral peak of the Cupid's bow is relatively easy to determine. It is located at the point where the ridge, which usually runs above the white roll, disappears from sight. Still, the precise point is not always clearly visible.

Since there is no width deficiency in the majority of unilateral clefts, this point can also be determined by using a caliper to measure the distance between the corner of the lip and the lateral reference point that indicates the peak of the Cupid's bow on the normal side. This distance is then transposed from the angle of the commissure on the cleft side, and the point can be marked without any risk of gross miscalculation.

By far the most difficult reference point to determine is that marking the nostril sill on the outer edge of the cleft. It must be remembered that, in the presence of a cleft, the alar base is subject to the distorted action of the facial muscles, which have lost their midline insertions on the nasal spine (see Chapter 6).

The alar cartilage is slightly everted because the deeper tissues remain anchored to the periosteum of the lateral maxillary process, and finds itself in a lower position than is normal due to the action of the sphincteric rings. These subsist despite the labial gap, as demonstrated by J. Delaire (1983). Thus, part of the cutaneous surface that is visible on the upper portion of the lip actually belongs to the nasal vestibule.

The usual tendency is to site the reference point for this nostril sill much too high. To avoid such a mistake, it is a good idea to grasp the nostril near the alar base and visualize the movement of rotation it will undergo once the cleft is repaired.

In most unilateral clefts where there is no cutaneous band, both sides of the cleft are identical in height. By comparing them with one another, the surgeon can avoid any gross error in plotting the location of the reference points.

Bilateral clefts

The same problems are encountered in plotting the reference points on both lateral borders. For the lower point that corresponds to the peak of the Cupid's bow, there is no normal width of tissue to serve as a guide. Hypoplasia of the whole area is far more pronounced, as is the convex curve of the white roll.

The ridge above this line is often less clearly defined. Extra caution is in order here, since the vertical height of the outer border of the cleft is often greater than that of its inner border due to hypoplasia of the prolabium. This is particularly noticeable in simple forms. The separation between the dry and moist zones of the vermilion can be of some assistance; however, the position of this reference point is often determined arbitrarily.

The upper point of the nostril sill is more easy to locate by following the method recommended for unilateral clefts.

Summary

To summarize, the reference points serve to determine the lengths of two segments:

1. The normal height of the lip between the reference point of the nostril sill and the lateral point that indicates the peak of the Cupid's bow in the case of unilateral clefts (4–3). For bilateral clefts, this normal reference does not exist. The height of the lip must be determined by using a caliper to measure the height of the outer border on a vertical line from the outer alar base. If the prolabium is severely hypoplastic, this figure may have to be reduced so that the calculations based on it will not lead to dissection of a triangle that is too big to be used on both sides.
2. The height of the cleft, which is measured exclusively on the inner border between the reference point for the peak of the bow and the point for the nostril sill. Indeed, the height of the cleft often differs from one border to the other, particularly when there is a cutaneous band (5–2).

This discussion demonstrates that, whichever the method applied, mistakes can still be made in plotting the reference points that serve as a basis for calculating the dimensions of the desired plasty.

This stage of plotting and placing the reference points tends to reflect the subjective aspect of the surgeon's art and, although surgeons sometimes show a certain reluctance towards mathematics, they should avail themselves more often of the precision it affords.

THE MATHEMATICAL BASIS OF THE MALEK TECHNIQUES USING EQUILATERAL TRIANGULAR FLAPS

When simple freshening of the borders was replaced by routine flap surgery, this was a giant step for cleft lip repair.

Despite its wide range of variants, this procedure is based on the principle of Z-plasty. According to this technique, additional length is gained between two points thanks to the dissection of two triangular flaps that share a common side. The common side corresponds to the segment that is to be lengthened, and the apices of the triangles are situated at each extremity of this length (Fig. 7.8).

Once the incisions have been made, inversion of the flaps results in inversion of the diagonals of the parallelogram initially traced. The long diagonal replaces the short and *vice versa*, so that the desired additional length is obtained.

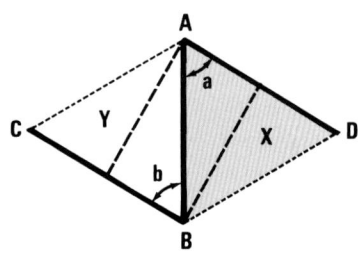
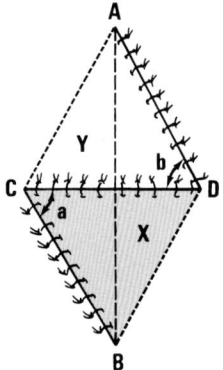

Fig. 7.8 Principles of Z-plasty based on two triangular flaps. Once the incisions have been made, the diagonals of a parallelogram are inverted to lengthen AB and shorten CD. The lengthening obtained is determined by the value of angles a and b.

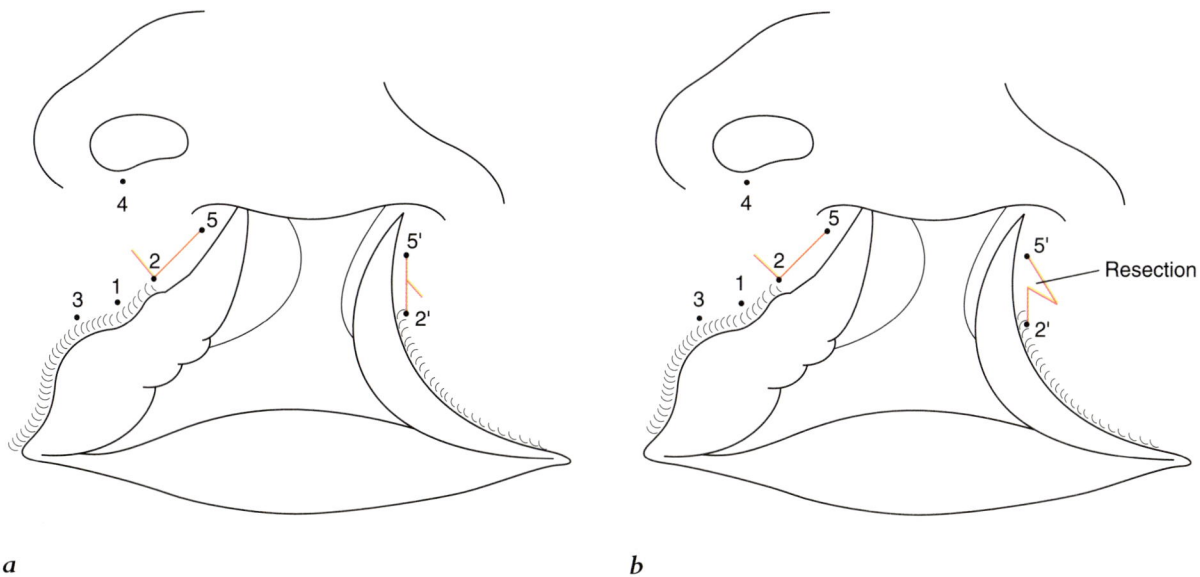

a   *b*

Fig. 7.9

a. When Z-plasty involves only part of the segment to be lengthened, adjustments are needed to allow rotation.

b. Resection of the angle on the line intersected by the plasty on one of the sides prevents distortion of the suture.

To increase lip length at the cleft that shows a deficit in height compared with the norm, the same principle is applied. However, Z-plasty only involves part of the height. Inversion of the flaps requires a certain number of adjustments and, as a rule, a triangular flap is elevated on the outer border and interposed between the lips of an incision made on the inner border. The customary design of a Z-plasty is not immediately recognizable from the outline of these incisions, but it is nonetheless a repair of this type.

The common medial segment of the plasty is divided to match the spread between the two borders of the cleft. On the inner border, the common side is normally extended by the edge of the cleft. On the outer border, the junction between the cleft and the side of the triangle that is not common is simply projected. It obviously forms an angle. Customarily, this angle is not taken into account but is merely represented by a dotted line (Fig. 7.9). Thus, there is always reasonably extensive resection of tissue from the outer border of the cleft.

Once the triangle is inserted into the cleft, the design does indeed correspond to that of a Z-plasty.

The correction of a deficit in lip height at the cleft is generally obtained by Z-plasty, whatever the specific procedure. A review of the various flap procedures follows (Fig. 7.10).

The Le Mesurier technique was the first to be used on unilateral clefts. The term of quadrangular flap plasty applied to this procedure has confused the issue. It was compared and contrasted with techniques developed later, which were described as triangular flaps. In actual fact, the inferior flap devised by Le Mesurier is also a triangular flap, characterized by a 90° angle at its apex.

The mathematical principle applied by Le Mesurier was not incorrect, and the measurements were accurate. However, this procedure is no longer used because it did not preserve the Cupid's bow (half of which was sacrificed on the cleft side), and therefore did not respect the width of the lip. Rotation of the flap was responsible for the elevation of the skin–vermilion line, which produced a replica of the lateral peak of the Cupid's bow (see Le Mesurier effect, p. 75).

In the Millard procedure, which is often mistakenly opposed to a triangular flap technique, there is

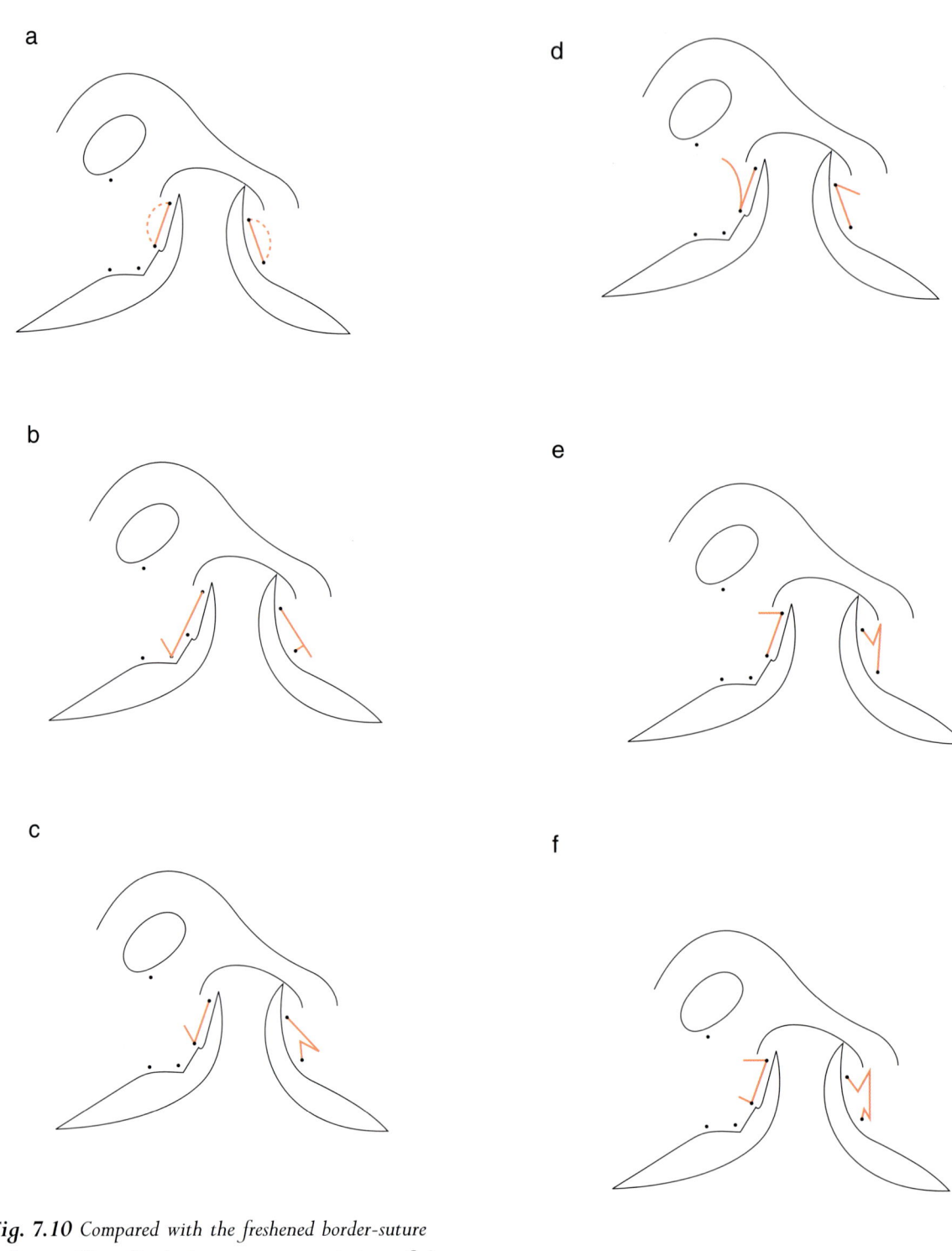

Fig. 7.10 *Compared with the freshened border-suture technique (Veau–Rose), there are many variations of the single or multiple flap procedure:*

a. Veau–Rose

b. Le Mesurier

c. Tennison, Randall, Malek, Skoog

d. Millard

e. Wynn, Malek-Tes

f. Double Z Trauner, Malek double Z

g. Willis, Skoog (upper flap inside the nose)

indeed a Z-plasty. First, a small triangular flap with a superior base is traced on the inner border by the curved incision. Second, a large triangular flap with a superior apex involves virtually the entire outer border. The Millard plasty can therefore be described as a particularly large inferior triangle plasty based on flaps of different sizes.

The Tennison procedure, which surgeons see as the prototype of triangular plasty, is characterized by dissection of a triangular flap from the outer border destined to be fitted into an incision on the inner border. The major technical difficulty of this procedure is in assessing adequate dimensions for the triangle and the inner incision so that the desired gain in lip height on the cleft side, corresponding to the value of the height on the normal side, is ultimately obtained. This problem explains why so many attempts have been made to give the procedure a precise mathematical basis.

In his seminal article (1952), Tennison gave a set of instructions but no mathematical explanation. His procedure, known as the stencil method, is strictly intuitive. There are no calculations involved. Briefly, a length of brass wire is used to measure the distance between the reference point for the nostril sill on the inner side of the cleft and the lateral point corresponding to the peak of the Cupid's bow on the normal side. The wire is then bent into three equal segments. The length of the inner incision is equal to one of these segments, therefore to one-third of the total length. Next, on the outer border, one end of the wire is placed on the upper reference point of the nostril sill and the other on the lower reference point of the cleft. The angle at which the wire is bent is then adjusted to suit the circumstances. Thus bent into shape, the three equal segments of wire are supposed to form the design of the incision on the outer border.

There is nothing precise about this method. It is hard to understand the renown built up around Tennison's name, which has become synonymous with the inferior triangle plasty although his procedure is difficult to follow and triangular plasties were described long before his method was published.

Randall (1959) attempted to give this method an authentic mathematical basis. He postulated that the height obtained was equal to the sum of the medians of the two triangles used in the plasty. In actual fact, the two medians are not on a straight line, except under certain conditions depending on the dimension of the triangles and the value of their angles. It is easy to see that evaluating the dimensions of triangles when only the medians are known can be a tricky problem, with a wide margin for error.

For these reasons, we have developed the method known as the inferior equilateral triangle (IET) technique.

Mathematical basis of the IET

First, we endeavored to establish a valid mathematical basis for the procedure.

The problem

Picturing the completed triangular flap technique, we can observe that two segments or heights are already known, according to our reference points:

- H' = the height of the lip at the cleft measured between reference points 2 and 5.
- H = the normal height of the lip measured between points 3 and 4.

Second, two angles are defined:

- Angle (A) corresponds to the angle formed by the incision on the inner border at the lateral reference point of the Cupid's bow with the medial side of the border.
- Angle (B) corresponds to the angle at the base of the triangle.

The shape is always an isosceles triangle since its two sides must be interposed between the lips of the incision on the inner border, which are necessarily identical (Fig. 7.11).

The values of angles (A) and (B) are essential in determining the additional length which will be gained by the Z-plasty, and the most important factor to determine is the value of their sum.

If only the value of angle (A) is determined at the start – in other words, if the inner border is incised first so that the incision forms an angle (A) with its edge – the geometrical constructions using the two known lengths H and H' clearly shows that an infinite number of isosceles triangles with a side corresponding to the

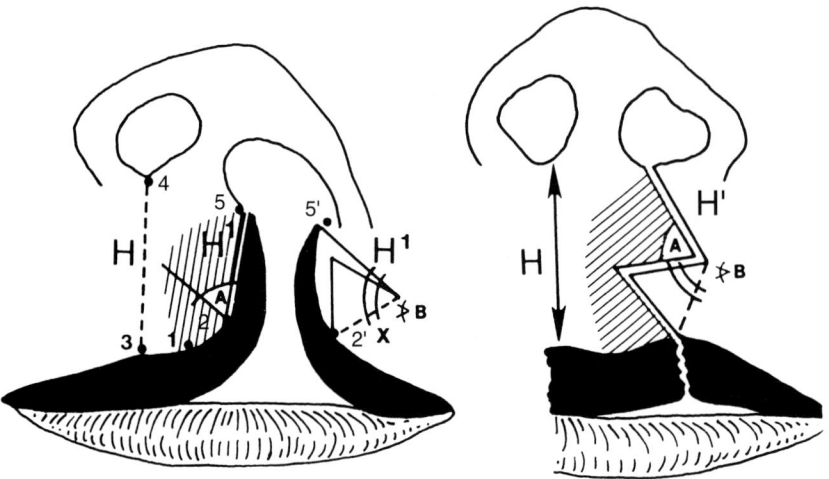

Fig. 7.11 Inferior triangle flap technique. Incisions on both borders, and finished plasty. The essential angles are (A) and (B), and the shape is an isosceles triangle.

length of the incision can be created to obtain the desired lengthening. Since no specific triangle is defined, it is difficult to decide which one to trace on the outer border (Fig. 7.12).

Conversely, if we start with an isosceles triangle traced on the outer border with a predetermined angle (B) established at its base, then only a single value for angle (A) can obtain the additional length

require. However, determining the dimensions of the plasty during the first phase of the operation again can be a practical impossibility (Fig. 7.13).

The solution

The sum of the angles (A) + (B) is given an arbitrary initial value. Since H and H′ are known, it is easy to determine the dimension of the base of the isosceles triangle, and a number of isosceles triangles can be obtained by varying the angle of the base (Fig. 7.14). However, there is only one equilateral triangle that provides the desired additional length.

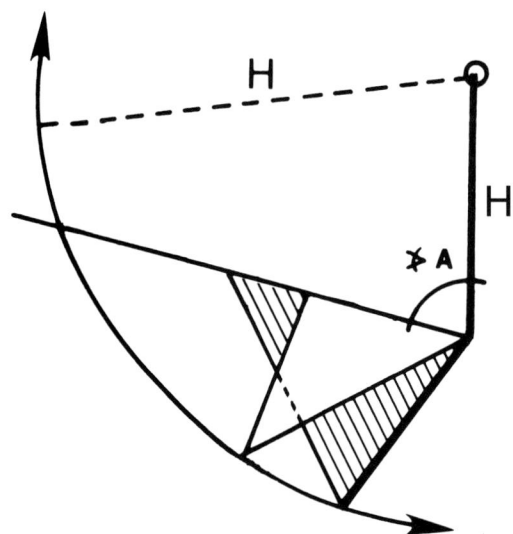

Fig. 7.12 If only angle (A) is determined (the angle formed by the inner border and its incision), the desired lengthening can be obtained by an infinite number of triangles.

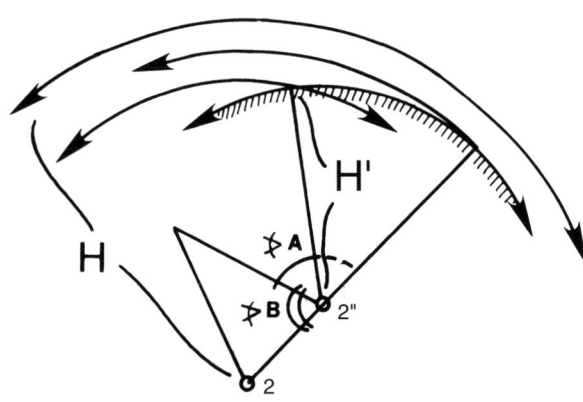

Fig. 7.13 If the angle (B) at the base of the isosceles triangle is predetermined, only one value of angle (A) permits the desired lengthening given by the intersection of two circles, one of radius H and center 2, and the other of radius H′ and center 2″. The calculation is not always possible.

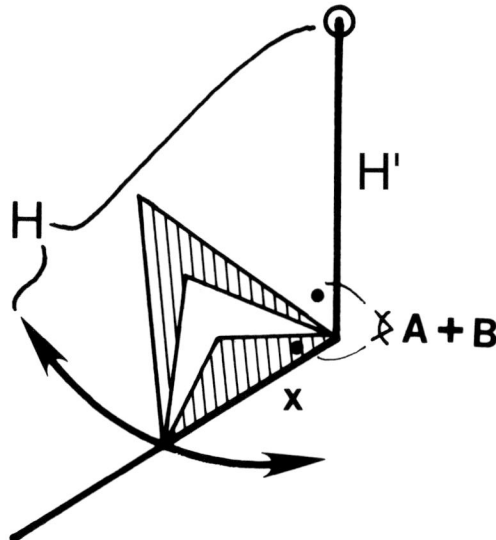

Fig. 7.14 *If the sum of the angles (A) + (B) is predetermined, a large number of isosceles triangles with identical bases can produce the required length, but only a single equilateral triangle can do so.*

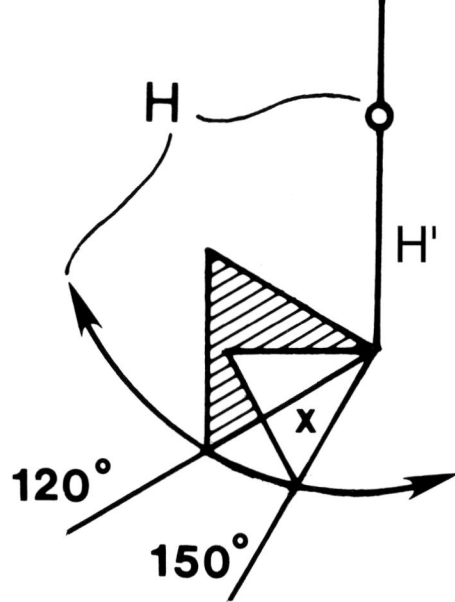

Fig. 7.15 *Since the angle at the base of an equilateral triangle is 60°, the combined sum amounts to 120° or 150°, depending on whether the value of 60° or 90° is attributed to angle (A). It is easy to see that a smaller triangle is obtained for the same length H if the 150° angle is used.*

If we choose to work with an equilateral triangle, this means that angle (B) (i.e. the angle at the base of the isosceles triangle) equals 60°. An equally arbitrary value of 60° can be attributed to angle (A). The incision on the inner border will then be made at an angle of 60°. Hence, the sum of these two angles equals 120°.

Under these conditions, the dimensions of the triangle can easily be calculated before surgery.

The same reasoning can be applied if a value of 90° is chosen for angle (A) (i.e. the incision on the outer border is made at a right-angle). Still using an equilateral triangle, the sum of the angles now equals 150° (Fig. 7.15).

In this case, the inner side of the cleft is incised closer to its free border. This allows more satisfactory opening or exposure of the lip near the skin–vermilion line, and permits better correction of its contour, which often presents a pronounced curve. The same holds true for the outer side, due to the rotation of the flap from the outer or lateral border.

On the other hand if, for an identical gain in length, we compare the dimensions of the plasties, the equilateral triangle with a sum of 150° (A + B)

produces a smaller flap than that obtained with 120°. This can present a considerable advantage in the case of severely hypoplastic borders where the calculations show that a very large triangle is needed to correct a significant difference between H and H'. This is why the angle of 150° is preferred and the 120° angle is only used to calculate the size of the triangle when

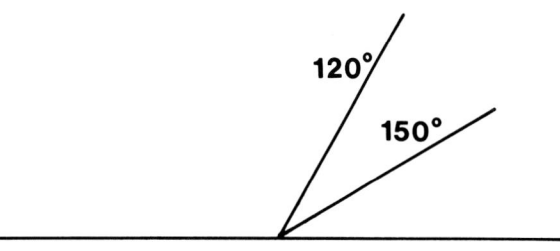

Fig. 7.16 *The pre-printed card used during the operation to measure the size of the triangle, with either a 120° or a 150° angle.*

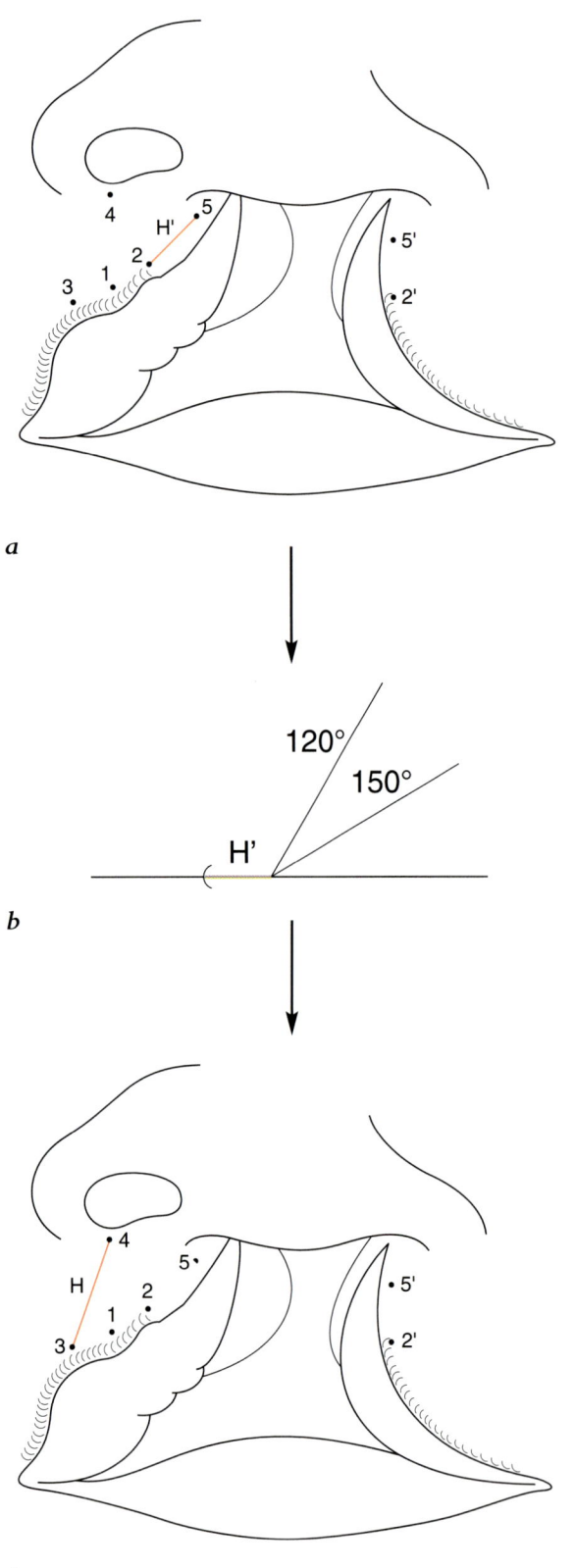

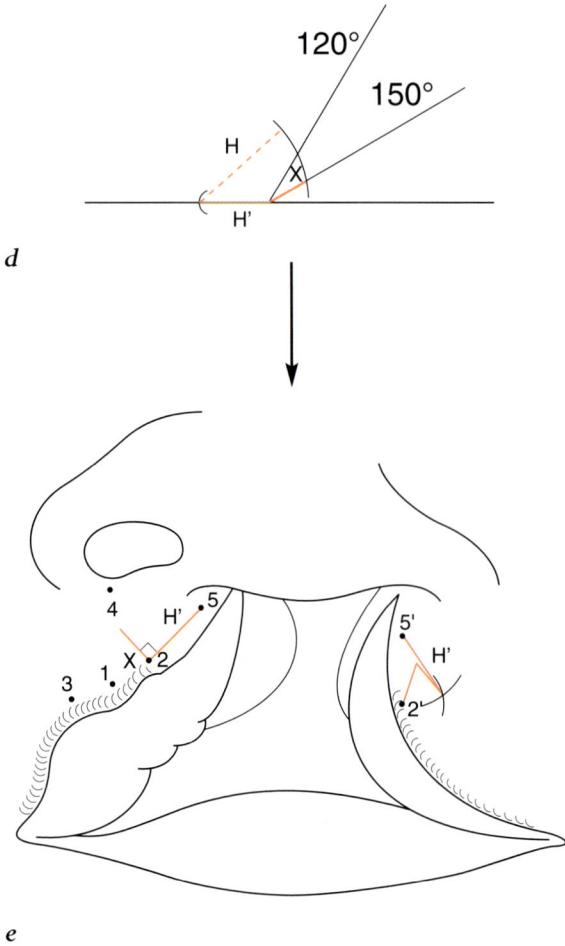

Fig. 7.17 *Operative sequences for measuring and design of the plasty in a unilateral cleft.*

a and b.   First, height (H′) of the cleft is measured and reported on the common side of the angles printed.

c and d. Then the height of the normal side is measured and, with a caliper, an arc of this value is drawn to cut the two other lines of the angles of the card. This determines the value of X, corresponding to the side of the future equilateral triangle.

e.   On the lip, on the inner border, a segment of value X is drawn at the inferior point of reference with an angle of 60° or 90° according to the choice made. On the outer border, first, from the superior point an arc of circle with a radius of H′ is drawn, then, from the inferior point another circle of the radius equal to X localizes the lateral point of the basis of the triangle. Finally, the equilateral triangle is drawn. After the incisions are made and the flaps put in place the height obtained is H.

hypoplasia is minimal.

These theoretical remarks may sound extremely complex, but they must be discussed in order to demonstrate the sound mathematical basis and the accuracy of our procedure. In practice, the procedure is quite simple to work.

Practical application of the IET

During the operation, it is very easy to calculate and trace the incisions. Necessary materials include a compass, pen and ink, and a sterile card on which angles of 120° and 150° with a common side are inscribed (Fig. 7.16).

Once the reference points are in place:

1. The height of the cleft is measured between points 2 and 5 on the inner border. The value of this height is transposed onto the common side of the two angles, from the apex (Fig. 7.17a and b).
2. From this point, the arc of a circle is traced with a radius of H – in other words, corresponding to the height of the normal side measured between reference points 3 and 4 (Fig 7.17c). This arc cuts the other sides of the angles and determines a segment with the apex, which corresponds to the base, or side X, of the equilateral triangle. The value of X that seems the more suitable of the two is chosen. Again, in the majority of cases, we opt for the segment on the side of the 150° angle (Fig. 7.17d).
3. A segment corresponding to the value of X is traced from the reference point on the inner border to form a right-angle with segment 2–5.
4. On the outer border, from point 5′ (reference for the nostril sill), a compass is used to trace the arc of a circle with a radius of H′.
5. From point 2′, a second arc is traced with a radius of X (base). The intersection of these two arcs gives the position of the outer extremity of the base of the triangle (Fig. 7.17.c). The apex is easy to locate because we are dealing with an equilateral triangle and the value of its side is known, and two arcs with a radius of X traced from each extremity of the base will intersect at this apex (Fig. 7.17e).

With experience, the measurements and the geometrical construction take very little time.

The mathematical precision of this method based

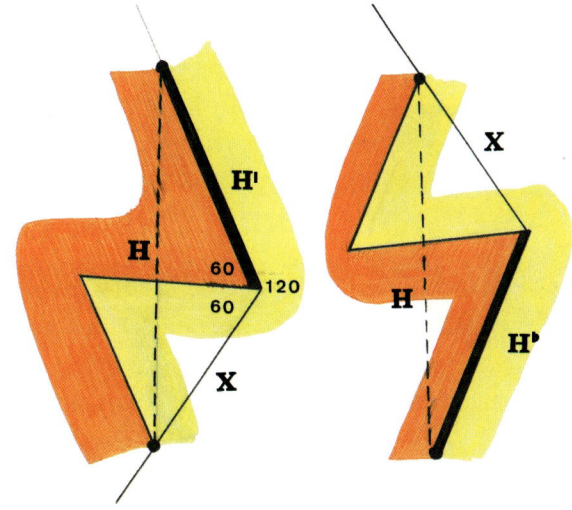

Fig. 7.18 *The 'reverse plasty' with the same measurement as the 'inferior' one.*

on an equilateral triangle flap permits variations such as the inverted triangle plasty, which is not suitable for primary repair, and the double Z-plasty, which has a number of advantages. It is our preferred technique when the degree of hypoplasia permits its use.

Inverted Z-plasty

With the inverted Z technique, the triangular plasty can be placed in the upper portion of the lip (Fig. 7.18).

The measurements are identical to those of the IET technique, but only the 120° angle is used (Fig. 7.19a). Since the dimensions of the triangle are known, it is traced on the lip in the following order:

1. On the medial or inner side, the incision starts at superior reference point 5 and forms an angle of 60° with the border (Fig. 7.19b).
2. On the lateral or outer border, the arcs of the two circles described earlier are inverted: the arc with a radius of H′ is drawn from point 2′; that with a radius of X from point 5′. Thus the base of the equilateral triangle is located beneath the alar of the nose (Fig. 7.19d).

The inverted orientation of the triangular flap

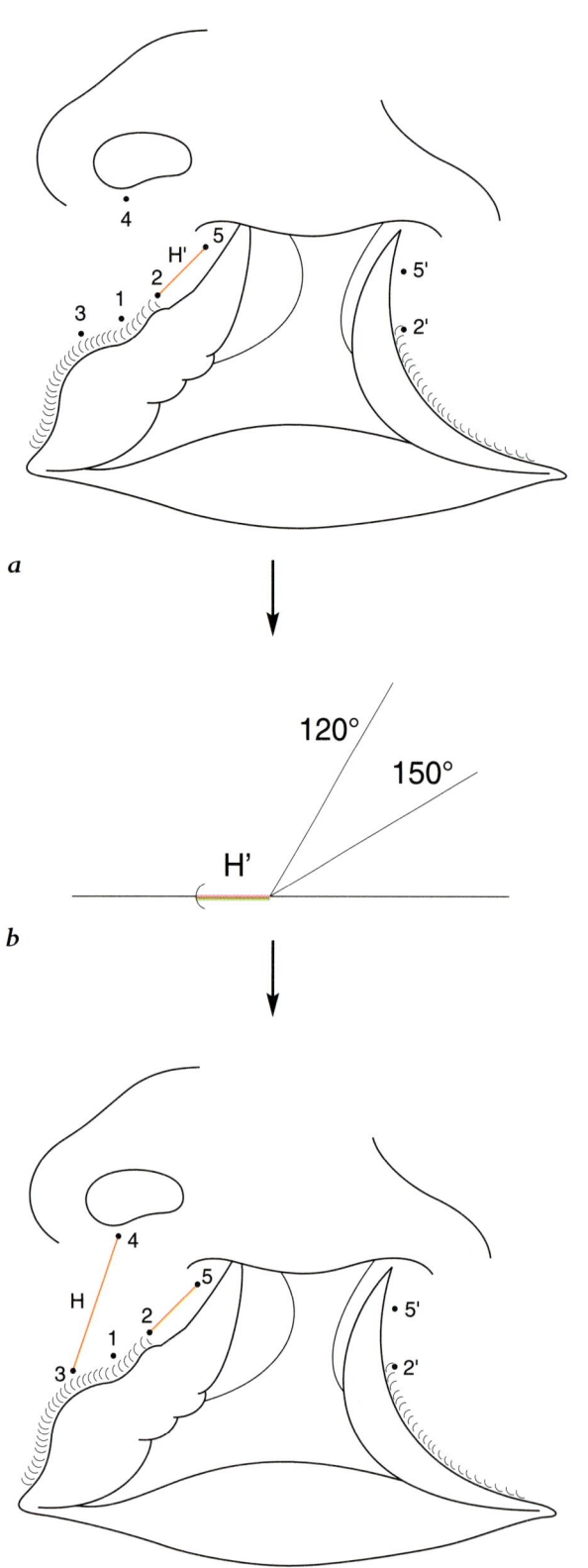

a

b

c

d

e

Fig. 7.19 *Operative sequences in a 'reverse plasty'.*

a and b. Measurement on the height of the cleft, reported on the common side of the angles.

c and d. Measurement of the normal height and calculation of X with the angle of 120°.

e.   Drawing of the plasty on the two edges of the cleft.

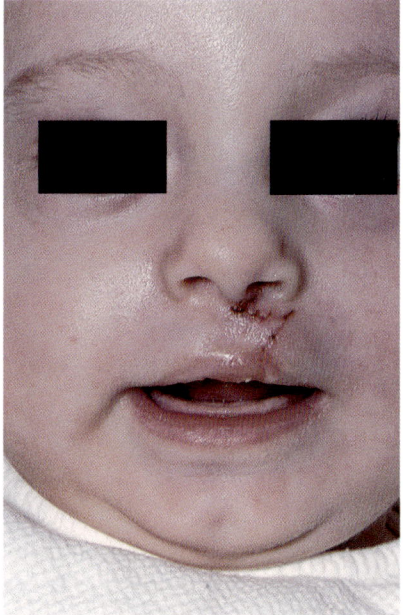

a

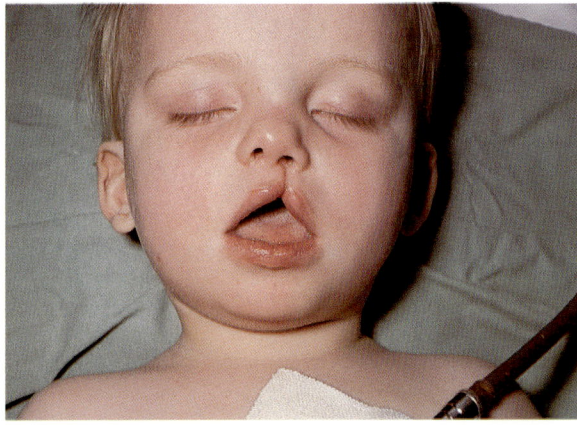

a

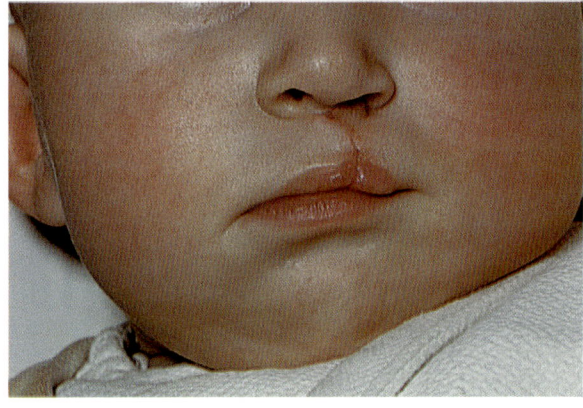

b

Fig. 7.21 *a and b. The same defects as in a 'reverse plasty' are observed with the Millard technique.*

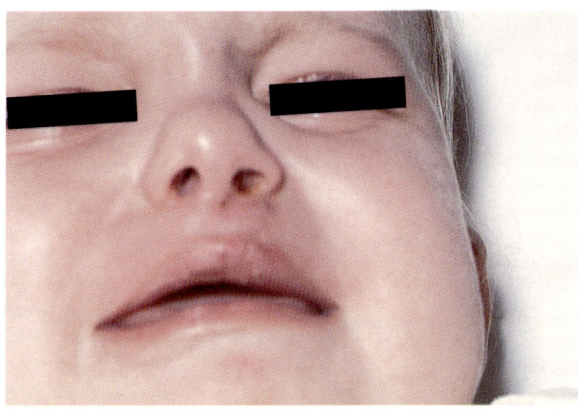

b

Fig. 7.20 *a and b. There is a good appearance for the nose with a 'reverse plasty' but the lip is not opened near the free border, giving the appearance of a notch.*

offers a significant advantage; its inclusion in the inner incision permits a good reinsertion of the alar wing, which was everted by abnormal muscle traction. The triangular flap adds tissue to the upper portion of the lip, which is often rather thin on the inner border at this level (Fig. 7.20a and b).

However, the inverted triangle technique does have its drawbacks. It does not open the lip near its free border, nor does it correct the pathological curve at the muco-muscular junction produced by the anomalous orientation of certain fibers of the orbicularis oris. This procedure therefore shares with the Millard technique the disadvantages of leaving a notch at the skin–vermilion line (Fig. 7.21a and b).

Double Z-plasty

The previous observations serve as a logical introduction to a discussion of the double Z-plasty, which

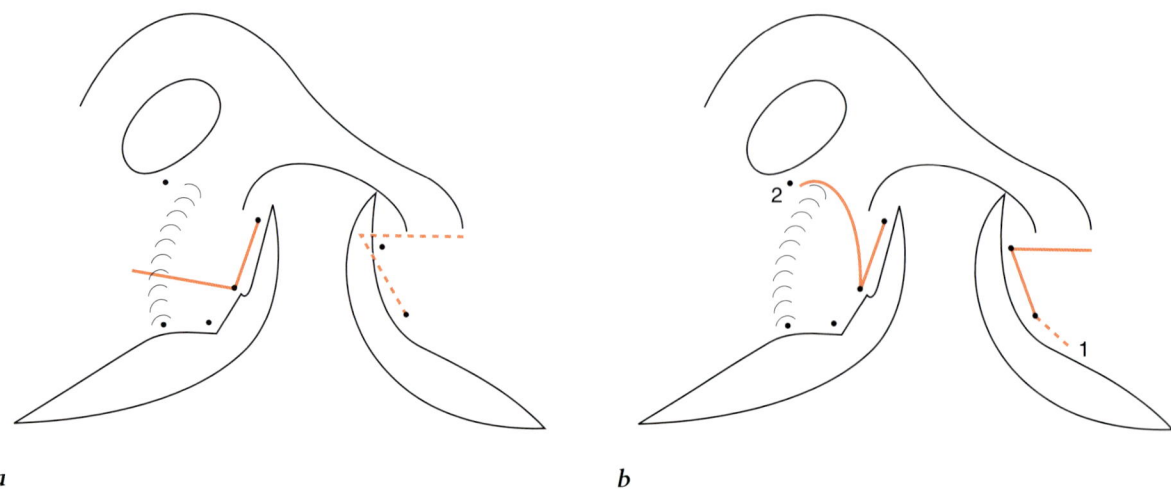

a   b

Fig. 7.22 *In cases with important hypoplasia, the use of a single triangular flap is impossible (a). With the Millard procedure (b) it would be necessary to enlarge the incisions on the outer edge (1) which will diminish the width of the lip and on the inner edge (2) which crosses the normal philtral crest.*

has a great many points in its favor.

If hypoplasia is severe, the measurements give an equilateral triangle of considerable size (even when a 150° angle is used). It may prove difficult, if not impossible, to trace such a large-sized triangle on either border. On the inner border, this would sometimes mean cutting through the philtral ridge on the normal side, which is likely to compromise the desired symmetry. In other cases, the triangle cannot be raised from the outer border without resecting a portion of the skin–vermilion line. This is to be avoided at all costs, since the width of the lip must be preserved. The Millard technique has the same difficulties (Fig. 7.22a and b).

In the field of plastic surgery, it is common knowledge that a large-sized Z-plasty can advantageously be replaced by a double Z-plasty. The double Z-plasty was first described by Collis in 1868 and, in 1955, Trauner proposed a technique quite similar to that we use. Our contribution is primarily in the mathematical accuracy of our procedure. We consider this to be an essential innovation, since it guarantees satisfactory symmetry.

Mathematical reasoning

If we take it that two equilateral triangle flaps are used (the first an inverted superior flap, and the second an inferior flap), then the two lengths H and

H′, known from the start, automatically appear in the final geometrical construction of the plasty (Fig. 7.23). Furthermore, we observe that two angles exist

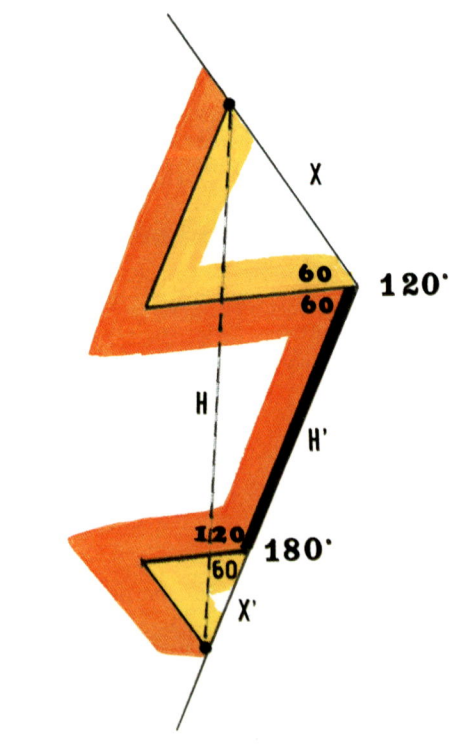

Fig. 7.23 *The geometrical construction of a double-Z plasty.*

that are contiguous to the angles of the base of each triangle.

The value of the angles of the base is 60°, since the triangles initially chosen are equilateral in form. If it is arbitrarily determined that the superior angle (formed by the incision on the inner border at point 5) corresponds to a value of 60°, then the sum of the two superior angles equals 120°. Likewise, if the inferior angle (corresponding to the lower incision on the inner border at point 2) is given an equally arbitrary value of 120°, then the sum of the two inferior angles equals 180°. Thus, the base of the inferior triangle will form a straight line with H′.

Therefore, we have an angle of 120° with, on one of its sides, a segment H′ starting at the apex. In addition, there is a segment corresponding to H, each extremity of which meets one side of the 120° angle.

The values of X (base of the superior equilateral triangle) and X′ (base of the inferior equilateral triangle) are determined by the position of these points, which mark off segment H. This position ranges between two extremes, if one extremity of segment H coincides with the extremities of segment H′.

Figure 7.23 gives a clear picture of these possibilities.

Thus, when H and H′ are known, if an angle of 120° is used, the dimensions of both triangles (superior and inferior) can be varied at will (Fig. 7.24a and b).

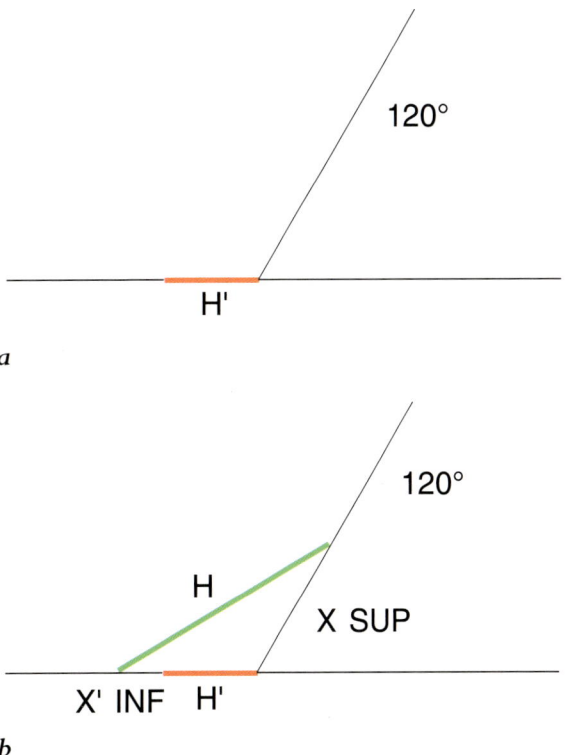

Fig. 7.24 *a and b   The two lengths H′ and H, with the angle of 120°, allow one to determine X and X′, which are the sides of the two equilateral triangles.*

Practical application of the double Z-plasty
In short, the desired lengthening can be obtained by a double Z-plasty based on two equilateral triangle flaps, which are measured according to mathematical principles and traced as follows:

1. The value of segment H′ is marked off along one side of the 120° angle printed on the sterile card (Fig. 7.25a and b).
2. The length of H is measured. The length of the side of each triangle is determined by transposing the two points of the compass to the sides of the 120° angle represented on the card (Fig. 7.25c and d).

As these two triangles are constructed, it is important to ensure that they are of adequate size. The triangle intended to furnish the superior flap should be the larger of the two. This produces the equivalent of an inverted plasty in the upper portion of the lip combined with a triangular flap near its free border.

The incisions are made on the inner (medial) and outer (lateral) borders.

On the medial border, the incision in the upper portion forms an angle of 60°. The lower incision forms an angle of 120° with this same border. These incisions are easy to trace, since they are parallel. The length of the superior incision equals X; that of the inferior equals X′ (Fig. 7.26).

On the lateral border, an arc of radius X is traced from reference point 5′. A second arc of radius X′ is traced from point 2′. The length of H′ (on the cleft side) is measured once more, and the tips of the compass are transferred, one onto the superior and the other onto the inferior arc. The latter point must not be located too close to the skin–vermilion line, to avoid creating the 'Le Mesurier effect' when the flap is rotated (see page 74).

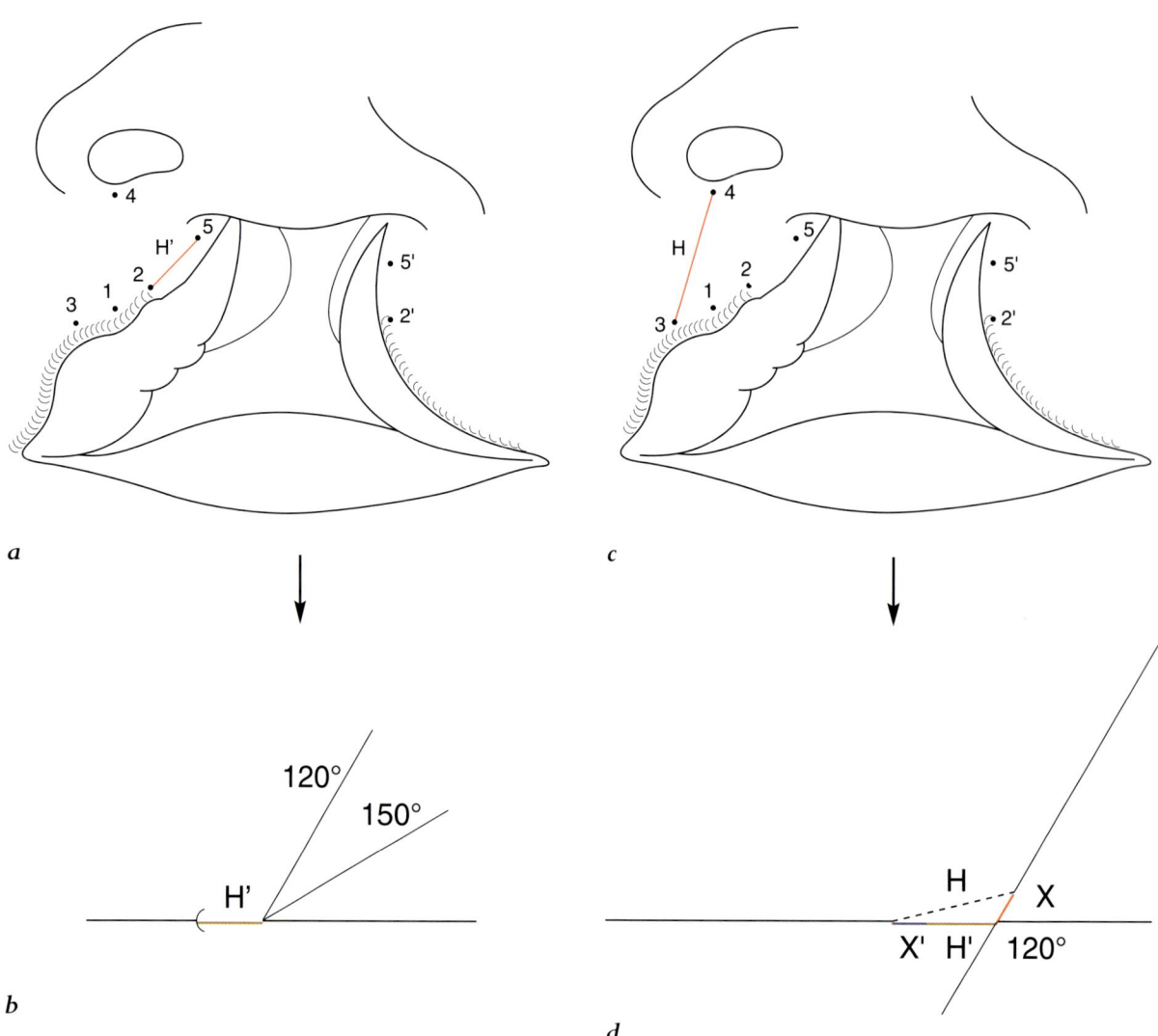

Fig. 7.25 *The operative sequences of a double-Z plasty.*
a and b. Measurement of the height of the cleft.
c and d. Measurement of the normal side. The length H is reported with a caliper on the card: the two points of the pins
lie on the two lines of the angle of 120°, determining arbitrarily the size of the two triangles, X and X'.

Lastly, the two equilateral triangles are drawn (Fig. 7.26).

Figure 7.27 shows an example of the double Z-plasty.

Conclusion

The description of these techniques may sound complex. It is easy to understand why they may inspire a certain reluctance in surgeons, who generally have little background in mathematics. However, the conviction that labial symmetry is an imperative should encourage them to adopt the most accurate technique from a mathematical point of view.

The time has come to cease those procedures that call for per-operative adjustments of the size of the plasty (Millard's 'cut as you go' technique), or those that depend on an initial choice of angle for the inner

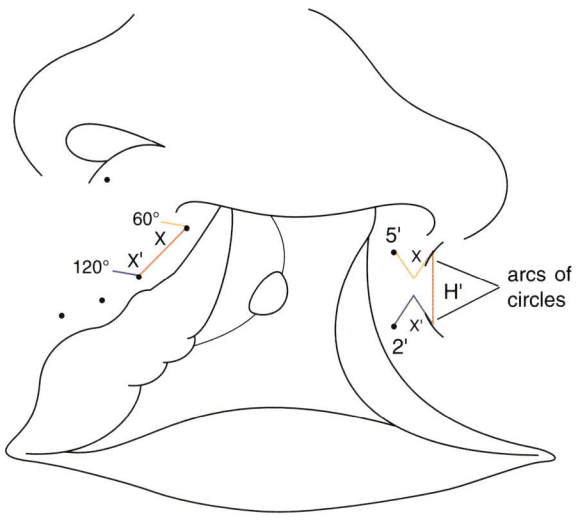

Fig. 7.26 *The drawing of the plasty on the lip.*

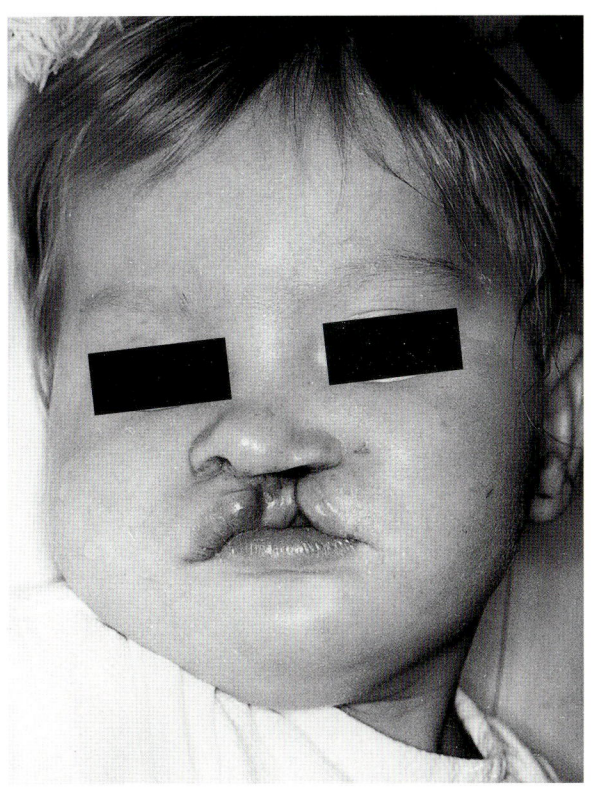

a

incision and therefore predetermine the subsequent phases of the operation. Such a *modus operandi* puts a great deal of pressure on the surgeon, and often produces disappointing results. Once the incisions are made, there is little leeway for adjustments.

If a triangular plasty is called for, why not apply the most accurate method from the start?

The Le Mesurier effect

The Le Mesurier effect is produced when the triangle from the outer border is rotated so that it can be inserted into the incision of the inner border. The rotation can lower the inner point of the triangle (destined to form the lateral peak of the Cupid's bow) relative to the level of the mucocutaneous ridge on the lateral portion of the lip. Thus, the skin–vermilion line may present the contour of a 'cocked hat', as Victor Veau used to call it, with a somewhat blunted superior angle. Although desirable in the context of a Le Mesurier repair (Fig. 7.28), which uses it to synthesize a Cupid's bow, this effect can become an intrusive defect when inferior triangular plasty is performed (simple or double Z) (Figs 7.29 and 7.30). It can spoil the results of surgery,

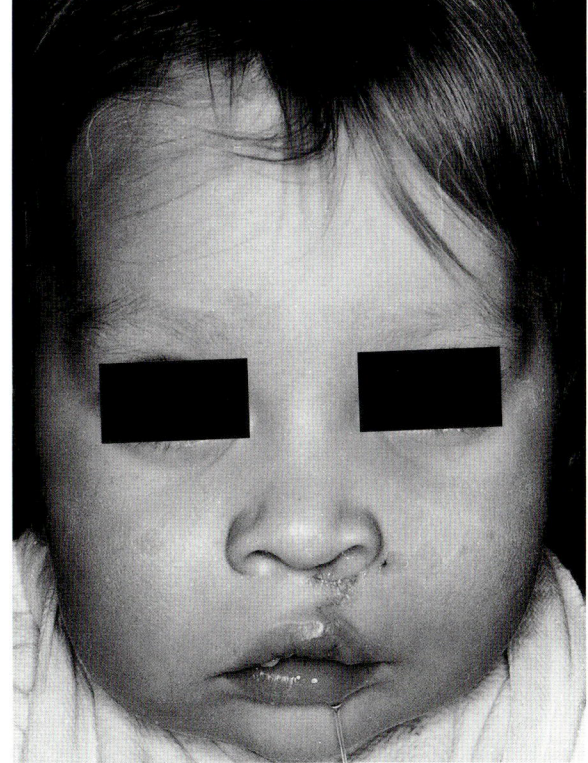

b

Fig. 7.27 *Clinical aspect of a double Z-plasty.*
a. Before surgery.
b. After a few days.

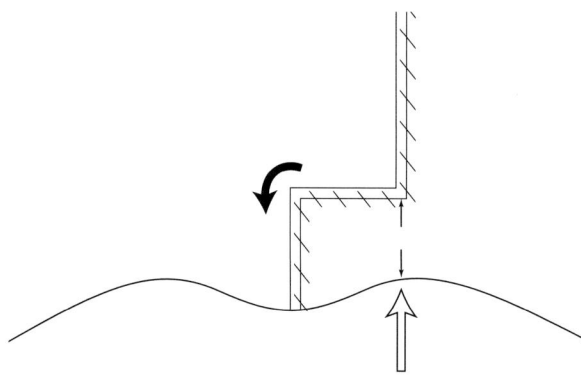

Fig. 7.28 *In the Le Mesurier technique, rotation of the flap elevates the skin–vermilion line to replicate a Cupid's bow.*

even when the measurements and technical skills are flawless.

To avoid this problem, rotation of the flap should be moderate, and the pedicle that attaches the flap to the rest of the lip should be relatively thick so that the skin–vermilion line will not be creased. In other words, the outer point of the base of the triangle should not be brought too close to the skin–vermilion line on the outer border.

When a double Z-plasty is planned, this defect can be prevented by creating a larger inferior triangle.

Lastly, the Le Mesurier effect may also occur on the inner border in double Z-plasty when the lower incision at 120° is made too near the skin–vermilion line of the Cupid's bow. When the underlying portion is rotated, it may produce a vertical furrow in the vermilion. In such cases, it is better to use a single flap plasty rather than a double Z (Fig. 7.31).

CHOICE OF TECHNIQUES IN BILATERAL CLEFTS

In bilateral clefts, the lip is split into three parts: the prolabium or premaxillary segment, and the two lateral portions.

As far as the lip alone is concerned, the gap may be identical on either side (symmetrical forms) or different (forms with a cutaneous band on one or both sides).

The shape of the prolabium or premaxilla varies

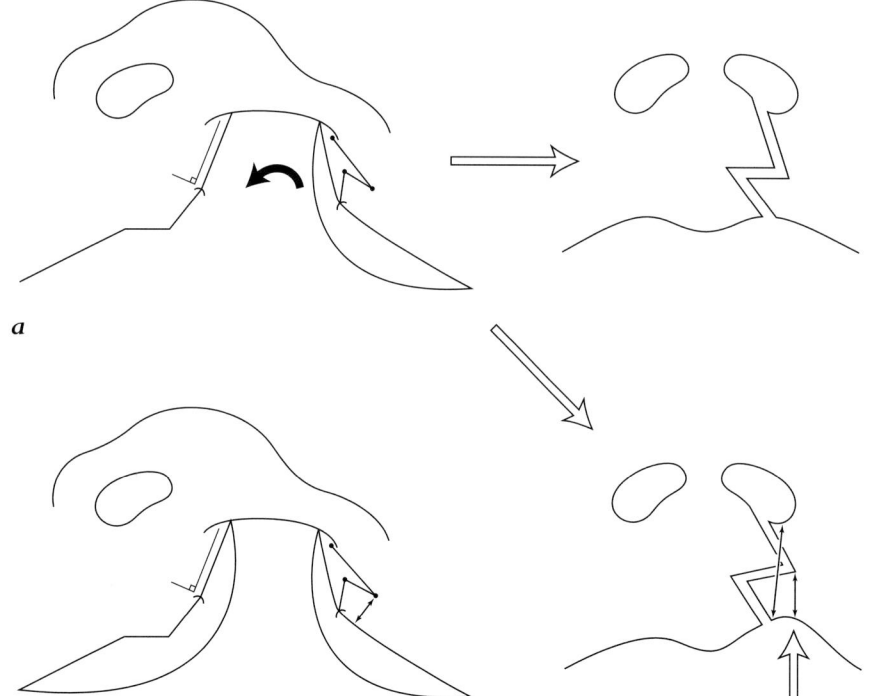

Fig. 7.29

a. *Normally, rotation of the flap has no repercussions.*

b. *If the outer tip of the base of the flap is advanced too close to the skin–vermilion line, the rotation involved is significant and produces a notch (the Le Mesurier effect).*

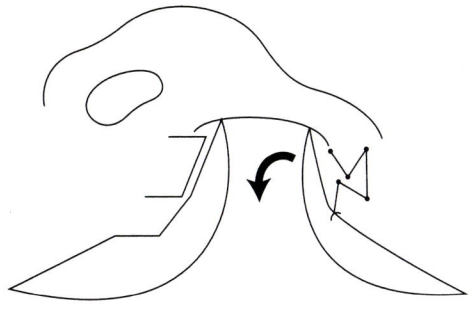

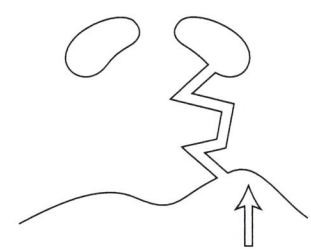

Fig. 7.30 There is an even greater risk in double Z-plasties, where the initial orientation of the inferior flap is different, and the rotation undergone considerable.

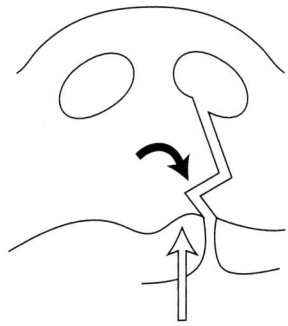

Fig. 7.31 The Le Mesurier effect can occur on the inner border, particularly in double Z-plasties.

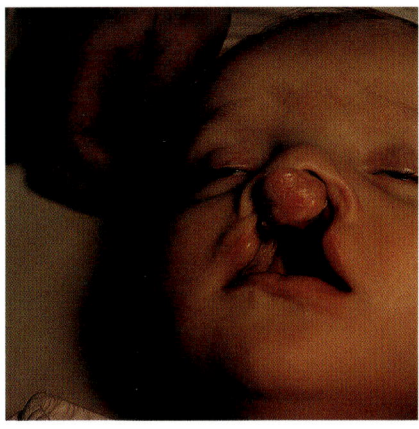

Fig. 7.32 Example of a complete bilateral cleft. The prolabium rests on the premaxilla, which protrudes considerably due to misalignment of the borders. The medial vestibule of the lip is virtually non-existent.

considerably from one case to another. As a rule, there is no sign of a Cupid's bow. The skin–vermilion line completely encompasses the cutaneous portion. The latter may present a transverse concavity or hollow akin to a philtrum without the ridges which usually border it. In most cases, however, it is convex on all sides and resembles a 'lens of flesh'. It rests on a more or less well developed premaxilla, over which it is extremely mobile.

Instead of a labial vestibule, there is merely a furrow, which is often inflamed or ulcerated. The medial frenum may be missing. The vermilion on the prolabium is quite a bit thinner than that of the lateral borders (Fig. 7.32).

On a histological level, the prolabium contains a few muscle fibers when it is totally isolated. There may be an abundance of subcutaneous tissue, which can give a good hold at the time of suturing. The prolabium has a good blood supply, particularly from the vessels that course down from the columella. The columella itself is unusually short due, firstly, to the undeniable existence of medial hypoplasia, which also

affects the nose and, secondly, due to the abnormal spread between the domes of the alar cartilages, which are pulled outward and downward by the traction exerted on the wings of the nose by the facial muscles.

These histological characteristics are even more obvious if there is no cutaneous band and if the bony borders are severely misaligned, which is the case for complete forms involving the bone structures.

Lastly, it is important to keep in mind that even the tiniest of prolabiums can spread remarkably once the cleft is repaired (Fig. 7.33). The height deficit, however, does not as a rule correct itself spontaneously.

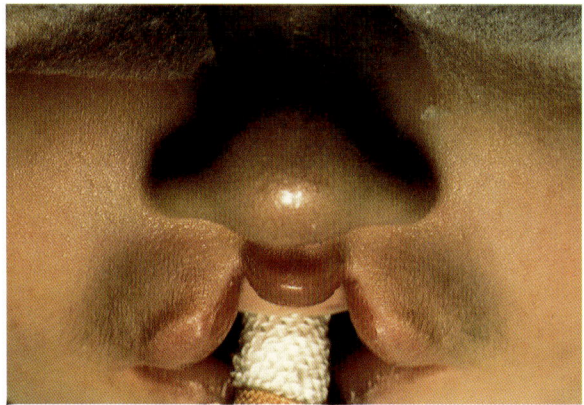

a

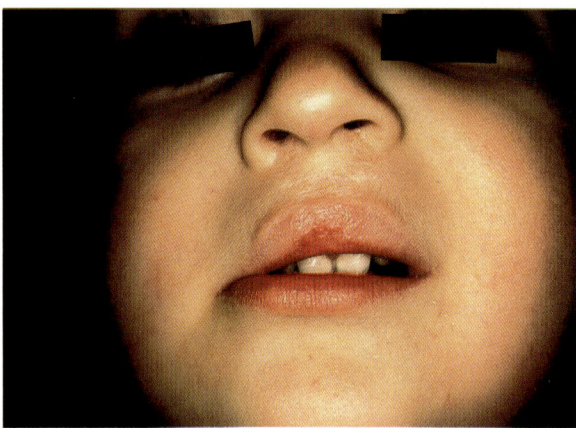

b

Fig. 7.33 *Even a particularly tiny prolabium can spread out to a striking extent after the two stages of cheiloplasty.*
a. Before surgery.
b. Several years afterwards.

Surgical repair

Surgery is always performed in two stages for a number of reasons, which we will stress repeatedly.

One reason is our consistent use of an inferior equilateral triangle plasty. If an attempt were made to close both sides during one and the same operation, the two transverse incisions might meet, thus creating an obvious danger of necrosis.

In asymmetrical total forms, such as those with a unilateral bridge, we customarily start with the more severely affected side. This is because, if the cleft is wider on one side, this would become even more pronounced if the other side were repaired first. Also, hypoplasia is particularly severe here, and calls for a large-sized plasty. It seems illogical to begin by lengthening the less hypoplastic side, since this would complicate the second stage of surgery.

We will take as an example lip closure in a symmetrical form.

Stage one
The essential step of placing the reference points is more difficult than in unilateral forms.

First, that medial portion of the skin–vermilion line destined to become the Cupid's bow must be delimited, bearing in mind that there is no sign of an angle or notch to identify it. Determining the midline calls for careful attention since the prolabium is highly mobile. If there is any trace of the frenum of the upper lip, it can help to locate the midline. If it is missing, there is always a faint groove between the prominences that represent the central incisors on the premaxilla.

Next, the lateral limits of the replicated Cupid's bow are marked. We have seen that the prolabium tends to stretch considerably in width after repair. Therefore, if the replica of the bow is too broad, the end result will be unattractive. Nonetheless, it is essential to preserve as much tissue as possible for use in secondary repair. In actual fact, the height of the lateral portion of the lip serves as a reference for the ideal height to be obtained. However, since the dimensions of the plasty are calculated on the height of the inner or medial border, it must not be too short. This would be the case if an attempt were made to preserve a large amount of the medial skin–vermilion line. It is all a question of judgement and of experience.

On the lateral borders the reference points are placed as described for unilateral clefts (Fig. 7.34).

Since there is no normal side, the value of H (normal reference), which gives the measurements for the flap, must be estimated arbitrarily. It may be taken for granted that H corresponds to the height measured on a line with the outer alar base in an area that is not affected by hypoplasia.

Once the reference points have been marked accurately, the incisions may be made.

The inner side of the lip must be adequately

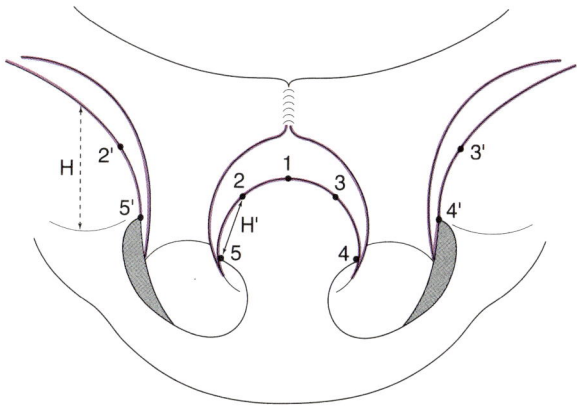

Fig. 7.34 *Placing the reference points in a symmetrical bilateral cleft. The normal height is measured on a line with the alar wing during the first stage of surgery.*

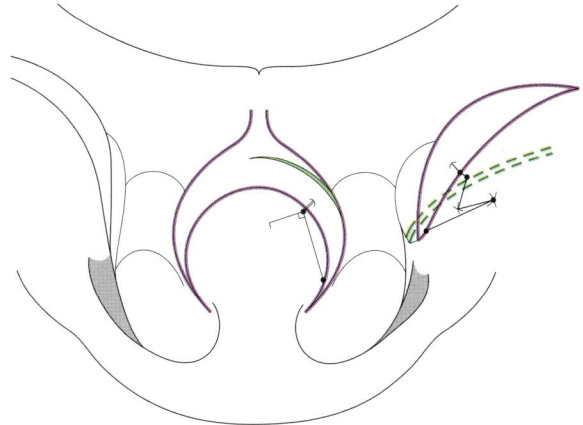

Fig. 7.36 *Pattern of incisions.*

exposed (its rounded contours and lens-shaped convexity have already been discussed). This is why an inferior triangular flap is always used. It should be calculated with a 150° angle, which gives a smaller flap and avoids an incision through the midline (Fig. 7.35). To prevent a V-shaped notch from appearing in the final skin–vermilion line, the incision must be made at a right-angle. To make room for this right-

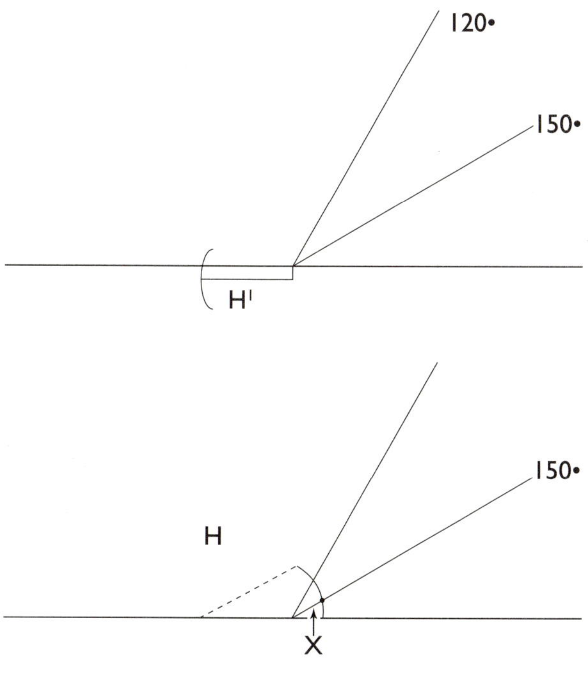

Fig. 7.35 *Measurements with a 150° angle.*

angled incision, the reference point on the cutaneous surface is shifted slightly beforehand.

The incision of the mucosa over the premaxilla is traced a millimetre or two from the furrow that marks the bottom of the barely-defined vestibule. It is extended beyond the midline (Fig. 7.36).

It is important to conserve all of the mucosa, including its underlying tissue on the inner border, despite the recommendations of Victor Veau, who rejected it as 'sterile' because it contains no muscle fibers. In actual fact, this mucosa proves extremely useful for the vermilion plasty described in a later section.

Stage two

The second stage of surgery is performed at least 2 months later.

The situation should be identical to that of cheiloplasty on a unilateral form. As already stated, the more hypoplastic side is corrected first in asymmetrical forms. The height obtained after the first stage of repair serves as the reference for the measurements (Fig. 7.37a).

The mucosal incision must extend beyond the midline to permit undermining of the tissues on the side already repaired. This determines the final results, i.e. satisfactory fullness of the lip at the midline and a good vestibule (Figs 7.37b, 7.38).

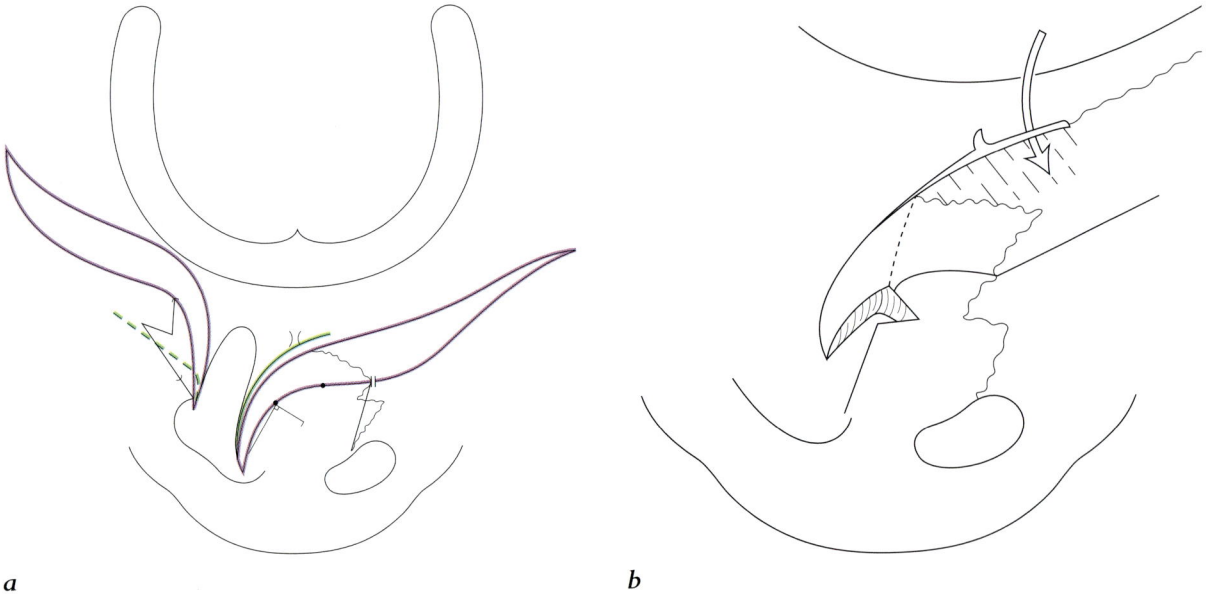

a   *b*

Fig. 7.37
a. Pattern of incisions during the second stage of cheiloplasty.
b. Incision of the mucosa, and extensive undermining on the first side repaired.

REPAIR OF THE VERMILION AND VESTIBULE

Repair of the mucosal portion of the lip, i.e. the vermilion (or visible part) and the vestibule (or hidden inner part), has always presented surgeons with a difficult problem.

Since the cleft leaves a gap of a certain width, the two sides must be drawn together for suturing. Whether the cleft is uni- or bilateral, the muscular and cutaneous elements are easy to work with ('uncannily elastic', according to Veau (1938)). The inner mucosa is the element that is in short supply. Therefore, the surgeon can only count on the mobility of the outer mucosa, which must be transposed towards the inner side without disfiguring the visible lip (as will be seen, there is a possible correlation between the transposition and the thickness of the vermilion). To carry out this transposition, the mucosa must be partially detached from the deep surface of the underlying muscle layer on the outer border of the lip.

Furthermore, as for the cutaneous portion of the lip, there is an initial height deficiency that must be corrected. As has been indicated, one or several Z-

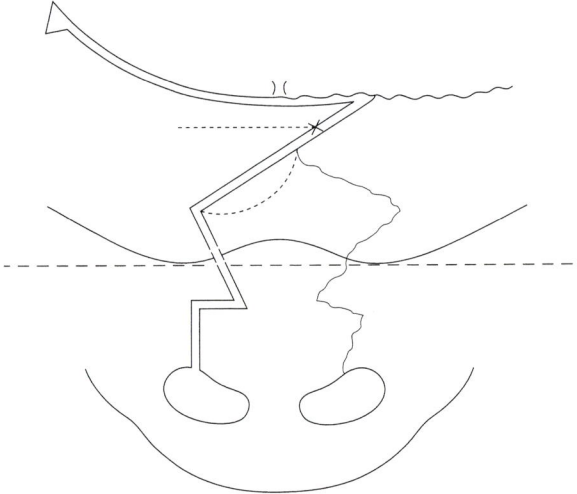

Fig. 7.38 *Final appearance of the cutaneous and mucosal incisions.*

plasties are used to lengthen the superficial layer of skin. The same procedure is required for the mucosa. However, since the tissues used are particularly pliable, mathematical calculations cannot be applied in preparing the flaps, which call for skillful adjustments that can easily be misjudged. Lastly, postoperative edema and the formation of scar tissue due to undermining can radically alter results that may have seemed quite satisfactory during surgery.

The sum of these unforeseeable factors explains the surgeon's difficulties.

Whatever the technique chosen for white lip repair, it is helpful to standardize the associated procedure, which involves the vermilion, the vestibular mucosa and the vestibular sulcus.

Unilateral clefts

The Z-plasty needed calls for use of a portion of the mucosal tissue from the borders of the cleft, which does not ordinarily enter into the width of the lip.

Several preliminary principles must be stated:

1. Despite Veau's recommendations to the contrary, the mucosa from the inner border, which he rejected as useless and even dangerous, can and should be used.
2. The frenum of the upper lip is always abnormally short. Certain specialists contend that it should be left intact (for fear of altering the fibro-skeleton of the lip, which might impair its mobility and subsequent growth). In actual fact, if the height deficiency is to be properly corrected, the frenum must be severed. In our experience, this has never produced undesirable aftereffects.
3. The mucosa of the flaps incised for plasty of the mucocutaneous lip must be completely detached, so that it will not check their rotation.
4. It is essential to reconstruct a deep vestibule. Flaps should not be elevated from the vestibular mucosa (to cover the inter-alveolar portion of the buccal plane, for instance), since they anchor the deeper level of the lip and thus reduce its mobility.

Vermilion incisions
Once the white lip and the muscular layer have been incised, a transverse incision is made which branches off to the deepest part of the vestibule (Fig. 7.39).

On the outer border, the incision is drawn slightly above the bottom of the sulcus so as to leave enough mucosa attached to the bone to permit suturing during the final stages of the operation. It must

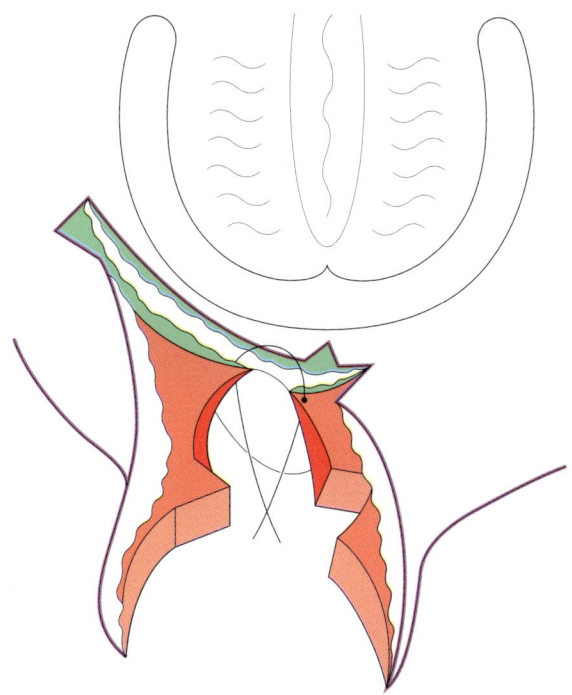

Fig. 7.39 *Treatment of mucosa in simple cleft: muscle layer reconstructed first, then cutaneous layer. Extensive undermining on both sides permits sectioning of vessels along cleft.*

extend reasonably far outwards, and must involve the underlying periosteum as well. This incision forms an angle with the incision continuing that of the margin of the lip. This angle also determines the angle at which the outer mucosa will be advanced into the inner incision. A small hemostat is placed at this point.

The corresponding incision on the inner border necessarily sections the frenum, which is usually short and hypertrophic. The inner incision must reach the bottom of the vestibule on the non-cleft side.

The muscle layer is undermined on both sides. This is where the blood vessels course along the borders of the cleft, and they must be severed and electrocoagulated. This step is extremely important. It permits transposition of the flap, and prevents the plasty destined to increase lip height from hindering opening of the lip.

After the stitch at the skin–vermilion line is positioned, the remaining steps concerning the vermilion are deferred until the end of mucocutaneous lip repair. Just below the skin–vermilion line, a length of suture material is attached to forceps to permit the traction needed for subsequent dissection of the vermilion (to avoid any risk of misalignment, the stitch at the skin–vermilion line itself is never used for traction).

While diverging traction is exerted between the hemostat at the angle of the incisions and the suture left just below the skin–vermilion line, the residual portion of muscle and skin and the mucocutaneous junction on each border are excised with fine scissors, together with about one millimetre of mucosa.

Next the mucosal layer is reconstructed. Before carrying out this procedure, the mucosa of the frenum which remains on the premaxilla should be sutured with a stitch or two. At this level, there is often a small arterial vessel which requires hemostasis.

Transposition of the outer mucosa

The next step concerns the transposition of the outer mucosa. It is often necessary to make an additional vertical back-cut in the mucosa on the outer portion of the vestibular incision due to the width of the gap, and despite the extensive undermining of the infraorbital fossa, which usually guarantees mobility of the entire lip mass (Fig. 7.40a).

Using absorbable suture material, a first stitch is placed in the outer mucosa a few millimetres above the angle. It must be anchored deep in the muscle layer for two major reasons; first, to prevent secondary ptosis of the mucosa, and second, to obtain a well-defined vestibular sulcus situated on the same level as that of the non-cleft side (Fig. 7.40b). The lower edge of the mucosa is then securely sutured to the mucosa remaining on the two bony segments. A good bite of the periosteum is taken to ensure a firm hold.

The transposition just described represents a first plasty, which is equivalent to a Z-plasty. A second must now be performed near the free border of the lip, both to complete reconstruction of satisfactory vertical height and to correct the convex curve of the free border, which is a consequence of hypoplasia (as stated previously, this hypoplastic deformity extends beyond the outer reference point on the

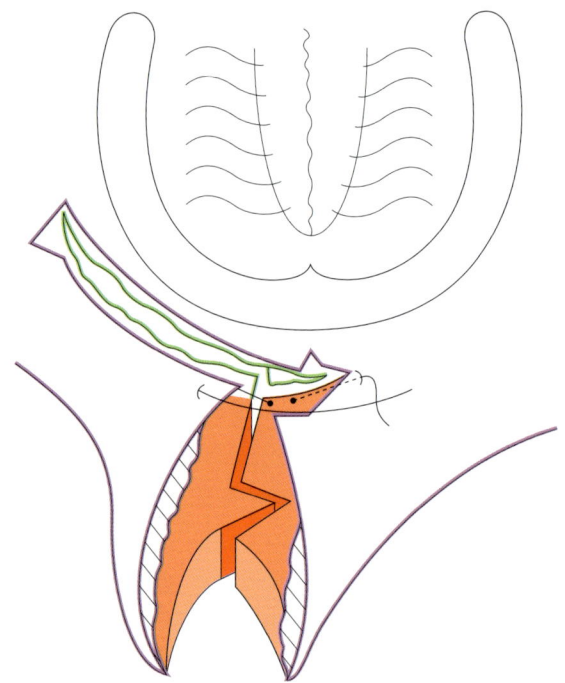

a

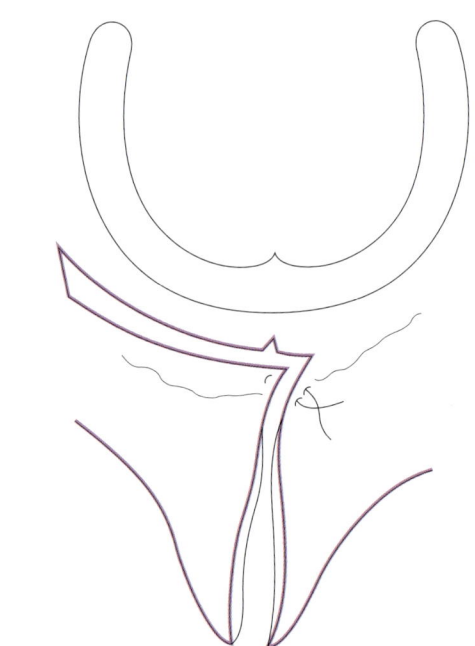

b

Fig. 7.40

a. *The vestibular tip of the outer mucosal flap is advanced towards the normal side beyond the sectioned frenum. A back-cut in the outer portion is often needed to facilitate transposition.*

b. *The anchoring stitch for the mucosa bites into the underlying muscle to obtain a well-defined vestibule and avoid ptosis of the undermined mucosa.*

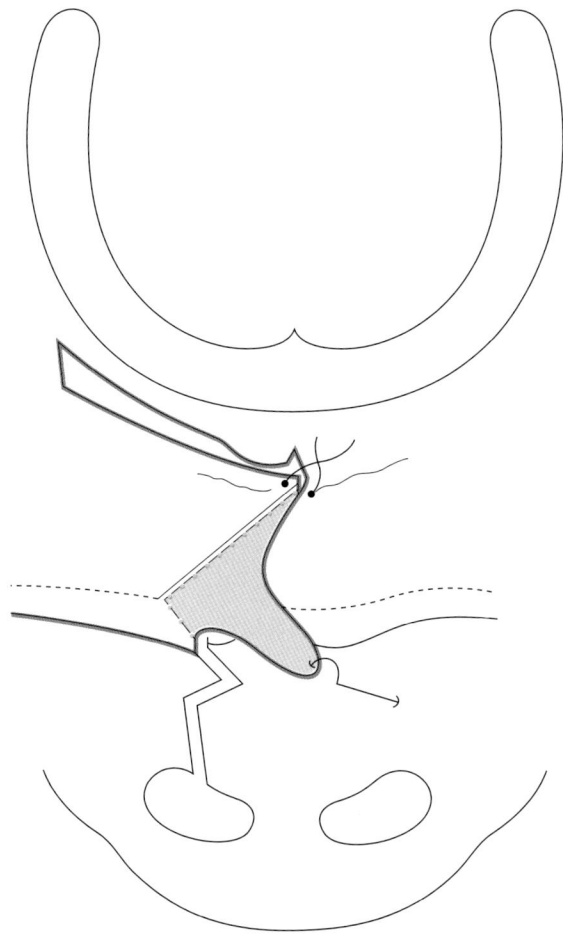

Fig. 7.41 *Extent of resection on the outer border: the oblique incision stops where the dry and moist zones meet. The tissue bordering the cleft is resected.*

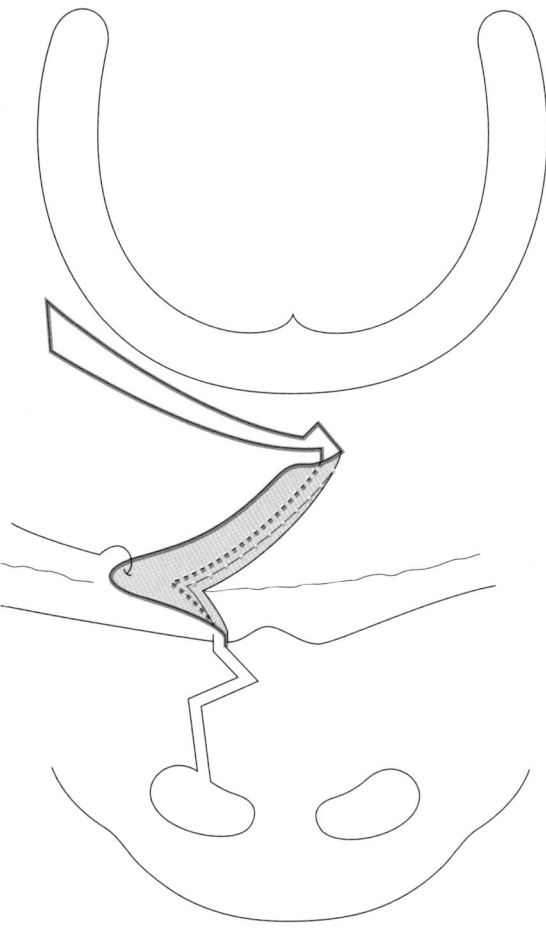

Fig. 7.42 *Resection on the inner border: only a triangle is retained for insertion into the counter-incision on the outer border.*

skin–vermilion line).

On the outer border, an oblique incision is drawn outwards to form an angle of approximately 40° with the skin–vermilion line. It should stop at the point where the dry and moist zones of the vermilion meet. This step is followed by resection of the turned-down portion of muco-muscular tissue (mucosa which originally bordered the cleft) along an oblique line that meets the mucosal angle of the vestibular sulcus (Fig. 7.41).

On the inner border, a triangular section of this muco-muscular tissue is retained. It is destined to be fitted into the incision on the outer border. The underlying portion of mucosa will be trimmed with scissors to match the slant of the outer mucosa (Fig. 7.42).

This second Z-plasty located below the skin–vermilion line achieves a suitable opening in the outer border. It prevents the development of a vertical irregularity in the vermilion, which frequently appears when the suture line of the vermilion is perpendicular to its free border. In this case, adjustments present a problem. Too much resection tends to draw the skin–vermilion line upwards (Fig. 7.43a), while too little tends to distort it in the opposite direction (Fig. 7.43b). When the lip is not open near the border or if vessels remain untouched a notch can appear (Fig. 7.43c).

Generally speaking, the fullness of the vermilion depends on how far inward the outer mucosa is displaced. Excessive inward displacement thickens the vermilion whereas too little or, worse still,

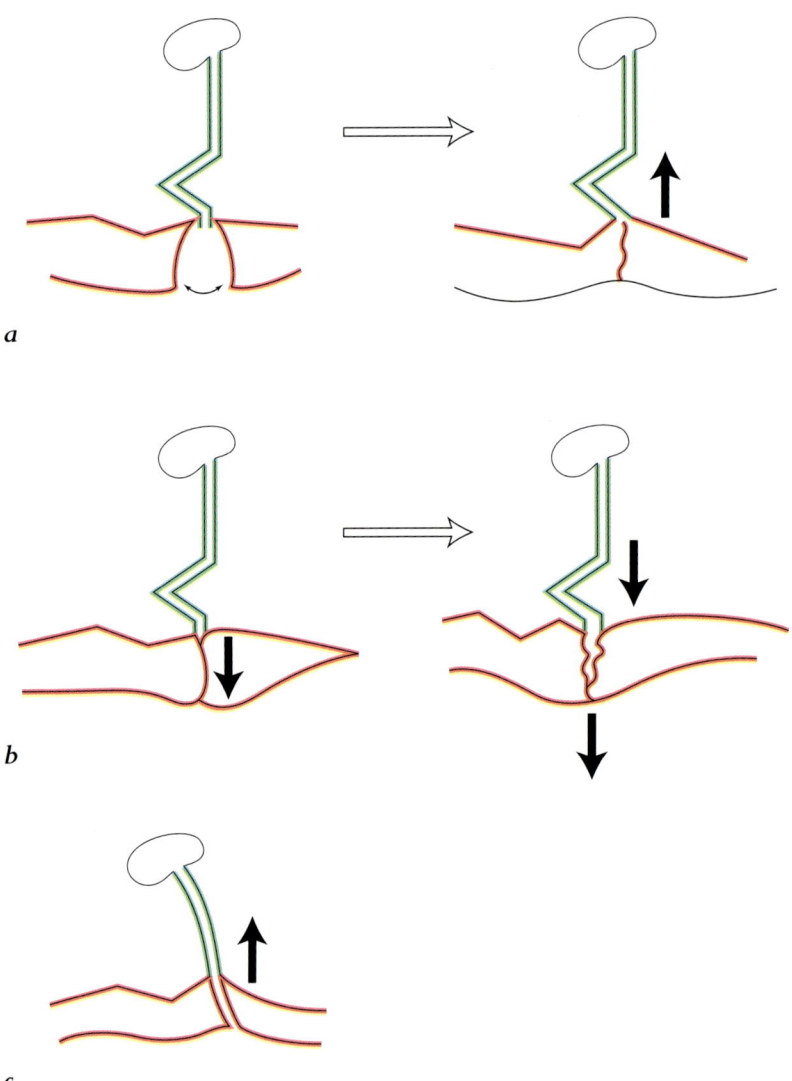

a

b

c

Fig. 7.43

a. *Excessive resection of the mucosa produces a notch in the skin–vermilion line.*

b. *Insufficient resection creates the opposite effect, a proboscis-like distortion.*

c. *A notch appears if the transverse incision of the lower portion of the lip is inadequate, or if the blood vessels are not sectioned.*

outward displacement makes it thinner (Fig. 7.44).

When the outer mucosa is transposed to the inner side, it causes the lower edge of the flap to cross the suture line of the nasal plane between the two alveolar borders. The mucosa detached from the muscle layer may seem at such a distance that healing is likely to be defective, but there are no real grounds for concern since the mucosa very quickly adheres.

To avoid ptosis of the mucosa and give a satisfactory depth to the vestibule, it is possible to make a stitch that takes a bite of lower mucosa and is threaded through the upper lip. This length of suture is knotted rather loosely around a cigarette roll of gauze to avoid leaving a mark on the skin. For the same reason, it is removed as soon as possible, about 48 hours after surgery (Fig. 7.45).

Bilateral clefts

Mucosal deficiency of the prolabium is a well-known finding. The vestibular sulcus is generally absent and if some trace is present, it is usually masked by ulcerated tissue. The vermilion is poorly developed compared with that of the outer borders.

For a long time, it was thought that no use could be made of the medial mucosa. To quote Veau (1938), 'the mucosa of the medial tubercle is the root of all evils, but the medial segment of the skin–vermilion line is highly useful'. Veau usually performed total resection of the inner mucosa, which he replaced with outer tissue. We have discontinued this policy, and have always been satisfied with the results.

Furthermore, we are opposed to one-stage

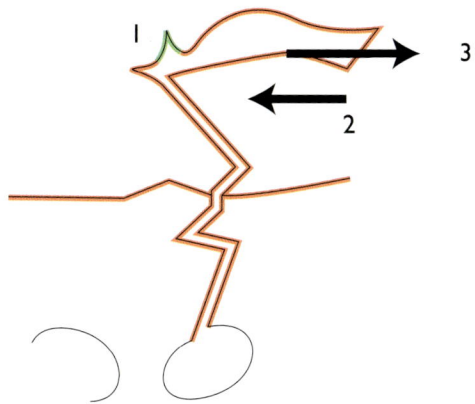

Fig. 7.44 *The fullness of the vermilion is affected by the direction in which the mucosa is transposed.*

1. The vermilion is thickened by sectioning the frenum.

2. The vermilion is thickened by advancing the mucosa inward.

3. The vermilion is thinned by displacing the mucosa outward.

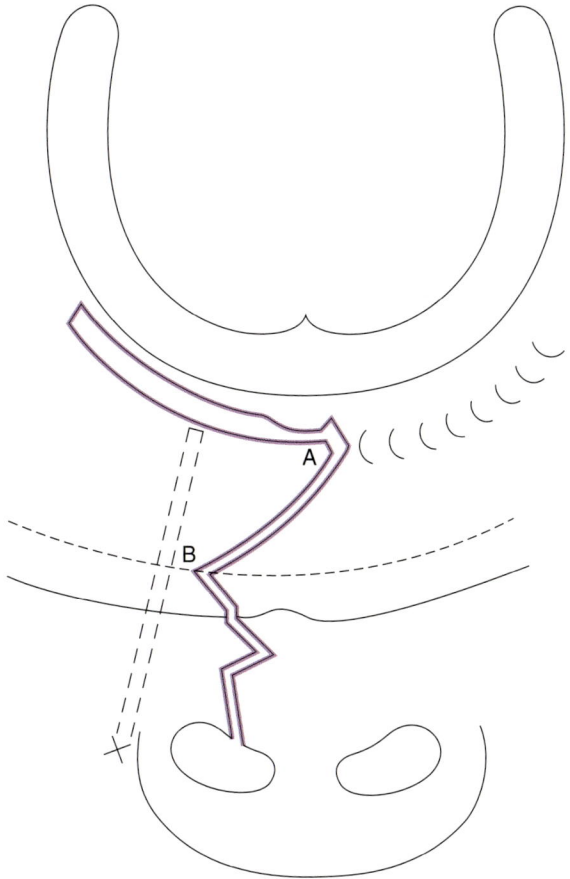

Fig. 7.45 *View of the final repair. The lip is shown in flat projection. Points A and B indicate the apices of Z-plasties: A = bottom of vestibule, B = transition between dry and moist zones of vermilion. The stitch transfixes the lip to speed healing and avoids ptosis of the mucosa.*

surgery, which corrects both sides in a single operation, and reiterate the main reasons:

- In complete forms, simultaneous correction requires a 'drawing the curtains' type closure of the lip to avoid endangering the blood supply to the premaxilla.
- Routine use of the inferior equilateral triangle flap is impossible, since it would isolate the lower portion of the prolabium and cause its necrosis.

Therefore, the same type of mucosal plasty is used for both uni- and bilateral forms, with the following adjustments for the latter:

1. During the first stage of cheiloplasty we section the frenum of the prolabium, which is quite conspicuous as a rule. The angle of the outer mucosa is advanced upwards to a considerable degree near the nasal level, where skin and mucosa meet on the opposite side of the cleft. The outer mucosa should cover the denuded portion of the medial tubercle as completely as possible.
2. During the second stage, the same maneuver is performed, now cutting across the mucosa that

was advanced during the first stage. In this way, it is possible to obtain a satisfactory vestibule in the central portion of the lip, which is not attached too close to the premaxilla. This procedure guarantees good results from an esthetic point of view, and re-establishes satisfactory lip dynamics. The mobility of the corrected lip contributes efficiently to returning the premaxilla to its proper position.

Hypoplasia of the medial mucosa is not responsible for the well known 'whistler' defect. This deformity occurs when the flaps of outer mucosa are not sufficiently advanced.

In bilateral clefts that have been repaired

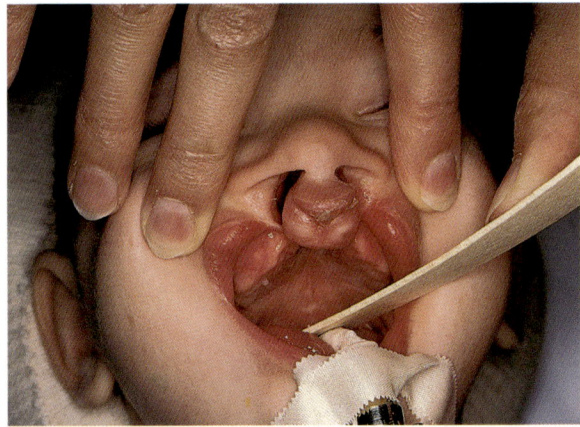

a

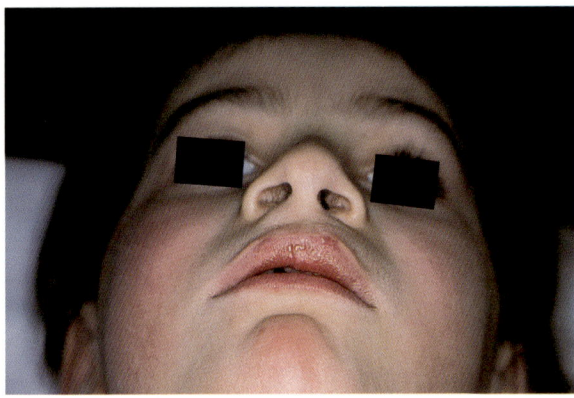

b

Fig. 7.46 a and b. *One of the major improvements in the treatment of bilateral clefts during recent years lies in the results obtained by the vermilion repair.*

correctly, medial tissues often show spectacular development. In our opinion, one of the major improvements in the treatment of bilateral clefts during recent years lies in the results obtained by vermilion repair (Fig. 7.46).

SUMMARY OF OPERATING PROCEDURE FOR SIMPLE CLEFT LIP

Unilateral clefts

The operation always follows the same order:

1. *Plotting and placement of the reference points*
   a. To prevent bleeding or contact with gauzes obliterating the reference markings during the operation, which presents a problem when the time comes for suturing, it is a good idea to make

a small puncture with the tip of a #11 scalpel blade to mark the two points that correspond to the nostril sill indelibly.

b. On the skin–vermilion line, the reference point should be shifted upward a bit so that the line itself can be outlined in ink for several millimetres. To ensure that the junction is clear-cut and perfectly aligned, the incision must cut across the line at a right-angle. Veau used to clamp a double needle across the mucocutaneous ridge, but this procedure has since ceased although the instrument itself can come in very handy.

2. *Calculation of the plasty*
   This is carried out using a card on which 120° and 150° angles are printed, and is followed by drawing the outline of the plasty on both edges.

3. *Infiltration*

4. *Incision*
   a. The cutaneo-muscular incisions must slice cleanly through the entire muscle layer without cutting into the mucosa. This is not a problem since the inner finger can easily follow the tip of the #11 blade (the lip is grasped firmly between the thumb and forefinger).

   b. The blade is held at a right-angle to the surface to obtain flaps of equal thickness; this guarantees the shape and solidity of the tissues so that the outcome after suturing corresponds to pre-operative calculations.

   c. The incisions are next made in the mucosa of the labial vestibule, leaving the portion of skin at the mucocutaneous junction of the cleft intact for the time being. The vestibular incision cuts through the underlying periosteum, but preserves enough tissue to permit easy suturing. The incision then branches off in a straight line to meet the apex of the cleft, provided the entire lip is not involved. On the inner plane, the incision necessarily sections the frenum of the upper lip, which is always abnormally short and thick, before meeting the back of the vestibule on the normal side.

5. *Undermining*
   a. Small, pointed scissors are used to separate the mucosa from the deeper muscle layer. A hemostat is placed at the angle of the junction between the vestibular mucosa and the mucosal margin of the cleft, and a skinhook (Gillies) is positioned in the

incision of the mucocutaneous ridge. If moderate diverging traction is exerted on these two instruments, it is easy to pass between them and penetrate the submucosal layer. This is clearly identified by the rounded acini of the labial salivary glands, which must remain embedded in the mucosa.

b. The blood vessels that course upward along the cleft are situated on this level. They 'lock' the height of the cleft borders. They must be located and sectioned after electrocoagulation, so that additional height can be gained by making zigzag incisions. For the same reason, the mucosa should be detached from the inner surface of the flaps. The latter are destined to undergo rotation, which must not be checked by non-incised mucosa.

c. Even in simple forms it is advisable to undermine the periosteum, so that it will be easier to advance the lip towards the midline and re-insert the muscle fibers.

d. Lastly, to improve the shape of the nostril, the outer alar base is undermined (particularly at the upper edge of the lip) so that it will not be pulled too far inwards when the muscle layer is advanced towards its point of re-insertion on the nasal spine.

6. *Suturing of the white or cutaneous lip*
   a. A few stitches with resorbable 5-0 sutures may prove necessary if the nasal floor is cleft. The first 6-0 nylon suture is placed at the site of the punctures that serve as reference points for the nostril sill. This suture is held taut with small forceps. Next, the muscle layer is closed using non-absorbable 5-0 sutures. A few stitches are placed at key points; at the extremities of the incisions and at the angles of the triangular plasty. The uppermost fibers of the muscle layer, which have been undermined on both surfaces, are attached to the lateral periosteum of the nasal spine of the maxilla with several stitches. They will add fullness to the upper portion of the inner border, which is often slightly sunken. Two stitches are placed on either side of the skin–vermilion line at the ends of the short segment previously incised, which is perpendicular to it. One of these is held by forceps for traction. It is not advisable to suture the mucocutaneous ridge itself, since the resulting traction

can cause misalignment of the vermilion border.
   b. Use 6-0 nylon for cutaneous suturing (absorbable sutures seem to be less well tolerated and tend to leave more traces). The sutures should not be pulled too tight.

7. *Incision and suturing of the vermilion and mucosa* are kept until last, and the steps involved are less methodically ordered (see previous section).

Bilateral clefts

For cheiloplasty in bilateral clefts we apply a certain number of set rules, which bear repeating here:

- We consistently use the technique of an inferior equilateral triangle flap. This is the best way to obtain satisfactory vertical lip height, even in those forms where the prolabium is severely hypoplastic. The favorable development, once both sides of the cleft are closed, comes as a particularly striking surprise in these cases. The calculations that serve as a reference are necessarily arbitrary, since there is no normal side to use for comparison. We calculate the height we intend to obtain on a vertical line at the level of the outer alar base. In the asymmetrical bilateral forms, the measurements are taken on the less hypoplastic side.

- As a consequence of our first rule, we never repair both sides during a single operation. This might endanger the blood supply to the lower portion of the prolabium, which would be left with a very slender pedicle.

- The prolabium must be preserved at all costs, and the same holds true for the central portion of mucocutaneous ridge it contains. This corresponds to the Cupid's bow, although the contours are not clearly marked. Resection of this portion would result in an excessively tight upper lip.

- During cheiloplasty, we do not attempt to correct the short columella. We thus avoid the formation of a scarline at the labio-columellar junction, which might compromise secondary repair. As already stated, we do not undertake any procedure involving nasal correction at this stage, other than the proper re-insertion of muscle fibers on the nasal spine.

- Although the muscle fibers of the prolabium are generally underdeveloped and sparse, if not absent, we do not attempt to suture the two portions of the orbicularis from the outer borders together. In any case, this would be totally against our principles, since we never perform surgery on both sides during the same operation.
- We find it wise to observe a waiting period between operations. A 2-month interval seems to suffice.
- In asymmetrical simple forms, it is better to start with the less affected side so that it will be easier to adjust the second plasty.

Operating procedure

The first stage of cheiloplasty follows, point by point, the procedure described for unilateral clefts.

1. *Plotting and placement of the reference points*
   Since there is no step in the mucocutaneous ridge to serve as a reference, the portion intended to correspond to the replica of a Cupid's bow is determined arbitrarily. Identifying its precise centre is a tricky procedure that calls for extra caution since the prolabium is extremely mobile. The frenum at the midline of the upper lip should be used as a guide. Although the future Cupid's bow should not be over-wide, it is essential to preserve as much tissue as possible. The reference points on the lateral border are placed according to the unilateral cleft procedure.

2. *Calculation of the plasty*
   Here again we use an inferior equilateral triangle with a 150° angle, as a rule, so as to obtain the smallest surface possible. The purpose is to keep the two transverse incisions from meeting or, even worse, overlapping once the two stages of the operation have been performed. Although the vascular supply to the isolated portion of the prolabium is no longer at risk thanks to the interval between operations, the esthetic result would not be satisfactory. The means of establishing the height measurement, which serves as a reference, have already been discussed.

3. *Incision*
   For the incision, the blade is held at a right-angle to the skin. It is important to conserve a good thickness of tissue for the flap that corresponds to the edge of the cleft. This tissue will be useful for vermilion repair. The incision should cut across the skin–vermilion line at a right-angle to avoid a step defect or similar misalignment.

4. *Undermining*
   This is performed next, with isolation of the nasal spine.

5. *Suturing*
   a. Muscle suturing follows the principles already described. The lateral muscle (detached on both surfaces near the upper reference point of the outer border) is anchored to the periosteum of the nasal spine. As already indicated, subcutaneous suturing with buried stitches is required due to the prolabium's paucity of muscle fibers.
   b. Cutaneous suturing comes next.
   c. The vermilion and the vestibule are repaired according to the procedure described in the previous section. The inner or medial mucosa is retained, despite Veau's recommendation to discard it.

Once this first stage of cheiloplasty has been carried out in bilateral forms, the impression should be that of an unoperated unilateral cleft, since the opposite side remains open. To avoid undue distress, the parents should be warned in advance that the first operation creates a new but temporary lack of symmetry.

The second stage of cheiloplasty takes place 2 months later, and bears an even closer resemblance to the procedure used for unilateral clefts. The method of plotting the reference points and calculating the plasty need not be repeated.

To permit proper repositioning of the medial portion, undermining will be reasonably extensive and will include any cicatricial adhesions on the repaired first side. Of necessity, the vestibular incision cuts through the preliminary work done on the vestibule during the first operation. Correction of the vestibule and of the prolabial vermilion represent by far the most difficult aspects of bilateral cleft repair since it is important to avoid producing a 'whistler' deformity, which is practically impossible to correct later on. However, we can safely say that the results of our techniques show spectacular improvement over those of more 'classic' methods.

AGE AT SURGERY

The ideal age for simple cleft repair is still the subject of much debate, and the date is often chosen in a purely arbitrary fashion. Thanks to the progress of pediatric anesthesia, surgery can be performed at a very early age. However, the pros and cons of early simple cleft repair do not clearly indicate the most desirable age for such surgery.

It is easy to understand why there is a significant psychological advantage to early surgery as far as the parents are concerned. Still, unlike more complex forms, the simple cleft is precisely the type that may not seem to call for urgent repair. Some parents postpone their visit to a specialist, and we occasionally see older infants who have not yet undergone surgery.

There is less of an argument with simple clefts for immediate correction of abnormal muscle insertions to prevent the deformities from being accentuated as time goes by. This is particularly true if the nostril sill is intact.

Delaying surgery has certain advantages. It allows time for the detection of associated malformations, and for an improvement in the infant's general state of health, bearing in mind that these infants are often premature. Also, during the first weeks of life the immune system depends on antibodies transmitted by the mother. An autonomous system does not take over until the age of about 2 months.

There may be feeding difficulties. Breast feeding can be allowed for the first few weeks, and it will be easier to suspend bottle-feeding in the days following surgery.

Tooth formation might be disrupted by surgery during the first weeks of life (Petit and Psaume, 1955). This argument has not been corroborated in simple clefts.

After consideration of the pros and cons, we have adopted the policy of operating on simple forms some time during the **fourth month**. Our strategy is based primarily on technical arguments. Surgery is far less difficult at 4 months than at a few weeks of age. The surgeon has better developed, more sturdy tissue to work with. Our anesthetists tend to agree, and the parents are usually willing to accept this waiting period, during which they can get over their initial shock and come to cherish their new baby. In simple bilateral forms, therefore, the standard age for surgery ranges from 4 to 6 months.

RESULTS

Esthetic result

It is extremely difficult to judge the results of lip repair in congenital clefts. Certain authors have worked out a grading system, which seems very artificial. The present day criteria of repair, which we have listed, can be examined one by one.

In actual fact, what counts most is the eye of others who, at a single glance, pass judgement on an esthetic result that is a combination of many factors. The important elements are:

1. Conspicuousness of the scar(s);
2. Symmetry of the face at rest;
3. Lip dynamics in such movements as speech, smiling and other expressions;
4. Contours of the upper lip in these different situations;
5. Arrangement of the teeth and position of the alveolar arch;
6. Symmetry of the nose and its aspect from all sides, particularly in profile; and
7. Tone of voice.

In addition to the eye of others, infants soon reach an age where they can study their own reflections in the mirror. The mirror, incidentally, can also attract the parents' attention. Although they quickly grow accustomed to the minor defects that still exist, they may be shocked by the inverted image reflected in a looking-glass.

Psychological repercussions

The psychological repercussions produced by the sequelae of a cleft are not easy to evaluate.

They are generally triggered by the environment. Other children who come into contact with the child, particularly at school, inspire the first questions and the first traumas. It is customary to observe the onset of psychological problems at about the age of 6 years, when the patient enters primary school. This is a ruthless age, when children come out with blunt and tactless comments to affirm their own identity.

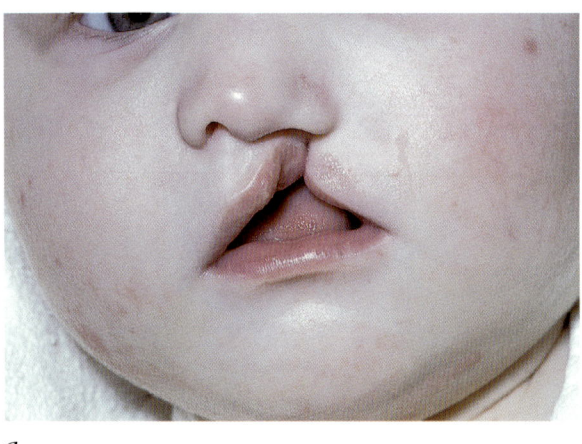

a

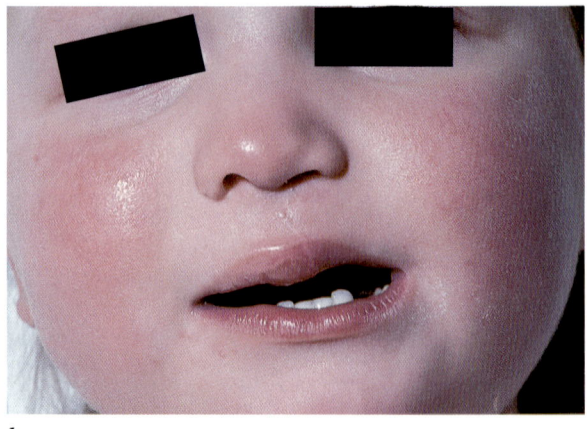

b

Fig. 7.47 *a and b Labial results (equilateral triangle flap technique). Notice correction of the extremely thin vermilion.*

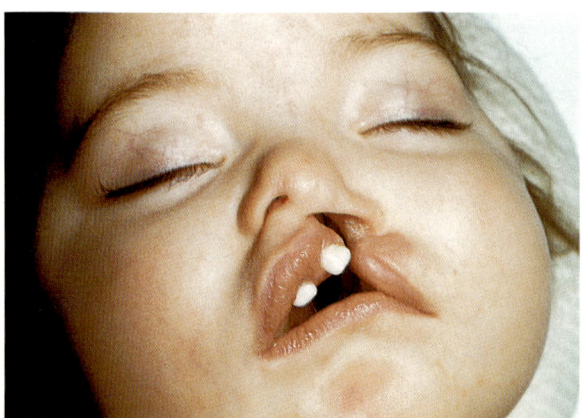

a

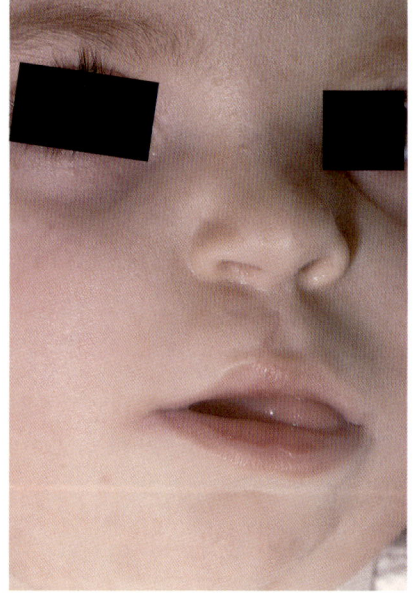

Fig. 7.49 *The inferior equilateral triangle technique generally preserves the philtral dimple.*

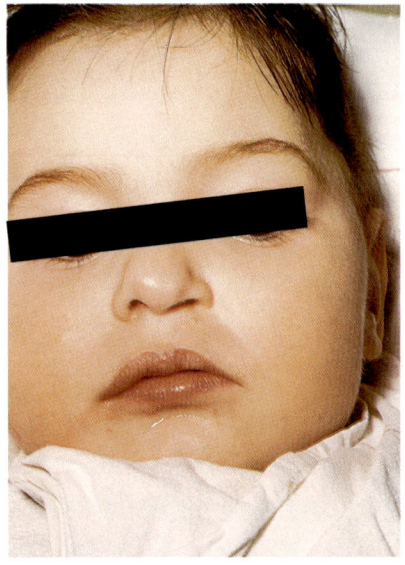

b

Fig. 7.48 *a and b Results on complete unilateral cleft, left side (IET).*

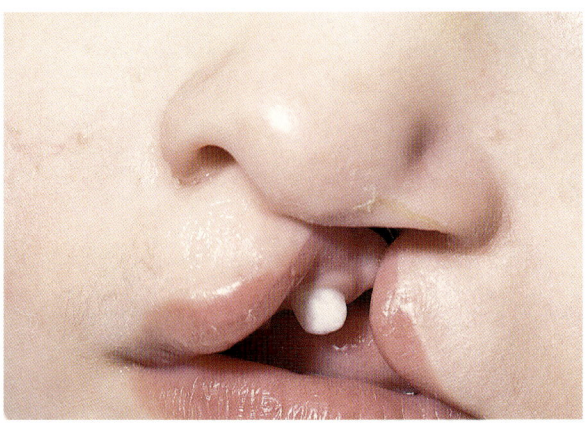

a

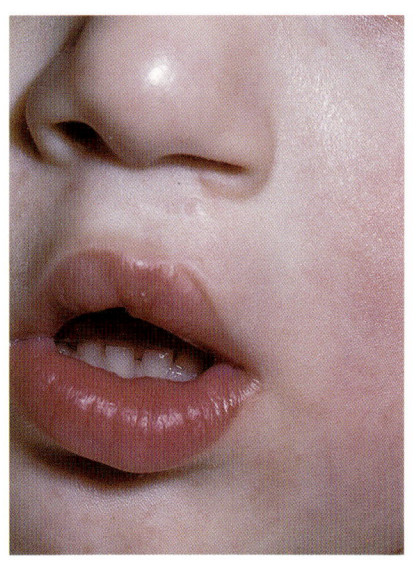

Fig. 7.50 *a and b Although the philtral ridge is absent, there is a nice pout near the free border of the lip.*

b

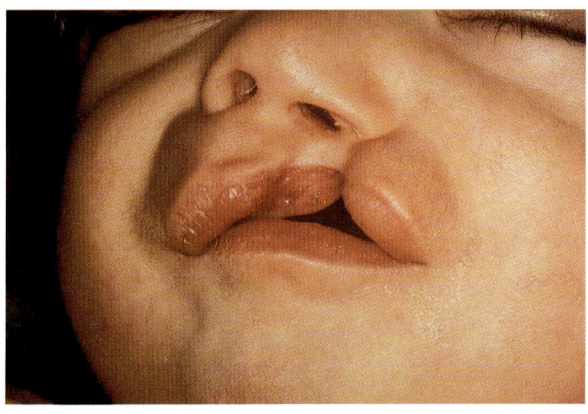

a

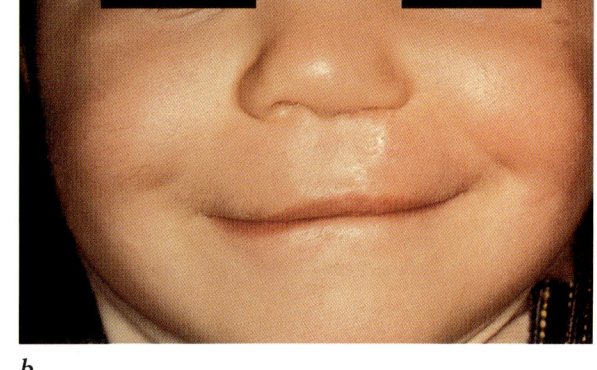

b

Fig. 7.51 *a and b Double Z-plasty provides good correction of a severe height deficit.*

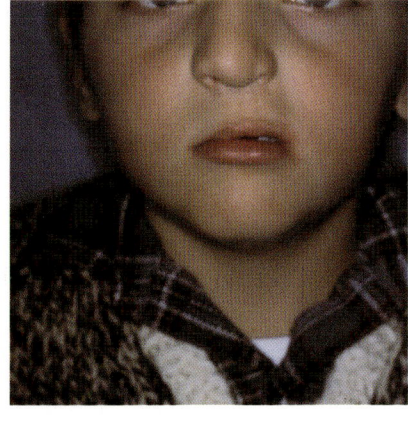

a

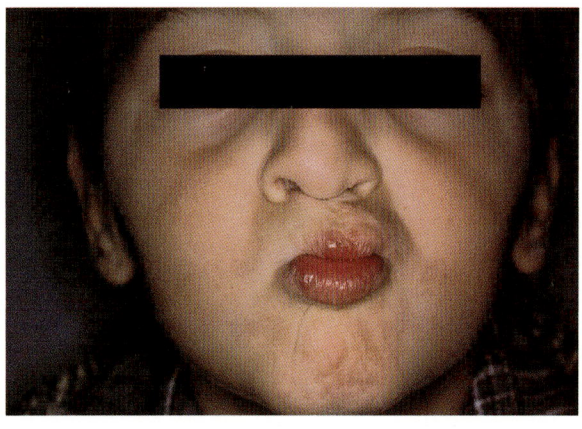

b

Fig. 7.52 *a and b Promising static results can prove disastrous from the dynamic point of view due to the unsatisfactory reinsertion of muscle fibers; for example, when the lip contracts as a sphincter.*

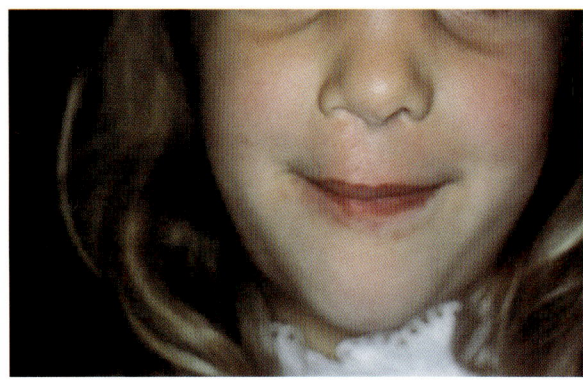

a

Fig. 7.53 a and b Double Z-plasty produces good
dynamic results.

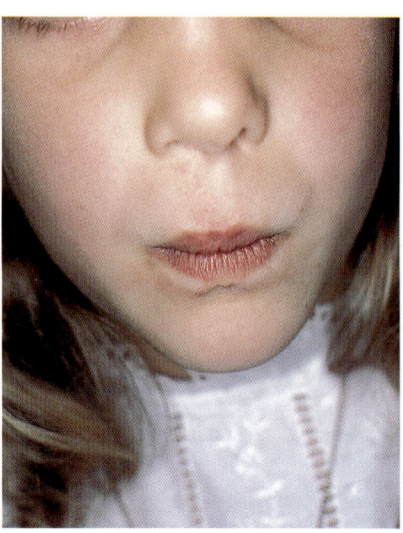

b

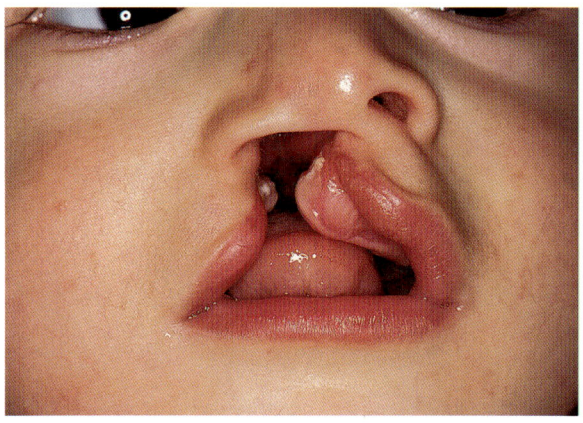

a

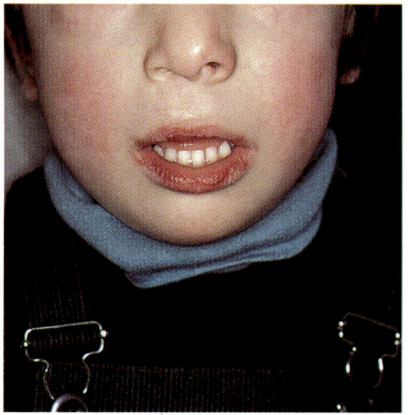

b

Fig. 7.54 a and b Results of double Z-plasty in broad unilateral cleft.

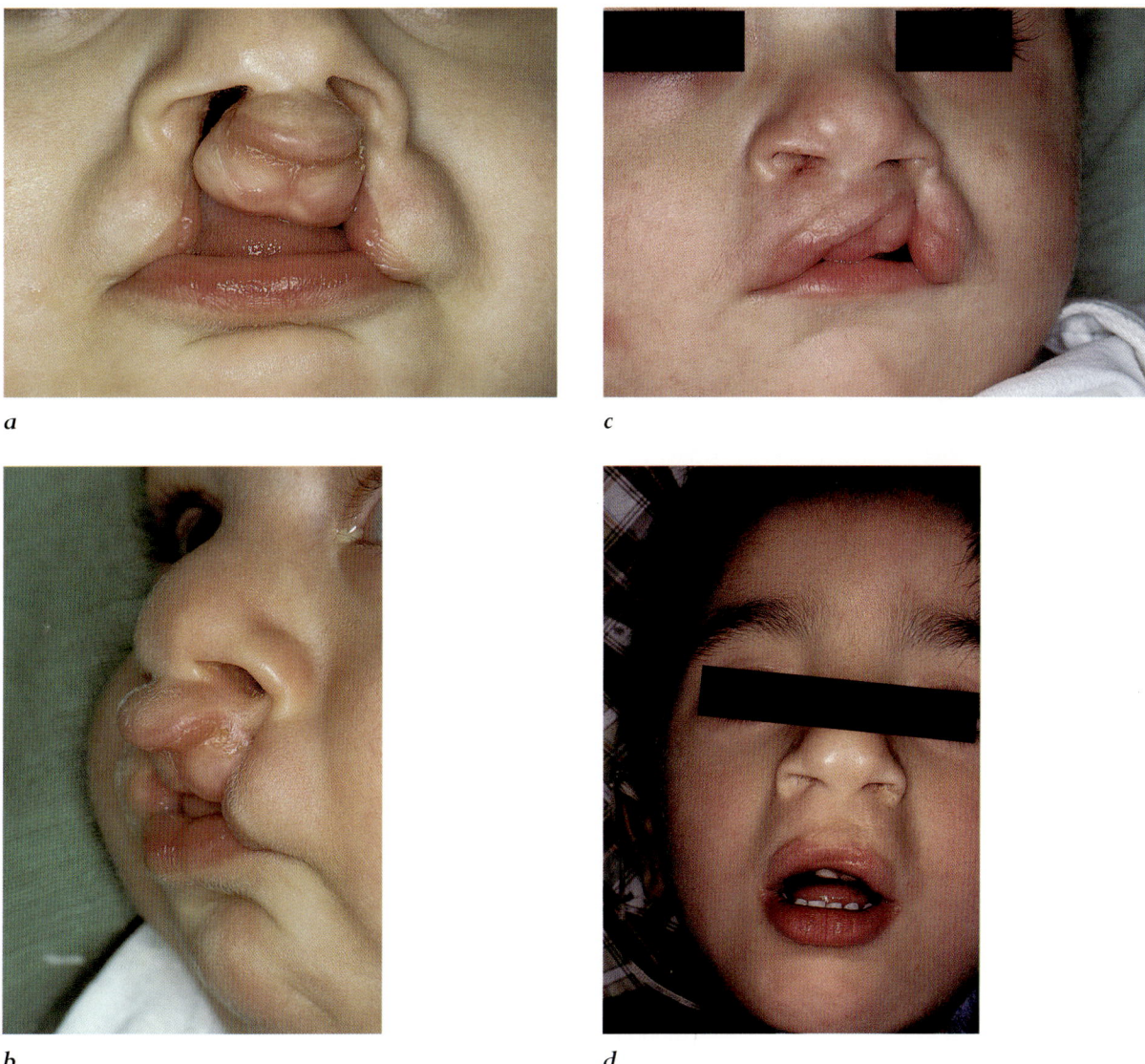

a

c

b

d

Fig. 7.55

a. Symmetrical complete bilateral cleft.

b. Three-quarter view showing misalignment of the borders.

c. After one side has been repaired, the appearance corresponds to that of a unilateral cleft.

d. Final results.

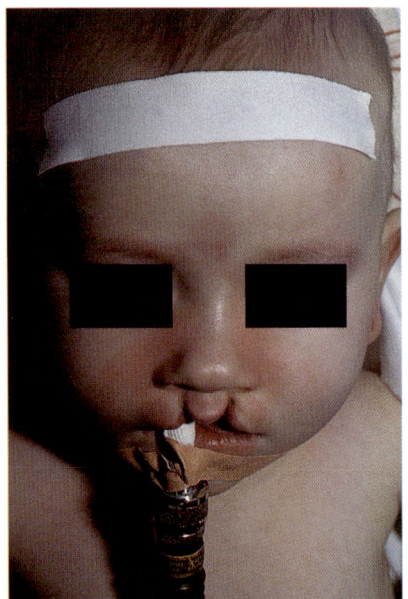

a

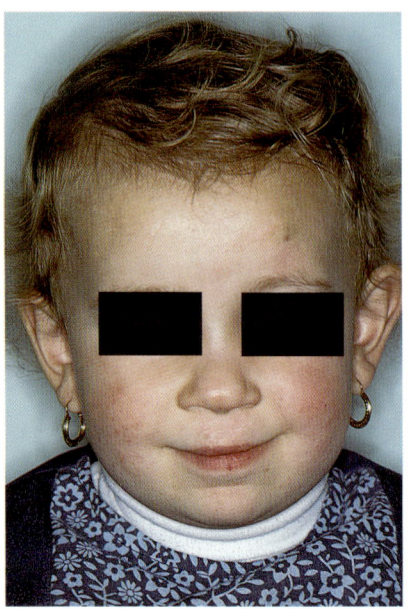

b

Fig. 7.56 *Simple bilateral cleft: before and after.*

8. Critical evaluation of the principal techniques

The author has described a method of lip repair that is called the equilateral triangle technique. I prefer it for an essential reason: to the author's knowledge, it is the only technique that uses mathematical precision to calculate the plasty needed to obtain good lip symmetry. This is a basic requirement.

This author finds it hard to grasp why other authors are less exacting about this goal and expose themselves to quite a few potential disappointments.

Nowadays, the techniques most commonly used world-wide are the Millard technique(s) and the triangular flap technique known as the Tennison operation. Neither of them allows for mathematical precision.

In the author's opinion, the case is clear: whatever the technique of repair, it must guarantee the symmetry of the lip.

Now that this essential prerequisite has been established, we can proceed to analyze the different techniques to determine whether or not they offer the advantages generally attributed to them. This is the purpose of the present chapter.

The techniques most frequently applied can be evaluated according to a certain number of criteria for lip repair.

UNILATERAL CLEFTS

Six criteria have been identified:

1. Height
2. Width
3. Contour of the skin–vermilion line
4. Eversion of the lip near its free border
5. Muscle on two levels:
   high – below the nostril sill
   low – near the free border of the lip
6. Nostril sill including the alar curve.

A rating system has been used to evaluate how well each technique meets the criteria listed above:

$$+ \ = \text{favorable effect}$$
$$\pm \ = \text{slight effect}$$
$$0 \ = \text{negative or no effect}$$

The results can be seen in Table 8.1.

Global evaluation of surgical results is not our goal; rather, we intend to judge and compare the procedures on the basis of the incisions involved.

Despite the wide range of techniques, it is possible to group the major procedures under simple headings.

Straight-line or curved incisions

These are the oldest techniques, based on suturing the freshened borders of the cleft (Fig. 8.1).

In France, the classic example is Veau's technique (1938). Veau, who established the major principles of satisfactory repair (transmitted to us by Petit and Psaume as of 1962), emphasized the importance of proper muscle suturing. He also advocated the resection of inner mucosa, which he qualified as 'sterile' because it did not lie over worthwhile muscle.

However, the freshen–suture technique does little to correct height deficiency except insofar as each border is resected on more of a slant. This

Table 8.1 *Ratings of techniques for repair of unilateral clefts*

| | Freshen–suture techniques | | | | Flap techniques | |
	Veau	Rose	Le Mesurier	Inferior triangle plasty/IET	Millard	Double flap
Height	0/±	±	+	+*	+	+
Width	0/±	+	0	+	+	+
Eversion	0	+	0	+	0	+
Muscle (high)	0	0	0	0	+	+
Muscle (low)	0	0	+	+	0	+
Nostril sill	0	0	0	0	+	+

*provided the method of measurement is correct

+ favorable effect

± slight effect

0 negative or no effect

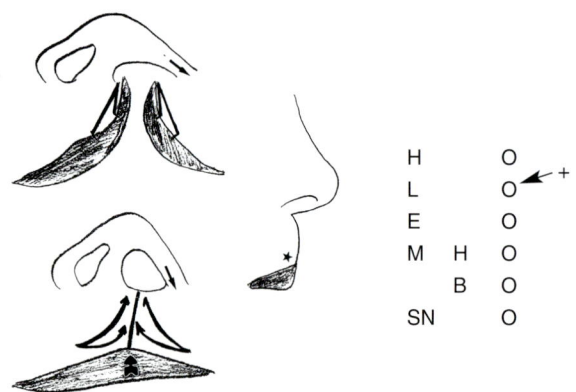

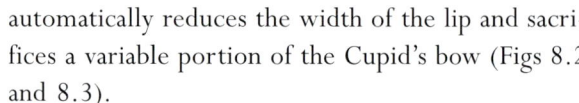

Fig. 8.1 *Veau: straight-line or curved incision techniques, based on suturing the freshened borders of the cleft.*

automatically reduces the width of the lip and sacrifices a variable portion of the Cupid's bow (Figs 8.2 and 8.3).

The curved incision popularized by Rose (1891) and Thomson (1912) palliates this defect to some extent. It produces a certain eversion of the free border of the lip, but does not obtain safe and simple correction of major height deficiency.

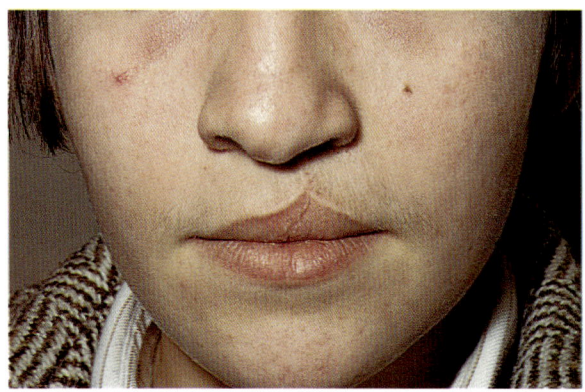

Fig. 8.2 *The freshen–suture technique does little to correct height deficiency.*

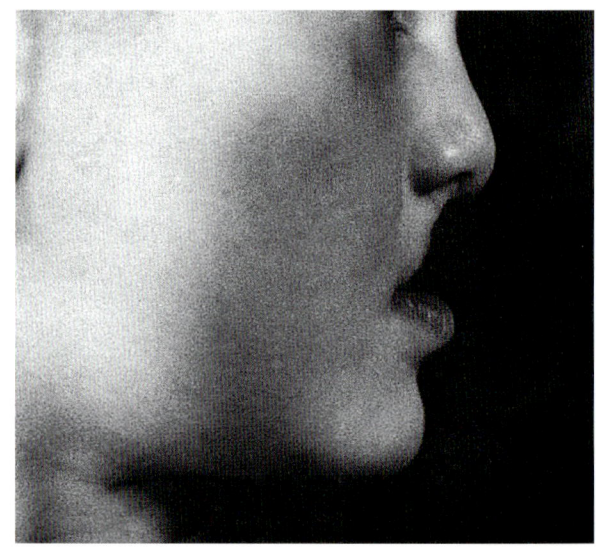

Fig. 8.3 *The resection automatically reduces the width of the lip and sacrifices part of the Cupid's bow.*

Whether straight or curved, this type of incision is not suitable for the correction of muscular lesions and totally neglects repositioning of the alar base.

Lastly, the contracture inherent in vertical scar lines can compromise the end result of a repair that was originally deemed satisfactory.

The ratings of these techniques are shown in Table 8.1.

Flap techniques

These are virtually the only procedures recommended since the 1950s. They are all based on the principle of Z-plasty (inversion of the diagonals of the parallelogram determined by the apices of the incisions). All Z-plasties therefore consist of two triangular flaps, which will be re-oriented in a new direction.

Rectangular flap procedure

The first technique to be described was the rectangular (quadrilateral) flap procedure. The flap is, in reality, a triangle, with a characteristic 90° angle opposite its pedicle.

This is the Le Mesurier technique, published in 1949 as a modified version of the procedure described by Hagedorn in 1884. A flap dissected on the outer border is introduced medially into an incision on the inner side, which includes an excised half Cupid's bow corresponding to the cleft (Fig. 8.4).

The originality of this procedure is connected with what we call the Le Mesurier effect: this term corresponds to the notch in the mucocutaneous line that appears at the point where the pedicle of the flap has been rotated. The Le Mesurier effect therefore reconstitutes or synthesizes the half of the Cupid's bow that was originally resected (see page 75).

The Le Mesurier technique does permit the height of the lip to be calculated, although not as accurately as it ideally should be.

It has often been suggested that this technique may lead to secondary lengthening of the lip, but there is no conclusive proof of this. The long lip probably corresponds to an initial defect, which becomes more conspicuous as the child matures.

The Le Mesurier technique presents the following disadvantages:

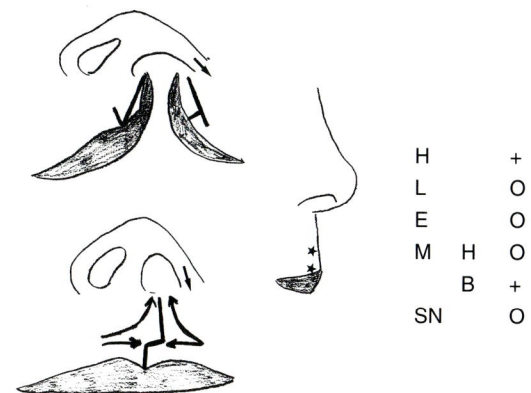

Fig. 8.4 *Le Mesurier: a flap dissected on the outer border is introduced medially into an incision of the inner side, which includes an excised half Cupid's bow.*

1. It does not preserve the total width of the lip. A portion of the Cupid's bow must be sacrificed.
2. Consequently, the mid-portion of the lip is off-centre. It is shifted towards the corner of the mouth on the cleft side (Fig. 8.5).
3. The lip is constricted near its free border. It droops somewhat, rather than presenting the desired eversion or pout (Fig. 8.6).

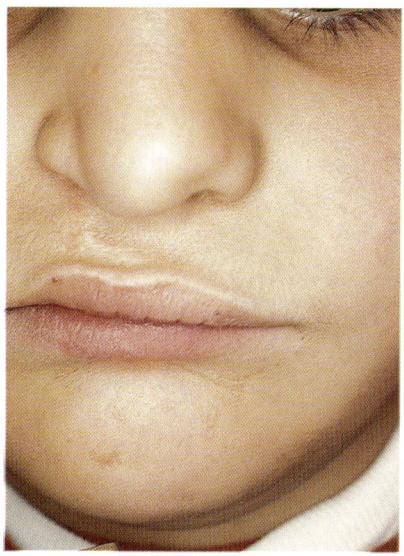

Fig. 8.5 *The mid-portion of the lip is shifted towards the corner of the mouth on the cleft side.*

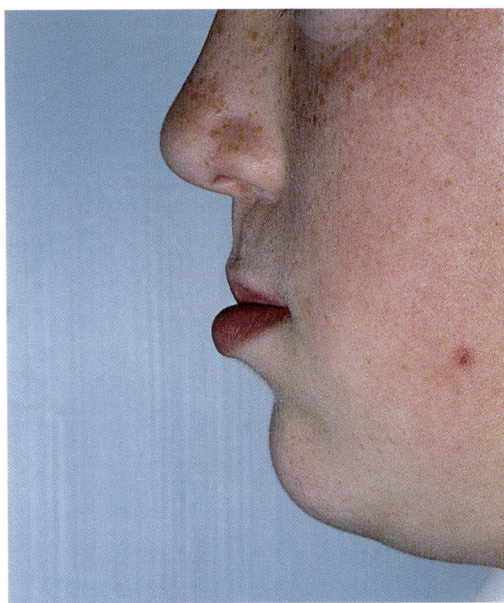

Fig. 8.6 *The lip is constricted near its free border and droops somewhat.*

4. Lastly, the upper muscle fibers just below the nostril sill are not re-oriented and eversion of the alar wing of the nose is not corrected.

An attempt has been made to spare the Cupid's bow by tracing more lateral incisions, but this modification transforms the procedure into a triangular flap plasty (with a 90° apex) without benefiting from the Le Mesurier effect.

Inferior triangle plasty

In techniques using an inferior triangular flap from the outer border, the inner-border is incised near its free border.

This procedure has been in use for quite some time. Jalaguier (1910) put it into practice, but it was unfortunately dropped by his pupil Victor Veau.

The name of Mirault is often linked to this technique, but wrongly so, since Mirault (1844) spoke only of vermilion flaps.

In 1930, Blair and Brown published a paper that has become the reference for this procedure.

In 1952, Tennison described his method for measuring the triangular plasty.

There is no mathematical basis to this method. It corresponds to a set of 'how-to' instructions, relying

on a stencil of brass wire. The length of the wire represents the distance measured from the upper reference point of the nostril sill on the inner border of the cleft to the lateral point for the peak of the Cupid's bow on the normal side. The wire is then bent into three equal segments, which are intended to form an equilateral triangle corresponding to the appropriate size of the flap. (The Tennison technique is also known as the 'stencil' method.)

One might well wonder how these instructions could ever produce satisfactory surgical results. Be that as it may, the procedure became very popular, since most surgeons were highly impressed by the fact that Tennison preserved the Cupid's bow. Moreover, the flap, which was often of considerable size, did obtain a good opening of the lip.

Names often undergo strange fates. For most authors, the Tennison technique corresponds to the inferior triangular flap procedure, although the measurements are not even remotely connected.

In 1959, Randall attempted to establish a mathematical basis for triangular plasty. He contended that the sum of the medians of the two triangular flaps lowered on the common side of the Z-plasty, which were continuous with one another, should correspond to the height of the non-cleft side. However, the line of these two medians is often angulated and, above all, constructing two triangles that share a common side thanks to two medians seems to present certain difficulties. Randall also set a limit on the length that should not be exceeded. Such recommendations are not in keeping with mathematical precision.

I will not review our own procedure, described in 1961 (see Borde et al, 1961). This has been discussed in the preceding chapters. We feel it is the only technique that guarantees mathematical precision and provides for simple per-operative measurements.

The advantages of the inferior triangle plasty are the same whatever the specific technique (Fig. 8.7); and the ratings are seen in Table 8.1.

Reverse incision techniques

These are techniques involving a more-or-less transverse incision of the upper portion of the inner border.

This allows its components to be lowered into their correct position. There are two possibilities:

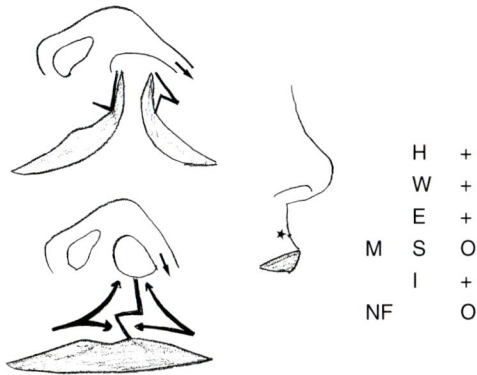

Fig. 8.7 *Inferior triangle plasty.*

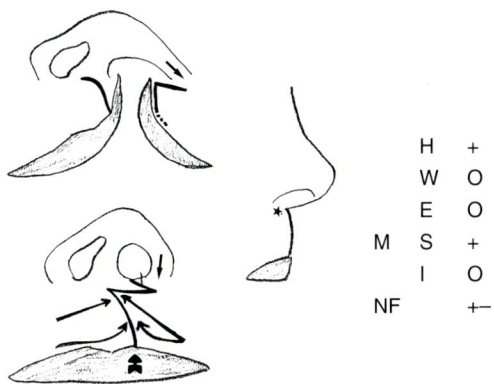

Fig. 8.8 *The Millard technique.*

1. A curved incision, i.e. the Millard technique.
2. Alternatively, the flap from the outer border is a true triangular flap. There are two techniques; the Wynn procedure, which is not widely used, and our technique, known as the inverted equilateral triangle (Malek).

The Millard technique

The Millard technique offers a number of theoretical advantages (Fig. 8.8). The scar replaces or follows the line of the philtral ridge on the cleft side, and the philtrum itself is not incised. The inclusion of almost the entire lip in the inner incision obtains a satisfactory orientation of that portion of the lip situated below the nostril sill and the columella. However, the lip is not adequately opened near its free border. Thus the mucocutaneous line still comes up too high on each border, giving the visual impression of a 'cocked hat' although, in moderate forms, the plasty does obtain a good lip height. This notch is even more conspicuous when the lip is moving (Fig. 8.9).

In forms that show considerable height deficiency, the only way to compensate for the shortfall of tissue is to extend the incisions in order to increase the dimensions of the outer triangular flap. This leads to resection of the mucocutaneous line, which sacrifices too much tissue from the width of the lip. In addition, muscle union in the lower portion is only fairly satisfactory.

The nostril sill is bolstered by the inner flap, but alar eversion is only partially corrected at best (Fig. 8.10).

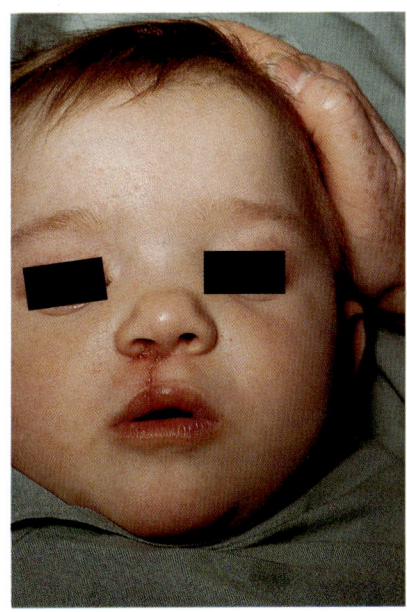

Fig. 8.9 *Millard: the notch is even more conspicuous when the lip is moving.*

Lastly, there is no eversion of the lip due to the absence of a Z-plasty near its free border.

To overcome these problems, Millard has suggested a certain number of refinements but, for the most part, the defects still exist. The use of a small triangular flap in the lower portion of the lip produces uncertain results, since no measurements are involved.

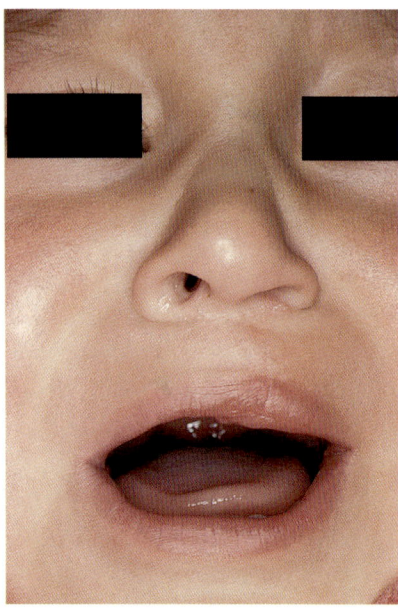

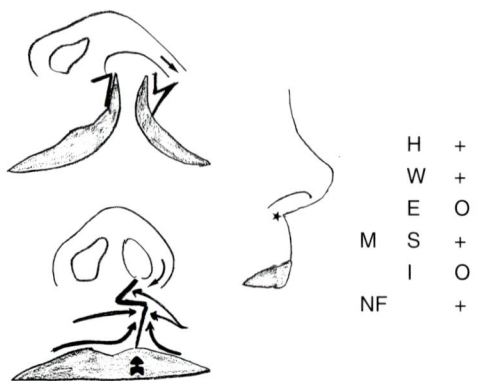

Fig. 8.12 *The inverted equilateral triangle technique.*

Fig. 8.10 *Millard: the nostril sill is bolstered by the inner flap, but alar eversion is only partially corrected at best.*

The inverted equilateral triangle technique (Malek)

When used in primary treatment, this method has the same drawbacks as Millard's technique: absence of opening in the lower portion of the lip. However, it does have the advantage of partially correcting eversion of the wing of the nose (Figs 8.11 and 8.12).

This technique is rated in Table 8.1.

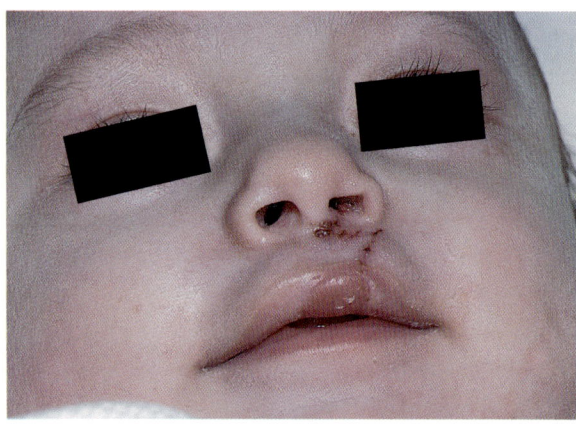

Fig. 8.11 *Inverted triangle: this has the advantage of partially correcting eversion of the wing of the nose.*

Double flap techniques

These are also known as double Z-plasties.

It is thought that Trauner was the first to propose this procedure, in 1955.

Collis, however, should not be cited in this context. The Irish surgeon is said to have described a double flap technique in 1868, but his superior flap was inserted into an intra-nasal incision above the base of the columella. Our focus here is the double flap procedure that exclusively concerns the lip – one superior and one inferior flap near the free border.

References to Skoog are equally inaccurate. To judge by his writings, Skoog (1958, 1969, 1974), like Collis, described the association of an inferior triangular flap with a superior flap, which was also intra-nasal rather than labial (see Chapter 7).

The double Z technique presents the following advantages:

1. It opens the lip quite satisfactorily on both the upper and lower levels, which permits suitable re-orientation of the muscle fibers, permits proper correction of the everted alar cartilage and creates a nice pout or eversion of the lip near its free border.
2. The double Z also restores good lip height, even in cases of severe deficiency, without sacrificing lip width, which is always to be avoided.

We have already seen that the double equilateral triangle, which we have devised, combines mathematical

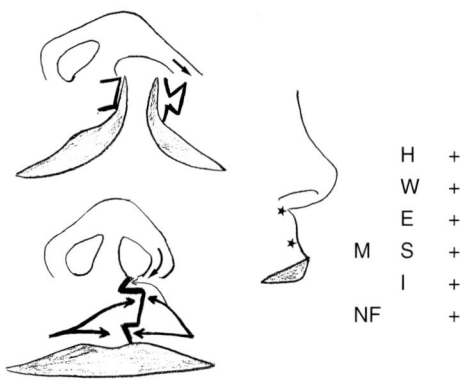

Fig. 8.13 *The double equilateral triangle combines mathematical precision and a technique that is easy to work with.*

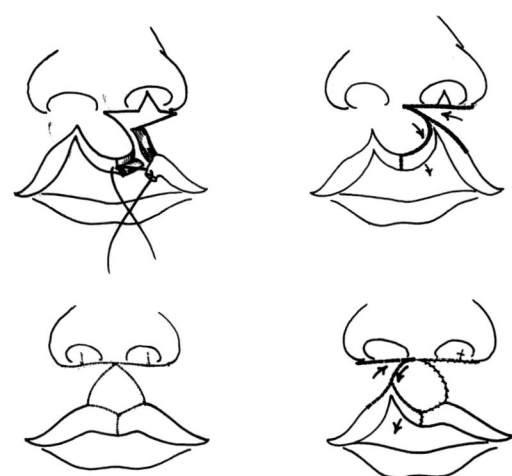

Fig. 8.14 *The Millard technique in bilateral forms.*

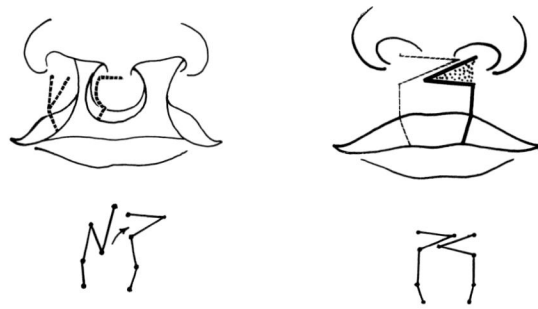

Fig. 8.15 *The Wynn technique.*

precision and a technique that is easy to work with (Fig. 8.13). The ratings are shown in Table 8.1. This should therefore be the preferred technique, especially for those severely hypoplastic forms that call for the calculation of a double Z.

BILATERAL CLEFTS

Innumerable techniques have been described for the repair of the bilateral cleft lip.

We automatically reject those that involve simultaneous correction of both sides in a single operation, for the many reasons already discussed (see Chapter 7). Nor do we retain those that attempt to lengthen the columella (Millard, 1958 or Wynn, 1965) (Figs 8.14 and 8.15). These procedures leave unattractive scars at the labio-columellar junction and, above all, compromise secondary surgery by cutting off nasal vascular supply to the prolabium.

Furthermore, the rounded contour of the prolabium, which frequently takes the shape of a convex lens, requires adequate opening with a downward rotation of the flaps as proposed by the triangular flap procedures (Blair–Brown, 1930). Straight-line (Veau, 1938) or curved incisions (Rose (1891)–Thomson (1912)) should not be used.

The equilateral triangle flap technique (Malek, 1983) meets all the demands of bilateral cleft lip repair.

LIP-ADHESION PROCEDURE

Recommended by many authors and, in particular, by Randall, the lip-adhesion procedure (or primary suture of the lip) is based on a certain number of theoretical arguments.

Closure of the two borders without using deep sutures is thought to reduce tension on the soft tissues when definitive repair is later performed. The reason given is that it helps to reposition or remodel the bone framework. By converting the lesions into those of a cleft with a band (or even a simple cleft), a better esthetic result might be expected, similar to that of 'minor' forms, particularly where the nostril contour is concerned.

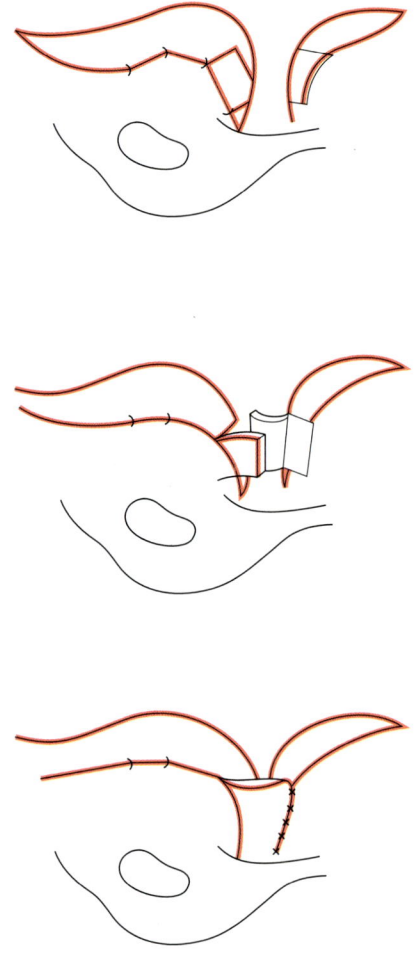

Fig. 8.16 *Lip-adhesion procedure, recommended by Randall. The flap excised from the skin of the outer border is folded back and sutured to a flap of equal thickness from the inner border.*

Lastly, in bilateral forms, protrusion of the premaxilla could be reduced if not corrected.

The lip-adhesion technique is recommended primarily for very wide clefts and for bilateral forms.

A relatively simple procedure, lip-adhesion does not create undue complications for subsequent cheiloplasty since no dissection is performed and the suture involves only tissue on the borders that will later be resected (Fig. 8.16). However, in our view it presents several serious disadvantages:

- It adds another step to the surgical agenda.
- It brings tension to bear on the bone structures at a very early age (it is performed in the first weeks of life), thus creating a major risk of displacement or collapse of the maxillary segments. It is in complete contradiction to our policy of primary veloplasty, which reverses the order of operations, since the tongue is not in a position to counter-act the new pressure created. Preventive use of a retained prosthesis does not necessarily have the desired effect (see Chapter 20).
- Despite opinions to the contrary, lip-adhesion can lead to troublesome scar formation.
- Lastly, the favorable effect on the appearance of the nasal structures has not been conclusively demonstrated.

In our opinion, the means to obtain better results can be found elsewhere.

III THE ISOLATED CLEFT PALATE

9. Anatomy and physiology of the normal palate

ANATOMY

The normal palate is composed of two parts; the hard palate and the soft palate.

The hard palate

The anterior part of the palate, known as the hard palate or palatal vault, is bony and solid. Its bone structure is comprised for the most part of the palatal shelves (palatine processes of the maxilla and of the palatine bone), which are joined on the midline. On the nasal side the suture line forms the nasal crest, which is attached to the vomer. The anterior third or upper part of the nasal crest rises to form the incisive crest, which is extended forward the edge of the maxilla by the anterior nasal spine.

Towards the back the vault is completed by the posterior nasal spine, formed by the shelves of the palatine bones.

On the midline, towards the front of the mouth, the incisive or anterior palatine foramen can be observed. It forms the posterior limit between a small, triangular bony segment and the rest of the palate. This triangular portion corresponds to the premaxillary segment, which is often called the primary palate (see Chapter 2).

The posterior or free border of the palatal shelves is notched on either side by grooves where the posterior palatine nerves and blood vessels pass between the palatine process and the wall of the maxilla (Fig. 9.1).

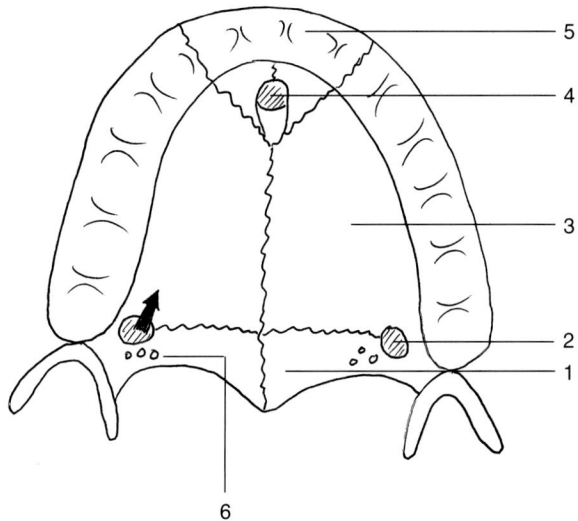

Fig. 9.1 *Skeleton of palatal vault, seen from below.*

1. *Palatal shelf of palatine bone*
2. *Posterior foramen for palatine bundle*
3. *Palatal shelf of maxilla*
4. *Anterior incisive foramen*
5. *Premaxilla*
6. *Lesser palatine foramina*

The hard palate is covered on the nasal side by mucosa of the nasal floor, which includes the postero-lateral and vomerine mucosa. On the oral side it is covered primarily by the highly characteristic mucoperiosteum, which is far thicker than its nasal counterpart. To be more accurate, as Veau

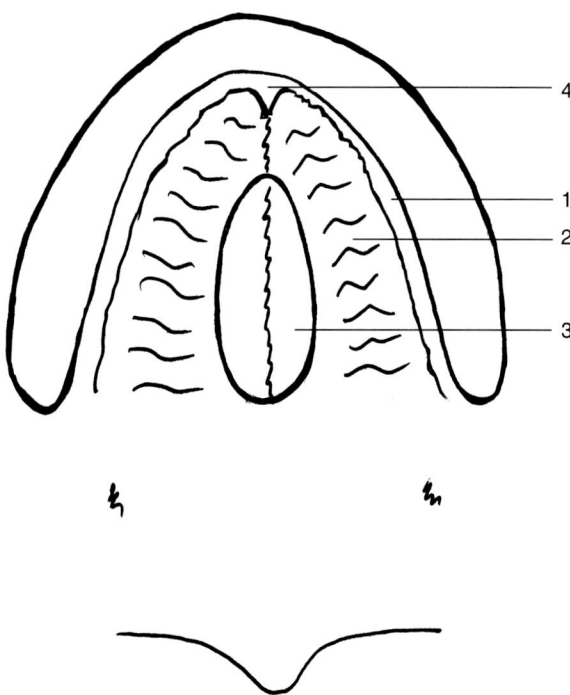

Fig. 9.2 *Aspect of mucosa covering palatal vault.*

1. Narrow, smooth gingival zone.
2. Palatine mucoperiosteum crossed by thick ridges.
3. Central zone forms a depression lined with smooth, thin mucosa.
4. Median lump or tuberculum.

pointed out, three distinct zones of oral mucosa can be identified (Fig. 9.2):

1. The outermost or gingival region adjacent to the teeth, where the mucosal layer is thin.
2. The middle area (palatine raphe), which is very prominent. Its surface is crisscrossed with rough, rasp-like ridges. The mucous layer is very thick and sturdy (fibro-mucosa), which enables the tongue to crush food against it.
3. The inner zone, where the layer is smooth and much thinner. It covers about one-third of the vault on either side of the midline. Together the two opposite halves form a central depression between the protrusions of thick mucoperiosteum, which sometimes leads pediatricians and parents to suspect the presence of a malformation.

As we will see, these latter two distinct zones play a major part in cleft palate repair. Only the thick middle mucoperiosteum contains the neurovascular bundle and heals at a satisfactory rate. However, raising a flap with a posterior pedicle from the mucoperiosteum is considered detrimental to growth. The thinner inner zone heals more slowly and offers less resistance to intra-oral pressure. On the other hand, it is very well vascularized by branches of the major or anterior palatine vessels. Dissecting a flap in this zone does not seem to produce the same iatrogenic effects.

At the foremost limit of the oral mucosa, immediately behind the incisive papilla, there exists a smooth median hump that corresponds to the incisive or anterior palatine foramen.

The soft palate

The second part of the palate is a mobile fibro-muscular structure known as the soft palate or velum. It is normally composed of two elements; the palatine aponeurosis, which constitutes a sort of fibrous skeleton, and the muscles proper. There are 10 of these, five on either side, and a brief run-down of their insertions follows.

The palatine aponeurosis is a very important structure, and the palatal muscles all insert into it directly or indirectly. It forms a fibrous quadrangle, which attaches anteriorly to the posterior border of the palatal shelves. Its posterior edge is curved and extends from the tip of one hamulus to the other. The muscles of the soft palate insert into both surfaces of the aponeurosis. Its lateral edges correspond to the fan-shaped expansion of the tendinous fibers from the tensor veli palatini muscle. The palatine aponeurosis is set on a plane that slants downward and backward at 45° because the line connecting the hamuli is lower than the posterior border of the palatal shelves. Presumably, the aponeurosis is not extensible. However, although its anterior border is anchored in bone, its posterior border can become mobile because its lateral extremities are attached to two elastic structures (the tendons and muscle fibers of the tensor veli palatini). Thus, the foremost portion of the soft palate that corresponds to the palatine aponeurosis can move up and down under the effects of muscle contraction and/or tongue pressure (Ruding, 1964) (Fig. 9.3).

a

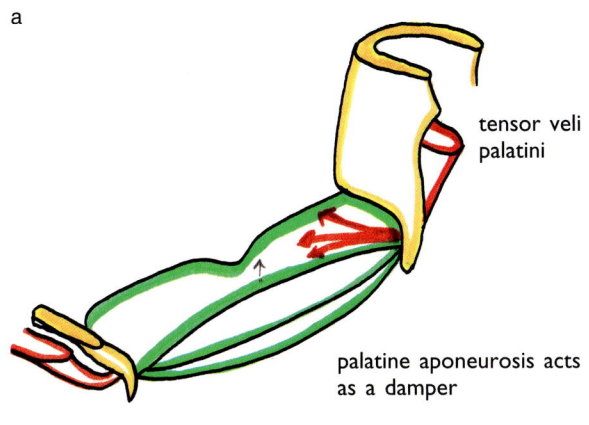

tensor veli palatini

palatine aponeurosis acts as a damper

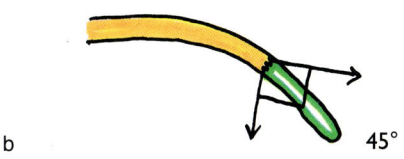

b   45°

Fig. 9.3 a. Palatine aponeurosis, a quadrangular structure fused on three sides. The posterior border shows a certain degree of mobility upward and downward. By regulating the tension of the fibers, the tensor veli palatini acts as a shock absorber. b. The palatine aponeurosis is set on a 45° slant compared with the skeletal plane of the vault.

The velar muscles can be divided into two groups on either side of the midline (Legent *et al.*, 1986): superiorly, the tensor veli palatini and the levator palatini; and inferiorly, the palatoglossus and the palato-pharyngeus. There are also two contiguous muscles that extend lengthwise along the midline within the fibers of the velum itself. These are the uvular muscles.

The superior velar muscles

The tensor veli palatini is situated outside the pharynx (i.e. exterior to the salpingopharyngeal bundle and to the superior constrictor). It arises from the greater wing of the sphenoid in front of and lateral to the spheno-petrosal fissure to which the auditory tube is attached, and from the antero-lateral wall of the Eustachian tube. Shaped like an inverted triangle, it narrows into a flat tendon that bends around the pterygoid hamulus at a right angle (there is a bursa between the tendon and the hamulus). A part of it then attaches to the adjacent border of the palatal

shelf, while the major portion expands into a fan shape before inserting into the aponeurosis. There, it connects with matching fibers from the opposite side. A certain portion of its deep-lying fibers inserts into the cartilage of the Eustachian tube (Fig. 9.4).

As its primary function, the tensor veli palatini contributes to opening the Eustachian tube. Its effect on the velum is still subject to debate (other than its role as 'shock absorber' for movements of the aponeurosis, which has already been described).

The levator veli palatini is oriented in the same direction as the Eustachian tube. Arising from the apical portion of the petrosal bone and from the cartilaginous wall of the Eustachian tube, it passes below the latter, where it forms a low ridge called the levator torus. The levator arcs inward and follows the lower curve of the medial ala of the pterygoid plate. Its fibers then fan out and interlace with fibers from the opposite side. Its action combines with that of the superior pharyngeal constrictor to close the velo-pharyngeal aperture.

Thus the superior muscles both insert at the base of the skull, from which they suspend the soft palate as if in a sling. The levator palatini lifts the velum (a valve mechanism that closes the oral from the nasal pharynx) and acts as a sphincter in combination with the superior constrictor.

The inferior velar muscles

These originate on the level of the soft palate and, unlike the preceding group, they therefore both arise and end in mobile structures.

The palatopharyngeus is a major muscle, both in its size and in the importance of its function. It is splayed into a double fan shape, and its upper insertions can be divided into three sets of muscle fibers:

1. The palatine or velar fibers, which join bundles of fibers from the opposite side and arise from the velum and the lower portion of the palatine aponeurosis.
2. Fibers that originate at the hamulus.
3. Fibers that arise near the opening of the auditory tube.

These fibers unite in a narrow bundle to form the arch of the posterior tonsillar pillar, which is set on a postero-inferior slant.

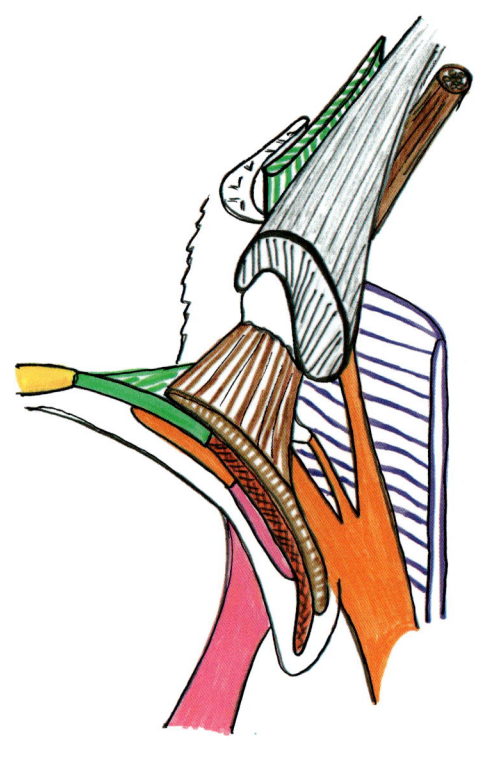

a

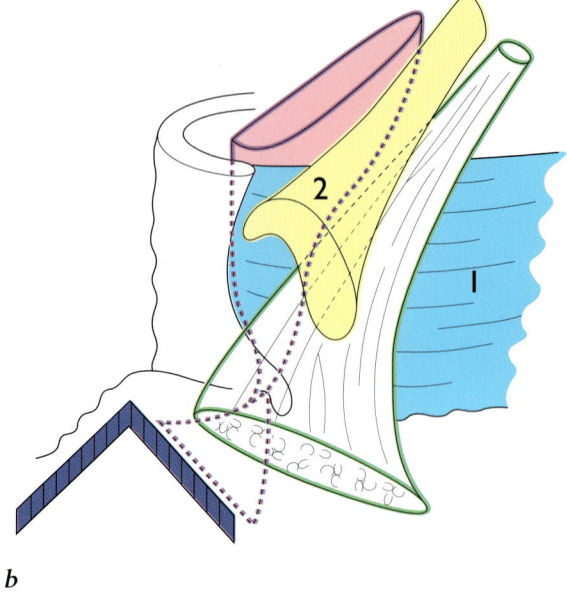

b

Fig. 9.4 *a. Internal view of the velar muscles. On either side there are two superior sets, two inferior sets and the uvular muscles.*
b. Relationship of the two superior muscles to the pharyngeal aponeurosis (1) and tubal cartilage (2).

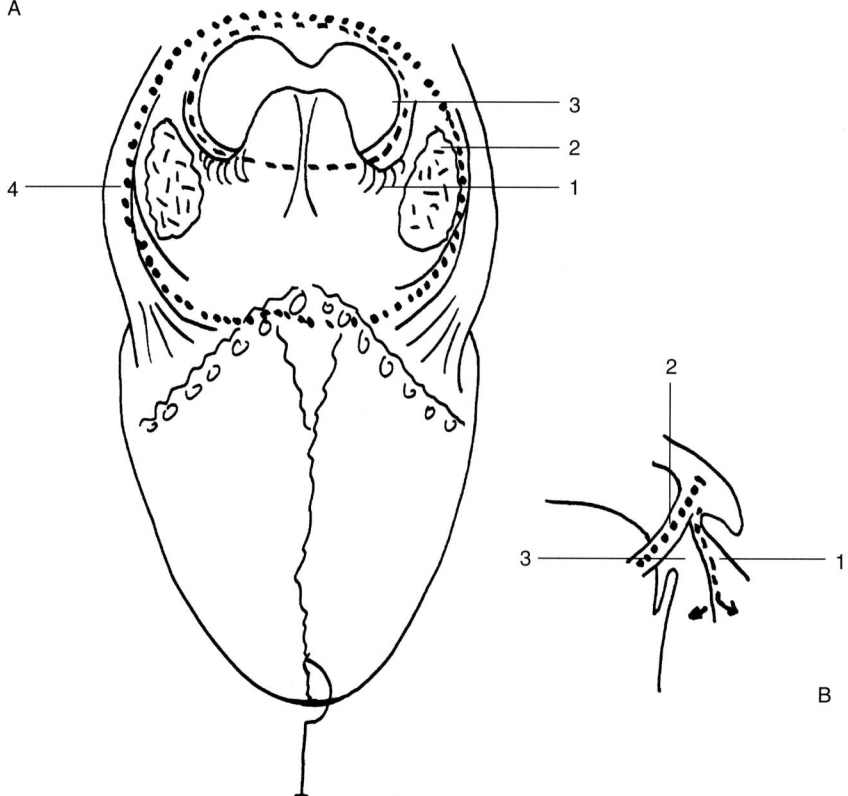

A

B

Fig. 9.5 *Oropharyngeal isthmuses: red, isthmus of the fauces; green, pharyngonasal isthmus.*

A. Base of the tongue, seen from above.
1   Lateral fold between tongue and epiglottis.
2   Tonsil.
3   Fold between pharynx and epiglottis. Posterior tonsillar pillar.
4   Anterior tonsillar pillar.

B. Location of isthmuses on profile view.
1   Posterior tonsillar pillar.
2   Anterior tonsillar pillar.
3   Tonsil area.

The palatopharyngeus ends in a fan shape on the thyroid cartilage and, principally, on the wall of the pharynx, where it connects with its contralateral. It delimits the **nasopharyngeal isthmus**, which separates the naso- and oropharynx. It serves to lower the soft palate and helps to lift the pharynx and the breathing apparatus. When the posterior pillars draw together, they function as a velar valve to prevent food from passing into the cavum during the swallowing process.

The palatoglossus is a more slender muscle that forms the anterior tonsillar pillar. It too originates in the anterior portion of the aponeurosis, then courses outward in an antero-inferior direction. It diverges into two parts; a sagittal bundle, which follows the lateral border of the tongue, and a transversal bundle, which attaches to the lingual septum. The arches of the palato-glossi on either side, together with the soft palate above and the base of the tongue below, form the boundaries of the **isthmus of the fauces**. This isthmus, which narrows when the palato-glossi lower the soft palate and lift the tongue, plays an extremely important role in the swallowing and breathing processes (Fig. 9.5).

The uvular muscles

The uvular muscles extend along the midline from the postero-superior surface of the palatine aponeurosis to the tip of the uvula and pass between the superior and inferior muscle groups. They serve to pull the soft palate taut and are believed to contribute to the dorsal erection of the uvula. This phenomenon flattens the upper surface of the soft palate against the superior constrictor. As my mentor Petit used to say, uvular repair is not merely a matter of surgical showmanship. On the contrary, its reconstruction is a necessity since the uvula functions as a valve when it presses against the narrowed opening of the nasopharyngeal sphincter.

Spatial geometry of the soft palate

The velum is not a flat sheet, as is customarily imagined (Fig. 9.6). Although this image does correspond, to a certain extent, to the anterior portion or aponeurosis, which stretches between the lower borders of the pterygoid processes and seems to extend the hard palate towards the back of the oral cavity, it is not true of the posterior portion. This section of the soft palate is, in fact, a thick, bulky layer produced by three rings or loops of muscle fiber that meet at the midline.

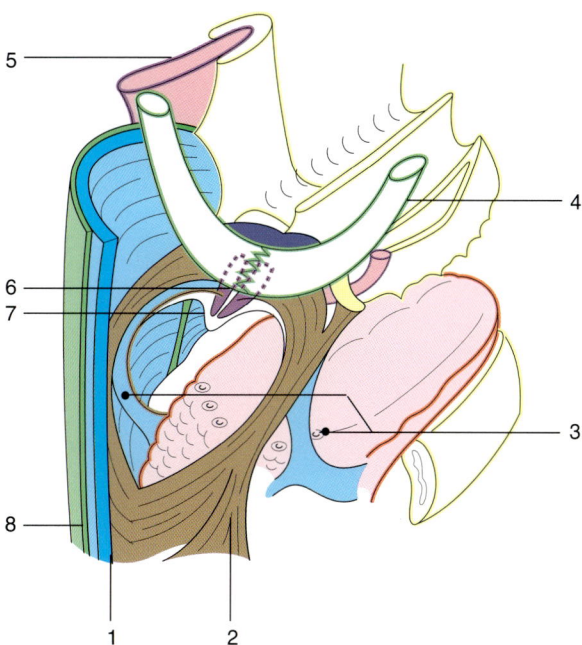

Fig. 9.6 *Postero-lateral view of the velar muscles (according to Legent et al., 1986), or spatial geometry of the soft palate. The two superior muscles are suspended from the base of the skull, and the two inferior muscles have mobile insertions. A dotted line marks the zone of contact between the velum and the superior pharyngeal constrictor.*

1. *Superior constrictor*
2. *Palato pharyngeal muscle*
3. *Palato glossus*
4. *Levator veli palatini*
5. *Tensor veli palatini*
6. *Uvular muscle*
7. *Buccinator*
8. *Aponeurosis of the pharynx*

The superior loop is formed by the mass of levator veli palatini fibers from either side. It opens in its upper portion at the base of the skull.

The two inferior loops are created by the palato-glossal and palato-pharyngeal arches. These are, respectively, the anterior and posterior tonsillar pillars. The rings they form open downward towards the base of the tongue and the pharynx. It therefore stands to reason that this portion of the soft palate cannot be seen as a flat structure.

Since these loops do not form a continuum, they alone cannot function as sphincters to close the orifices

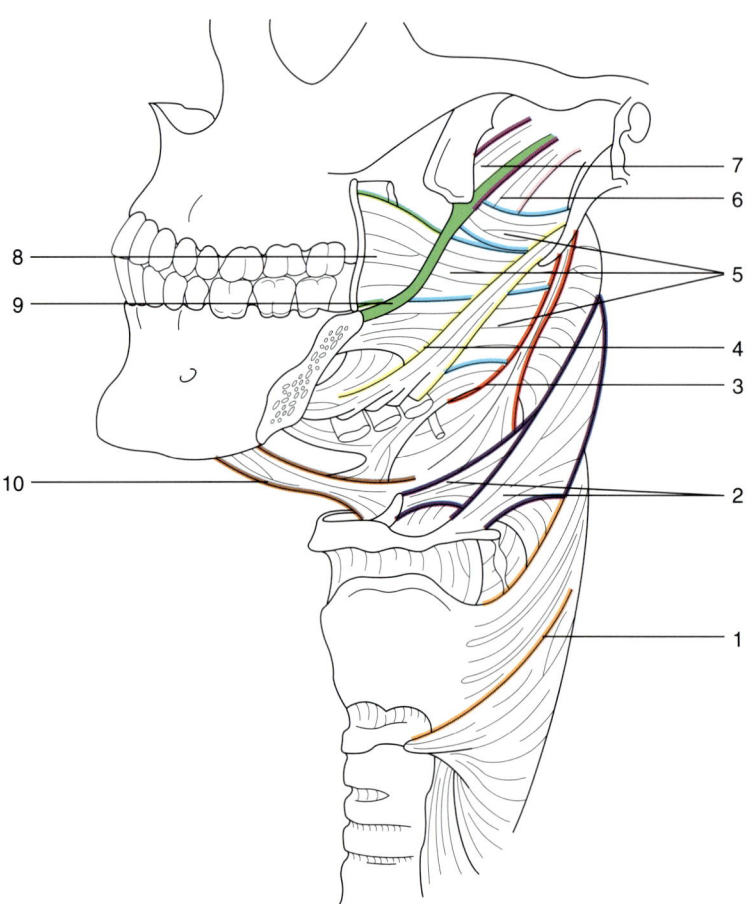

Fig. 9.7 *Muscles of the pharynx.*

1. *Inferior constrictor of the pharynx*
2. *M. hypopharyngeus on middle constrictor*
3. *Stylopharyngeus*
4. *Styloglossus*
5. *Superior constrictor of the pharynx*
6. *Levator veli palatini*
7. *Tensor veli palatini*
8. *Buccinator*
9. *Pterygomandibular ligament*
10. *Genioglossus*

of the naso- and oropharynx. The sphincteric mechanism must be completed by the action of two additional components; the superior pharyngeal constrictor and the base of the tongue. Their role will be developed in the section on physiology, and will help to explain how the soft palate functions as a valve.

The superior pharyngeal constrictor (Fig. 9.7) does not number among the muscles of the soft palate. Nevertheless, it is relevant to this particular section because it contributes to the formation of the 'nasopharyngeal sphincter' (Whillis, 1930), which is also comprised of velar muscle. It is a broad muscle in the shape of a groove. Its uppermost fibers insert into the posterior borders and hamuli of the medial alae of the pterygoid process, and it also occasionally attaches to the pharyngeal tubercle of the occipital bone. This muscle normally presents a free upper border, which may at times split into two strands if the occipital insertion exists. This border and the lateral fibers of the levator veli palatini cross each other to form an 'X'.

When the superior constrictor contracts, it draws the wall of the pharynx and the upper surface of the soft palate together. Contact between these two elements is therefore established. On one side, there is the soft palate. As the muscles that compose it contract, it thickens and forms a bend (probably due to the effect of levator palatini and uvular muscles contractions). On the other side, the wall of the pharynx moves forward to meet the velum. At times, a transverse ridge is visible on a level with the atlas. Known as Passavant's ridge or bar, it is not a constant finding and its origin has not yet been clearly identified. Certain specialists believe that it corresponds to a thickening of the transverse fibers of the nasopharyngeal sphincter, which would therefore play the major functional role. Others contend that it is a horizontal fold in the muscle tissue produced by the occipital insertion, which occasionally occurs and causes the fibers to bulge by restraining their upper portion. Still others identify it as the point where the first fibers of the middle pharyngeal constrictor overlap with the lower fibers of the superior constrictor.

Closure of the nasopharynx is therefore obtained by contact over a broad surface, which results from simultaneous contraction of the levator palatini and

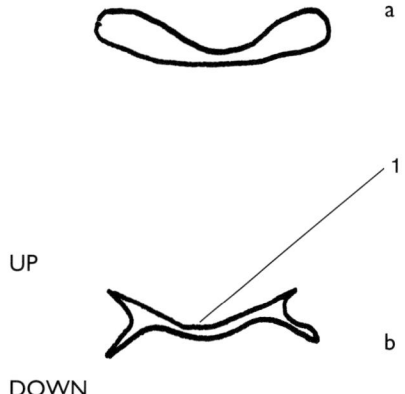

levator is a well-known anatomical fact. In addition, tongue pressure flattens the portion of the soft palate that corresponds to the uvula and its base against the pharyngeal wall, thus creating a tight seal that prevents the reflux of food into the nasal fossae during the swallowing process.

This nasopharyngeal closure has been observed thanks to a variety of techniques. Naso-endoscopy is particularly instructive. As Pigott (1969) has demonstrated, it helps to explain why air escapes into the nose during speech (velopharyngeal insufficiency) (Fig. 9.8).

Fig. 9.8 *Closure of the nasopharynx viewed by naso-endoscopy (Pigott, 1969): a. without and b. with the contraction of the palatopharyngeal muscle.*

1 Convexity due to the uvular muscles

superior pharyngeal constrictor. As the loop formed by the levator tightens, it facilitates closure. This supposes a certain independence of the muscle from the pterygoid plate on which it lies. Transverse mobility of the

Nerve and blood supply of the palate

The motor nerve supply to the tensor veli palatini is provided by branches of the trigeminal nerve. The other muscles are supplied by the IXth and Xth nerves, which enter from the rear (Fig. 9.9).

The vagus nerve also participates via the pharyngeal plexus, which includes the glossopharyngeal nerve, the pharyngeal branch of the vagus nerve and sensory branches.

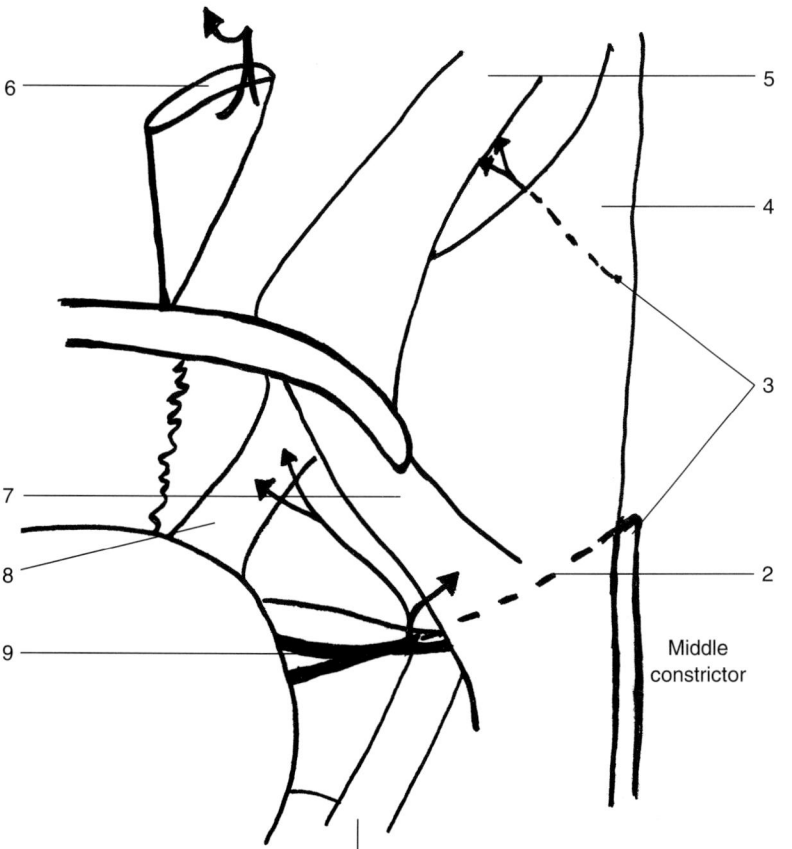

Fig. 9.9 *Motor nerve system of the palate (Broomhead, 1951).*

1.   *Stylopharyngeus*
2.   *Nerve to middle constrictor*
3.   *Nerve of LP from pharyngeal branch of vagus (X)*
4.   *Superior constrictor*
5.   *Levatro palatini*
6.   *Tensor palatini*
7.   *Palatopharyngeus*
8.   *Palatoglossus*
9.   *Glossopharyngeal nerve*

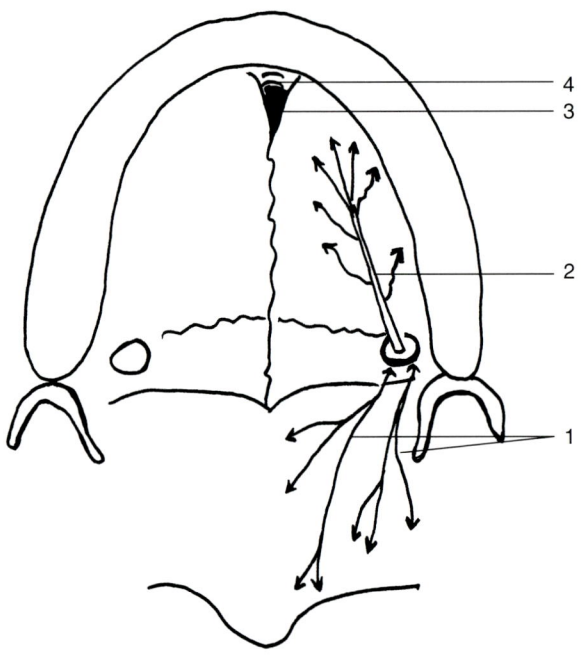

Fig. 9.10 *Sensory nerve system of the palate (Broomhead, 1951).*

1. *Lesser palatine nerves*
2. *Greater palatine nerve*
3. *Anterior* ⎫
   Incisive ⎭ *foramina*
4. *Primary palate*

The smaller palatine nerves furnish the sensory nerve supply of the velar mucosa and glands, which are said to make up half the volume of the soft palate. They emerge through the lesser palatine foramina behind the palatal shelves and may contribute to the motor nerve supply of the uvular muscles.

The anterior and middle palatine nerves supply the fibro-mucosa (Fig. 9.10).

The palatal arteries are, in brief:

• Soft palate: a branch of the ascending palatine artery and the smaller palatine artery.
• Hard palate: the posterior palatine artery as well as branches from the tonsillar and ascending pharyngeal arteries.

PHYSIOLOGY

The mechanisms of the palate and the aero-digestive tract are among the most complex in the human body, and it is essential that the members of the multidisciplinary team responsible for treating cleft palate anomalies be well versed in this field to enable all concerned to offer a valid contribution to discussions of the clinical or para-clinical data concerning each case. A joint decision can then be reached on therapeutic measures adapted to the needs and concerns of each specialist.

It is true that the medical curriculum does not generally cover these aspects, unless certain highly specialized fields of study are included. Their complexity may account for this omission. Nonetheless, they can be presented simply and concisely.

Two preliminary points must be noted. First, why do the respiratory and digestive passages intersect? The study of embryology provides part of the answer. During the first months of embryonic development, the palate gradually forms a horizontal partition, which splits the cephalic extremity of the digestive tube. The nasal fossae, above, are separated from the oral cavity, below. The airway develops from the anterior wall of the digestive tube as a diverticulum oriented in an antero-inferior direction, and it will therefore be located in front of the future esophagus. A section of the original tube remains to become the pharynx. It is gradually bent at a right angle to the uppermost or oro-nasal portion (Fig. 9.11).

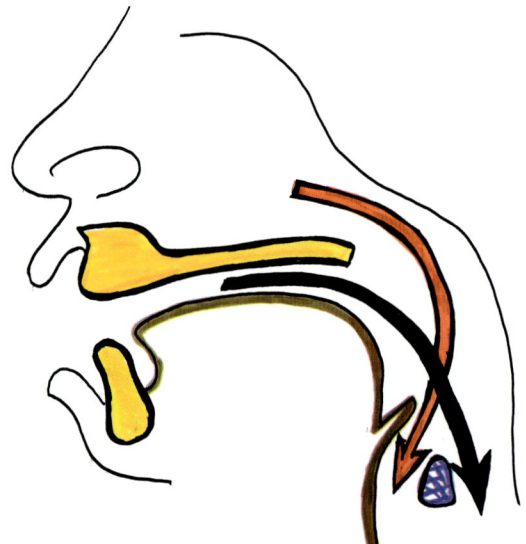

Fig. 9.11 *Intersection of the aero-digestive tracts. Development of the airway from the anterior wall of the digestive tube and the right-angled bend of the original tube explains the configuration of the pharynx.*

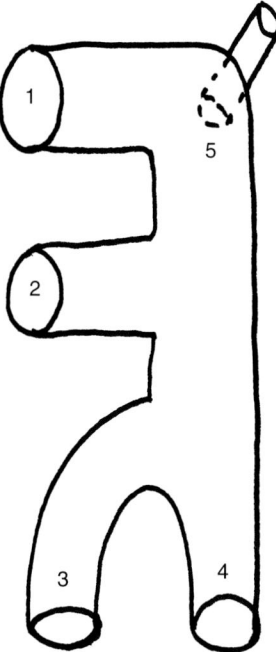

Fig. 9.12 Five ducts open into the pharynx, each with its own individual closing mechanism:

1. *Nasal fossae*
2. *Mouth*
3. *Trachea*
4. *Esophagus*
5. *Eustachian tube*
   (According to Lespargot, 1987).

These steps of development show why the air and food passages intersect and explain their final positions. There are therefore five ducts that open into the pharynx; the nasal fossae and mouth in the antero-superior portion, and the larynx and esophagus in the lower portion. Each duct has its individual closing mechanism at the point where it joins the pharynx in order to ensure the alternate separation or communication between the airway and the digestive system (Fig. 9.12).

Second, the palate contributes to both systems of upper occlusion, those of the mouth and of the nose. The airway opens or shuts as it moves down or up, and this process is visualized by the movement of the protruding thyroid cartilage known as the Adam's apple beneath the skin of the neck. Glottal closure provides an additional safety device to close off the airway.

The palate can therefore:

1. Ensure complete occlusion of the nasal fossae (in conjunction with the superior pharyngeal constrictor). As seen earlier, by establishing contact between the two loops, it functions as a true sphincter during the swallowing process when the airway moves upward.
2. Close the mouth in a normal fashion during breathing (by closing the isthmus of the fauces in combined action with the base of the tongue) when the airway moves downward.

The palate also plays a major role in the hearing process, since the superior muscles control the opening and closing of the pharyngeal orifice of the Eustachian tube, and it is involved as well in the production of speech. By regulating the opening and closure of the nasal fossae, it modulates the volume of resonance in sounds produced by the larynx.

Finally, the velum is the seat of highly developed nerve endings, which trigger a certain number of physiological reflexes (for example, the stimulation of peristaltic contractions in the digestive tube or the reflex of nausea induced by untimely stomach contractions). The palatine fibro-mucosa, in conjunction with the tongue, also represents one of the organs of mastication and taste.

A more detailed analysis of the soft palate's role in certain vital functions is presented in the following discussion (Fig. 9.13).

The swallowing process

During the swallowing process, the nasopharynx is closed as a vital physiological phenomenon is brought into play.

When the airway rises, it causes the laryngeal orifice to close. Virtually all the elevator muscles come into action, raising the hyoid bone and thereby simultaneously elevating the base of the tongue and the whole infra-hyoid system.

The tongue presents a certain degree of elasticity. When elevated, as described above, it comes to rest against the roof of the mouth. Its shape changes as it presses against the hard palate and the aponeurosis.

The lingual contractions that serve to move food towards the back of the mouth cause the tongue to rotate around the hyoid bone as it rises. This modifies

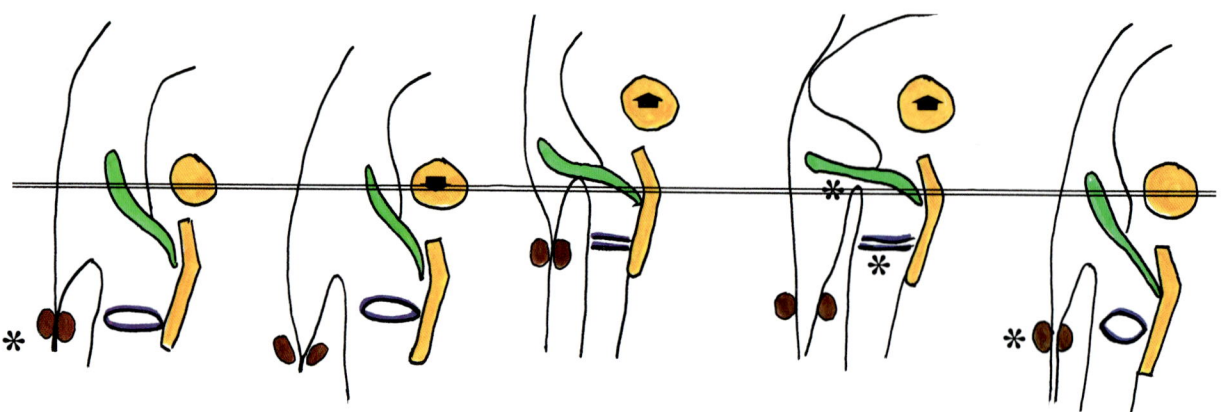

Fig. 9.13 *Different stages of the swallowing process, with elevation and descent of the airway and successive phases of laryngeal reflex (A. Lespargot, 1987).* ● *represents the hyoid bone situation.*

the orientation of the epiglottis, which shifts from vertical to horizontal. The epiglottis caps the upper opening of the larynx and closes it by flattening itself against the contour of the interarytenoidian ridge. Shaped like the peak of a roof, the epiglottis prevents swallowing the wrong way by diverting the bolus to the sides. As a last safety device, the glottal sphincter is closed.

On a higher level, closure of the nasopharynx, which is also a necessity during swallowing, is effected in the following manner (Fig. 9.14):

1. The anterior half of the soft palate, comprising the aponeurosis and the insertions of the inferior muscles (palatoglossi and palatopharyngei), is lowered as its muscles contract and contribute to

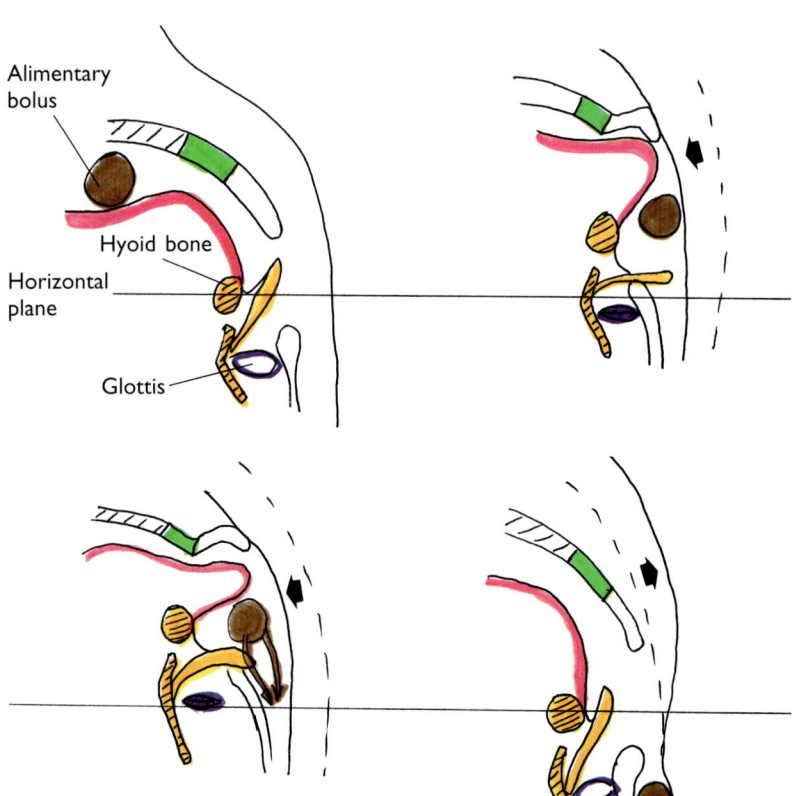

Alimentary bolus

Hyoid bone

Horizontal plane

Glottis

Fig. 9.14 *Mobility of the soft palate and tongue during normal deglutition, demonstrated on profile videofluoroscopy.*

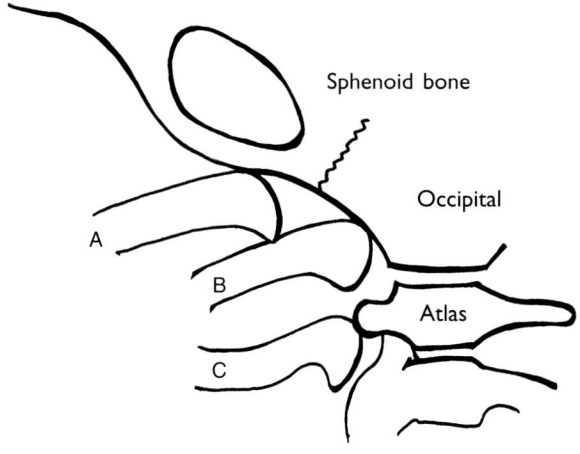

Fig. 9.15 The zone of contact between the velum and the posterior wall of the pharynx varies with age.

A. *Infant: corpus of sphenoid bone.*
B. *Older child: occipital tuberosity.*
C. *Adult: anterior arch of atlas.*

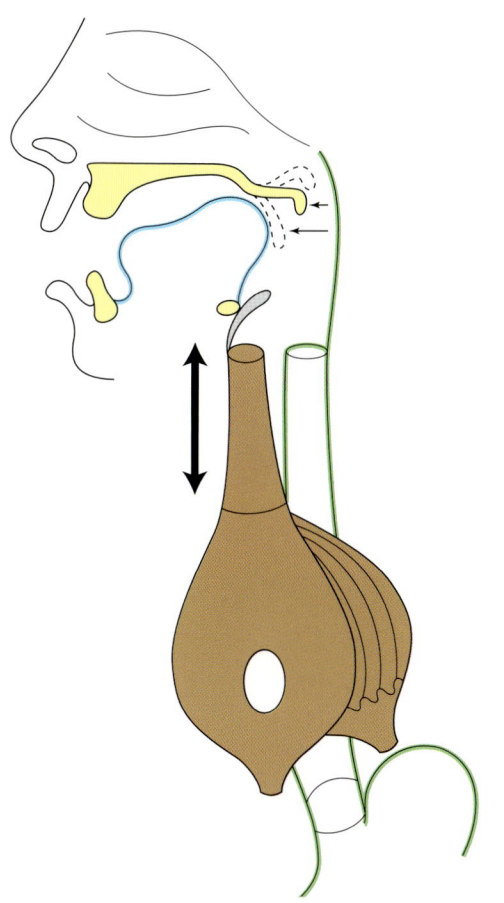

Fig. 9.16 Diagram of the respiratory tract: elevation or descent of the aero-digestive tube closes or opens the orifice of the pulmonary bellows.

the elevation of the hyoid bone. In a sense, the hard palate is extended towards the rear as this portion of the soft palate, which displays a certain mobility (Rabischong, personal communication), is lowered and stretched taut. The anterior part of the velum offers resistance to the mechanical pressure of the tongue as its surface scrapes the palate and contracts to propel the bolus towards the pharynx, somewhat like a paddle-wheel.

2. The posterior half of the soft palate, comprised primarily of levator palatini fibers, rises to meet the superior constrictor as the latter contracts and moves forward. The level it reaches may vary (Fig. 9.15). It seals the nasopharynx. We have seen the role of the uvula in producing air-tight sphincteric closure (clearly visible on naso-endoscopy and X-rays). Tongue pressure reinforces the tight seal. This contact between the base of the tongue and the palate is what triggers the peristaltic system which begins with contractions of the middle and inferior pharyngeal constrictors. Their action on the progression of the bolus is relayed by esophagian peristalsis.

During the dynamic phase of swallowing, the Eustachian tube is held open by contraction of the tensor and levator palatini (described earlier). The levator torus lifts the posterior edge of the tubal cartilage, while the tensor draws the anterior rim of the cartilage downward.

Breathing

During breathing, the nasopharynx is open.

Unlike during swallowing, the airway is in a low position, the hyoid bone and tongue are no longer raised, and the levator muscles are all relaxed. The inferior muscles of the velum (the palatoglossi and palatopharyngei) are passively attracted downward and lower the soft palate, which is flattened against the base of the tongue. The velum contributes to moving the tongue forward by narrowing the isthmus of the fauces as the palatoglossi draw together (the parachute mechanism, described in Chapter 15). The superior constrictor relaxes. The nasopharynx is therefore open.

The absence of superior palatine muscle contraction results in closure of the Eustachian tube when its elastic cartilage rotates.

Air circulates freely in and out during both inspiration and expiration (Fig. 9.16).

Phonation

During phonation, the nasopharynx is closed to a greater or lesser degree.

Sounds are generally emitted during the phase of expiration. The position of the airway corresponds to that indicated earlier, with the tracheolaryngeal section in a low position.

It is important to have an elementary background on speech and its development among normal children, and this is provided in collaboration with M.-R. Mousset (1989).

A few general remarks on phonation

A distinction must be made between the phonatory system, which permits the production of sounds and speech, and the more complex function of phonation, which calls on both neurosensory and neuromotor systems as well as on hearing perception. Phonation is a servosystem of the cybernetic type, with a potential for constant adjustment.

The voice, which transmits speech, depends first and foremost on the respiratory system. Speech production requires:

- The pulmonary bellows, which provide an airstream that is under pressure during the phase of exhalation.
- The larynx (voice-box), where sound originates when air passes through the vocal cords causing vibration.
- Resonating cavities (pharyngeal, oral and nasal), which filter and amplify sound produced by the larynx.
- Organs of speech (articulators), which are mobile.

The soft palate controls access to the nasal resonating cavity; the jaws, tongue and lips alter the shape of the oral resonating cavity; and the tongue and lips command 'points of articulation' at which consonants are produced by the narrowing or temporary blockage of the air passage, particularly within the mouth.

The role of the soft palate in the phonatory system

The soft palate plays an active role by shunting air into the proper resonating cavity. When the soft palate is relaxed, the airway towards the nasal cavity remains open. When it contracts it shuts off this airway, thus forcing the air to pass through the oral cavity.

In almost all languages, the nasal resonating cavity is only put to occasional use (it permits the production of such nasal consonants as [n], [m], etc.). Otherwise, access to the nasal cavity must remain closed in perfect co-ordination with the other organs of speech. Any malfunction of the soft palate creates an impression of nasal distortion. When the soft palate functions properly to close the nasal passage, the flow of air exhaled is shunted towards the oral cavity with the pressure necessary for clear speech production. Any leakage lowers the pressure and makes speech less intelligible. The velopharyngeal closing mechanism differs from that described for the swallowing process.

It has been seen that, during exhalation, the nasopharynx is open and the airway is in a low position. In this situation, nasopharyngeal closure without elevation of the airway is linked to muscle action that does not cause the laryngotracheal system to rise.

The superior constrictor intervenes by reducing the diameter of the nasopharynx. At times, Passavant's ridge is visible. The anterior half of the soft palate remains lowered, and the posterior pillars draw together. The posterior half of the soft palate is the portion that rises to meet the back wall of the pharynx, and contraction of the uvular muscles contributes to the formation of a posterior bend at the base of the uvula. This elevation of the soft palate can be attributed primarily to the levator palatini muscle. The muscles are in a constant state of tonic contraction during the entire phase of speech production. When the diameter of the pharynx is reduced, slight oscillations of the soft palate suffice to close the nasopharynx. The process involved functions as a valve mechanism, which opens and shuts far more rapidly than the sphincteric contraction that occurs during swallowing.

Where speech is concerned, the open/shut mechanism must be prepared to function in a fraction of a second.

The role of the articulators

The articulators modify the shape, volume and cross-section of the opening in the oral resonating cavity.

The mandible or lower jaw permits anterior widening of the oral cavity. The vowels are classified as 'open' ([a]) or 'closed' ([i], [u]), depending on how far the jaws are spread. The tongue can divide the oral space into a double cavity, which multiplies the possible types of resonance and creates the range of vowels. The lips can be more or less rounded, which creates an additional source of resonance and contributes to greater variety in the quality of vowel tone.

Consonants are specific sounds produced when the lips or tongue close or narrow the oral cavity, and there are two categories: plosives and fricatives.

Plosives (for example, [p]) involve three consecutive steps:

1. Occlusion. The lips meet and are relatively tensed. The soft palate rises to close the nasopharynx. After the airstream produced by exhalation enters the oral cavity, the mouth remains tightly closed.
2. Impounding or holding. The air present in the oral cavity is impounded under pressure for a few hundredths of a second. The flow of pulmonary air is stopped.
3. Plosion. The articulators (lips for [p]/[b]) suddenly relax, releasing the impounded air with a slight (ex)plosion.

The velum remains in a raised position if the consonant is followed by a vowel as in the syllable [pa]. The consonant or phoneme [p] is classified as a bilabial plosive.

In most languages there are a number of additional points of occlusion (Fig. 9.17), including those between the tip of the tongue and the alveolar ridge ([t]/[d]), and between the back of the tongue and the velar region ([k]/[g]) etc. In certain languages (such as Arabic), other points of occlusion exist – for example, between the tongue and the posterior region of the soft palate. This is similar to that of [k], but produces a radically different sound.

Fricatives belong to another category of consonants. The articulators are narrowed rather than closed at a specific point, and the passage of air through the restricted zone produces a certain amount of friction. The most common zones affected are those between the lower lip and upper incisors (the labio-dentals, [f] or [v]), between the tip of the tongue and the alveolar ridge (the tongue is hollowed

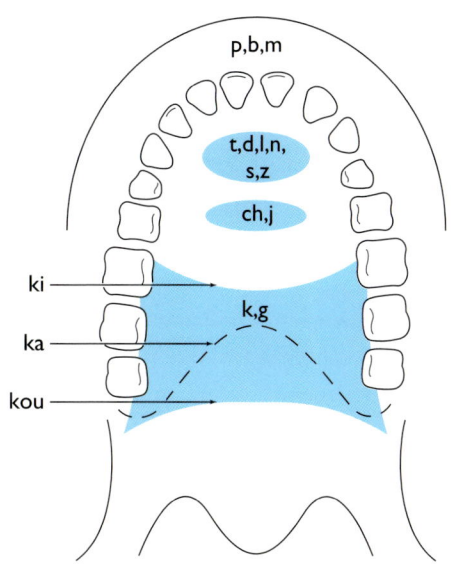

Fig. 9.17 *Zones of contact between the tongue and the palate or pharynx determine the 'points of articulation' for production of plosive consonants.*

into a narrow runnel which projects air against the front teeth, [s]/[z]), and between the tongue and the anterior portion of the palate (-sh- or [ʃ]).

As is the case for plosives, the articulation of fricatives involves three phases: catastasis, impounding and metastasis. However, the impounding phase is different. It is mute for plosives but audible for fricatives, since it produces the characteristic sound of friction or sibilance.

The soft palate helps to build up the necessary pressure within the oral cavity before the air stream reaches the restricted zones.

The development of normal phonation

From the moment of birth, the breathing apparatus, articulators and resonating cavities are ready to function. Sound is produced in the larynx when the infant cries.

At a very early stage, brief random vocalization begins. Sounds are low in volume, and tend to have a neutral quality which resembles that of the vowel [e] (as in 'bed'). These vocal emissions, automatically amplified by the resonating cavities, are often interspersed with glottal stops (plosions produced by the opening/closing mechanism of the laryngeal sphincter or vocal cords). This is the way the infant learns to co-ordinate the larynx and breathing, simultaneously learning to control air pressure to obtain the required volume.

Towards the age of 2 months, a period of vocalizing usually takes place that focuses more specifically on the soft palate. This is the cooing stage, dominated by the use of central or back vowels like [u] (as in 'put') between voiced consonant sounds (involving vibration) articulated by the back of the tongue and the velum. The isthmus of the fauces as a whole participates; the tongue, velum, uvula and pillars of the fauces, which draw together and vibrate like vocal cords under the pressure of the pulmonary wind supply. At this stage, hearing has a role to play in a servosystem of the cybernetic type. Only considerably later, as of the second half of the first year and for a period averaging 2 years, does the infant gradually learn to master the articulators in order to imitate sounds of the language heard.

As of 6 months of age, the introduction of babbling marks a significant step. Babbling is characterized by the association and repetition of vowels and consonants. This phase coincides with intense mandibular activity. During teething, the infant often chews a finger or teething ring. If laryngeal vocalizing and chewing activity happen to coincide, they often set off a long stream of cooing interspersed with pseudo-consonants, which sounds like a sequence of syllables.

This period is very important because it occurs immediately prior to the acquisition of syllabic speech structures. It is characterized by intervals of vocalizing that combine jaw activity sometimes with the lips and sometimes with the front or back regions of the tongue.

When vocalizing involves a certain degree of muscle tone, it sounds as though the infant is uttering a syllabic sequence(*pa-*, *ta-*, *ka-*). This stage is highly important to the parents, who imagine that they are actually hearing their child speak for the first time. Stimulated by parental feed-back, they encourage the infant to keep on vocalizing by repeating the sounds made.

These intervals of pseudo-speech or baby-talk would probably not be possible were they not preceded by an earlier period of building up the muscle tone of the soft palate through contractions that control oral air pressure.

Babbling undergoes considerable evolution. The vocalizing produced during the first 6 months is similar whatever the native language, but it becomes differentiated as of the eighth month. It is then possible to recognize the specific patterns of the language spoken in the infant's environment, because vocalizing is remodeled by hearing perception.

The infant gradually drops the use of glottal stops, which are meaningless sounds. In attempting to imitate the elements of the language heard, the infant also switches from back to front sounds, which imply greater involvement of the lips and tongue. The child is now beginning to acquire the skills of meaningful language.

Hearing

The palate contributes to the hearing system because the superior palatine muscles regulate the opening and closing of the Eustachian tube. The latter establishes communication between the middle ear and the nasopharynx, and permits air pressure to be equalized on both sides of the eardrum. This enables the tympanic membrane to vibrate more freely with the transmission of sound waves.

- When the velar muscles are slack, the tubal orifice is closed. This is the case during breathing. The airway is in a low position, and the tubal cartilage is vertical.
- When the superior muscles contract (during the swallowing process), the tubal orifice is opened. The bony portion of the tensor veli palatini forms a wall, which maintains the antero-posterior orientation of the anterior section of the tubal cartilage. The latter is drawn downward by the slender strand of muscle fibers which insert into it. When the levator palatini contracts, it pulls away from the medial pterygoid plate in a posterior direction. Its volume changes (torus) and the levator lifts the lower section of tubal cartilage, which opens the Eustachian tube (Fig. 9.18).

TONGUE

In a study of the physiology of the aero-digestive tract, and particularly of the palate, it would be a serious oversight to omit the tongue.

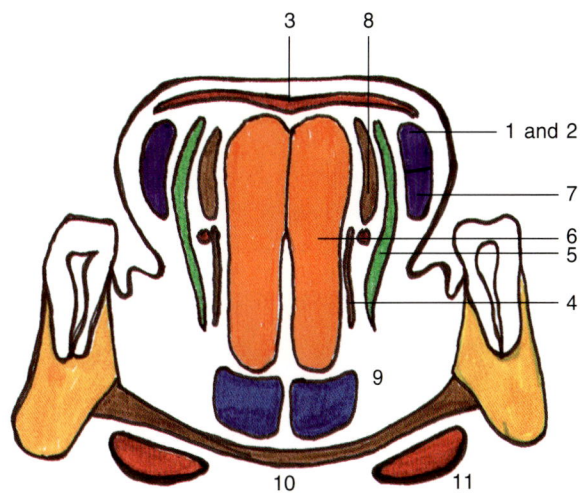

Fig. 9.19 *Muscle structures of the tongue (the intrinsic muscles and muscles of the floor of the mouth).*

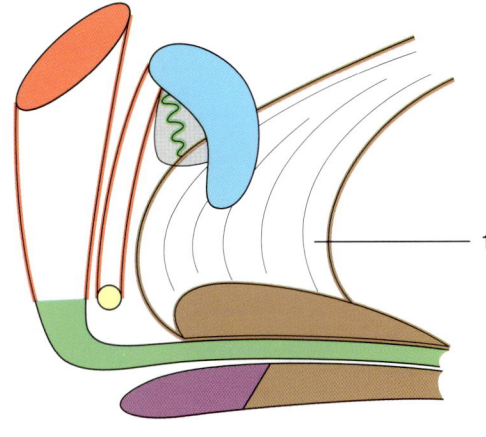

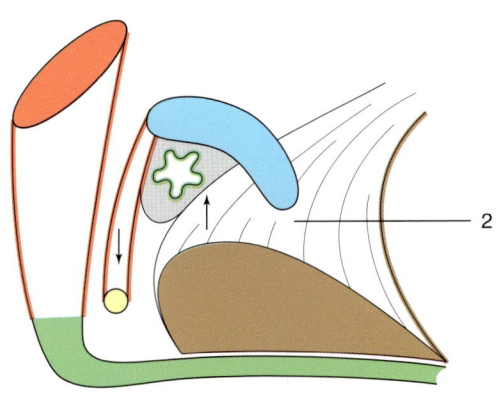

Fig. 9.18 *Opening/closing mechanism of the pharyngeal orifice of the Eustachian tube.*

1.   Levator veli palatini
2.   Torus of the levator veli palatini

The tongue is a highly specific organ in the human species and it fulfills a number of fundamental roles:

1. In the morphogenesis of the oral cavity, which has the palate as its roof.
2. In the sucking/swallowing process, where the tongue regulates positive and negative pressure within the oral cavity and propels the bolus of food towards the pharynx and esophagus after a potential chewing phase.
3. In breathing, where the tongue maintains patency of the airway.
4. In phonation, where it contributes to the production of speech.

The tongue is composed of 17 muscles, including one single muscle and eight pairs (Fig. 9.19). The muscles of the floor of the mouth are included among the neck muscles (digastricus, stylohyoideus, mylohyoideus, geniohyoideus).

The intrinsic muscles include:

1 The palatoglossi
2 The amygdal glossi or tonsillar muscle
3 The superior lingualis muscle with transverse lingualis fibers
4 The inferior lingualis muscles
5 The hyoglossi
6 The genioglossi – inferior, middle and anterior fibers (Fig. 9.20)
7 The styloglossi
8 The pharyngoglossi (fibers of superior pharyngeal constrictor).

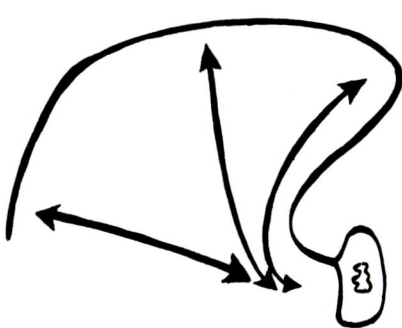

Fig. 9.20 *Radiating pattern of genioglossi muscle fibers.*

Body of the tongue					
Muscles		**Motions**			
		Backward	**Downward**	**Upward**	**Forward**
Isthmus of the fauces	Palatoglossus (+tonsillar muscle)	+			
Tongue	Superior lingualis (with transverse fibers)		+		
Tongue	Inferior lingualis		+		
Tongue	Hyoglossus		+		
	Genioglossus				
	Anterior	+	+		
	Middle				+
	Inferior			+	+
	Styloglossus	+		+	
	Pharyngoglossus	+		+	

Floor of the mouth (neck)	
Geniohyoid	
	Elevate the hyoid bone and the aero-digestive tract
Mylohyoid	
	Lower the mandible
Digastric + stylohyoid muscle	
Muscles under the hyoid bone	Lower the hyoid bone and the aero-digestive tract

Fig. 9.21 *Chart indicating the action of different intrinsic muscles and the movements they govern.*

A reminder of each muscle's major function is listed in Figure 9.21.

The extrinsic muscles are mainly those belonging to the floor of the mouth:

9   The geniohyoid muscles
10   The mylohyoid muscles
11   The digastric muscles.

They also include the supra- and subhyoid muscles, which modify the position of the hyoid bone and, therefore, of the tongue. For a detailed description, anatomical studies should be consulted. The most important points to remember are that:

- The suprahyoid muscles elevate the hyoid bone and lower the mandible.
- The subhyoid muscles lower the hyoid bone and the aero-digestive tract.

In particular, the hyoid bone can only move up and down and shows no sagittal or transverse mobility. This factor permits a better understanding of physiology at the aero-digestive junction.

10. Pathological anatomy and physiology in isolated cleft palate

BONE STRUCTURE

The bony palatal vault is only affected in cases of complete cleft.

In complete clefts of the isolated palate (known as bilateral), the gap in the bone structure extends as far forward as the incisive or anterior palatine foramen. The palatal shelves are underdeveloped and steeply angled. The width of the cleft varies; it is linked to the degree of hypoplasia, but also to the widened gap between the maxillar tuberosities. This is a result of lingual pressure, since the tongue tends to penetrate into the cleft, and the outward (lateral) pull of the divided muscles of the soft palate.

The lower edge of the vomer forms a straight line. It is generally perched above its normal level, but the angle of the palatal shelves may partially or totally mask its abnormally high position. Towards the front of the oral cavity, the palatal shelves fail to fuse together and the lower border of the premaxillary segment is attached to the vomer on a rather steep incline.

The increase in the distance between the tuberosities is a commonly acknowledged concept since Brophy's publications on the subject. Veau, who rejected the latter's therapeutic approach (Brophy advocated osteotomy of the palatal shelves so that they could be drawn together and more easily sutured edge to edge), did not accept this factor and discarded it.

Hypoplasia of the shelves is most pronounced towards the back of the oral cavity. The palatal shelf of the palatine bone is the least developed, with a gap in the posterior nasal spine that nonetheless remains visible. The greater palatine foramen is located in a more anterior and lateral position than normal.

In less severe cases of isolated cleft palate, the length of the gap in the hard palate varies. It must be pointed out that the gap in the soft tissue does not always correspond precisely to that in the bone. A layer of mucosa can extend forward and conceal a longer underlying cleft in the bone structure, which may reach as far as the anterior palatine foramen (sub-mucosal cleft) (see Anatomo-clinical forms, Chapter 3).

Near the midline, the border of the bony cleft may present either a sharp angle or a rounded curve, no doubt related to penetration of the tongue over a certain length of time.

MUSCLES AND MUCOSA

The cleft palate causes major anatomical disorders, to which Veau devoted a thorough study.

All the muscles that normally comprise the soft palate can be found along the borders of the cleft. The origins of the superior muscles are the same, but the volume of their fibers, their orientation and terminal insertions are modified. In the case of the inferior muscles, it is their origin that differs.

The palatine aponeurosis is, of course, missing at the midline. Laterally, it subsists only as a small fibrotic bundle. The aponeurotic insertions of the tensor veli palatini are more oblique than usual, and their fibers extend along the edges of the bony cleft.

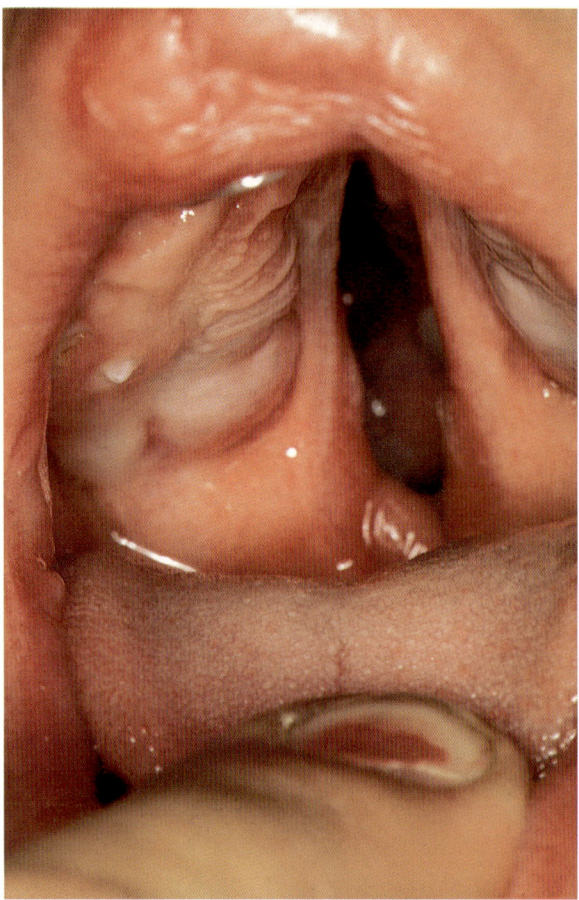

Fig. 10.1 *Contour of the 'muscle of the cleft' bundle on the borders of the cleft.*

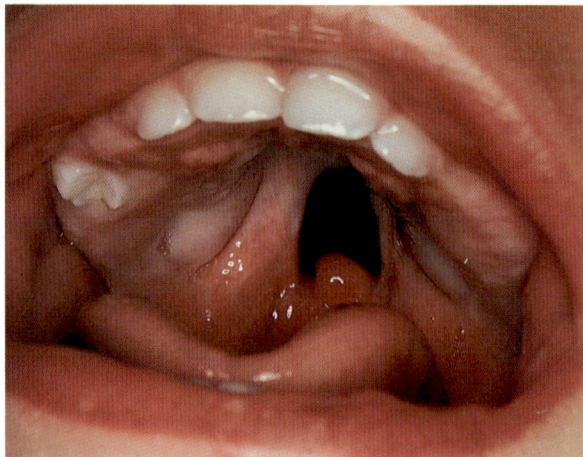

Fig. 10.2 *Medial orientation of the two half-uvula.*

Thus, the palatal muscles can only insert into the few remaining fibers of the palatine aponeurosis and into the adjacent bone.

The two major muscles of the soft palate – the levator veli palatini and the palato-pharyngeus – do not join on the midline. Their fibers run parallel to the margins of the cleft, and have therefore lost their original transverse orientation. The most anterior portions are, in fact, perpendicular to their normal direction. They form a visible bundle of variable size along the border of the bony cleft, which Veau called the 'muscle de la fente', or muscle of the cleft (Fig. 10.1). Ruding offers a plausible explanation for this phenomenon. He believes that closure of the bony palatal cleft, which occurs in all normal embryos, takes place in an antero-posterior direction. As the bones fuse, the muscular portion of the palate is displaced

towards the back of the oral cavity; the uvula is formed last of all, once the muscles have achieved their full development. Arrested development explains the direction and insertion of the fibers, which closely attach the to half-vela in an anterior position.

The tensor veli palatini tendon, after its passage along the bottom of the hamular groove, can only insert into the bony hard palate. In the presence of a cleft, therefore, its origin and its insertion are both immobile. Its fibers affect only the movement of the Eustachian tube, and cannot act as 'shock absorbers' once the soft palate is repaired.

The free borders of the two half-vela are generally not properly aligned, and the two halves of the uvula converge towards one another. Active contraction of the divided fibers of each part of the uvular muscle may be responsible for this orientation (Fig. 10.2).

The overlying mucosa is also altered.

In the soft palate, a difference in color between the nasal and oral mucosa can be observed at their pathological meeting point on the margins of the cleft. Oral mucosa is paler, while nasal mucosa is redder. The dividing line is visible, but is not always sharply delimited. It forms a spiral on the free border of the half-velum; this can be attributed either to the predominance of the traction exerted by the inferior muscles or to a greater development of the levator veli palatini fibers. When the margin of the cleft is

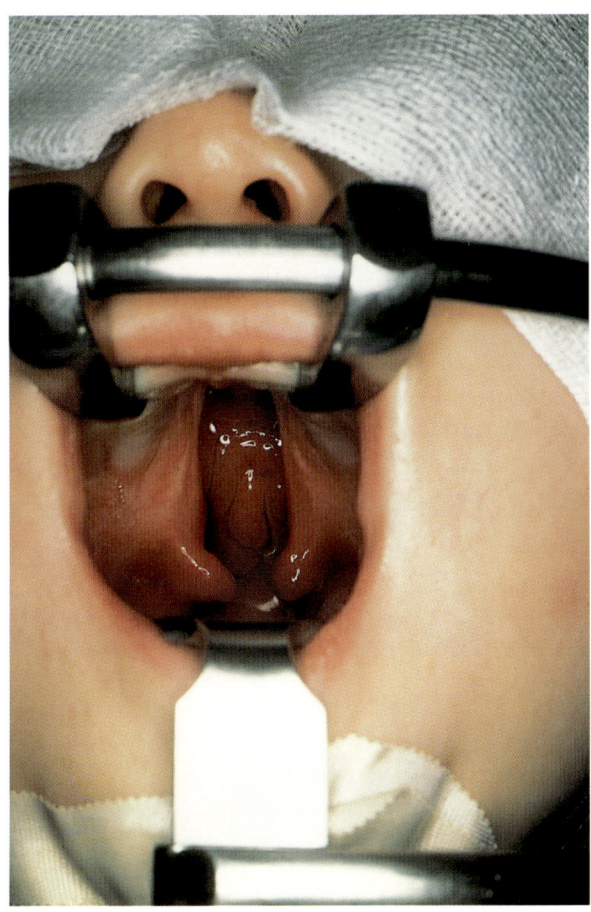

Fig. 10.3 The dividing line between paler oral and redder nasal mucosa forms a spiral along the border of the cleft.

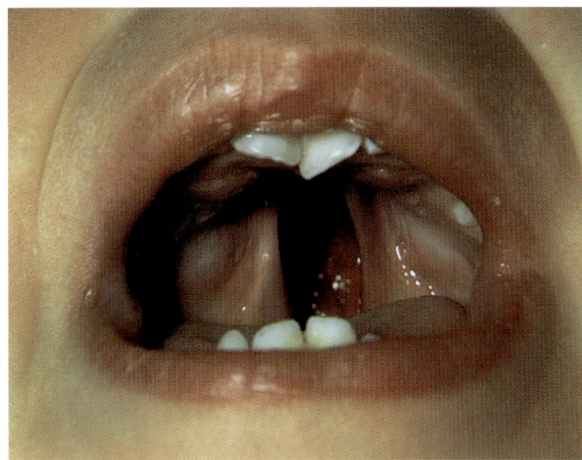

Fig. 10.4 On the right side of the cleft, the sharp furrow marking the separation between the mucoperiosteum and the inner layer of mucosa extends outward below the posterior borders of the palatal shelves.

incised, the blade of the scalpel should follow this line (Fig. 10.3).

The arches of the two velar pillars are left intact.

On the hard palate, the furrow that separates the thick fibro-mucosa from the thin inner layer can be detected. When the soft palate structure is well developed, this furrow can run quite deep. There may be considerable umbilication where it meets the two halves of the posterior nasal spine, and this can create operative problems, which are discussed in a later section. The furrow may also extend outward at a right angle directly below the posterior borders of the palatal shelves (Fig. 10.4).

At the summit of the vault, the lower edge of the vomer is visible. It is covered with nasal mucosa, but sometimes presents a lengthwise band of paler

mucosa which might be mistaken for the oral variety. There is no embryological explanation for the existence of this band of atypical coloration, which is probably the result of metaplasia secondary to irritation of the vomerine mucosa.

Finally, the presence of the cleft reveals structures usually masked by an intact soft palate. This is the case for the pharyngeal mucosa. Embedded in the membrane of its upper portion is a rosy, carpet-like area. This is the nasopharyngeal tonsil, site of the adenoids, which are composed of radiating folds of lymphoid tissue.

The lower edge of the vomer is also visible, as are its two alae, which are covered with smooth mucosa. The alae are joined with the sphenoid corpus. Behind them there is often a blind recess, which shows up on profile MRI views. This is on the same level as Rathke's pouch, which corresponds to the junction between the ectoderm and the endoderm of the embryological foregut or stomodeum.

Laterally, it is possible to detect both Rosenmüller's recess behind the torus of the levator veli palatini, and the opening of the Eustachian tube. The mucosa surrounding this orifice presents a mass of closed follicles known as the tubal tonsil (Rouviere, 1943) (Fig. 10.5).

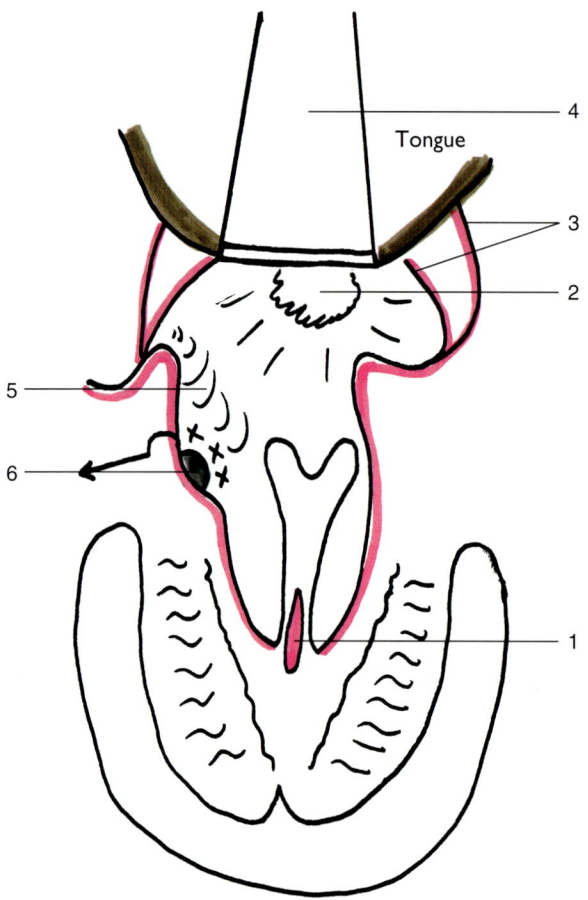

Fig. 10.5 *Different aspects of velar and pharyngeal mucosae as they appear after mouth-gag is installed for surgery.*

1.   *Sometimes oral mucosa band*
2.   *Pharyngeal bursa*
3.   *Anterior and posterior tonsillar pilars*
4.   *Metal (mouth gag)*
5.   *Rosenmüller fossa*
6.   *Eustachian tube aperture with adenoids surrounding and tubal tonsil*

PHYSIOPATHOLOGY OF THE CLEFT PALATE

Cleft palate is responsible for some major physiological disorders. The pharynx communicates more extensively with the nasal fossae and the oral cavity, and the complex mechanisms of swallowing, breathing, hearing (via the Eustachian tube) and speech are therefore impaired. The anatomical lesions also lead to new muscle action and interaction.

It is during the first days or weeks of life that these major functions are established through learning experience and practice. This is the period during which 'integrated circuits' are set up within the nervous system. Their loops are composed of centripetal circuits, which transmit impulses to the central nervous system, where stimuli undergo analysis (unconscious, to begin with). Responses are then dispatched to the effector motor systems on the periphery. The neurological phenomenon of habituation to directions which are 'signalled', so to speak, explains why these original circuits continue to be chosen more rapidly and more readily later on. Therefore, functional anomalies are very quickly established and soon become automatic reflexes, which prove difficult to eradicate after surgery.

Moreover, the absence of efficient contractions on the part of the palatal muscles is responsible for their lack of development (rather than hypoplastic malformation itself, as is often mistakenly thought), and can eventually result in irreversible degeneration. Veau laid a great deal of stress on this aspect of palatal malformation.

These facts justify performing surgery on affected infants as soon as possible. All the necessary precautions must be taken concerning the anesthetic and surgical risks of an early operation, but, thanks to improved techniques, the danger is minimal nowadays.

Sucking/swallowing disorders

Sucking becomes difficult, if not impossible, when the oral cavity and nasal fossae communicate on a permanent basis. This is because the oral cavity must be tightly sealed so that contractions of the tongue can create negative pressure and generate some degree of aspiration towards the front of the mouth and the lips.

In cases of posterior cleft palate, the lingual mass occupies the rear of the oral cavity and stops the gap in the roof of the mouth. Thus, aspiration can be achieved in that portion of the oral cavity situated in front of the tongue. This is not the case, however, for anterior or complete labio-palatal clefts, where there is permanent communication with the nose.

Since sucking is so difficult, the hole in the nipple of the baby bottle must be considerably enlarged so that the contents can flow freely.

The infant can sometimes manage breast-feeding, provided the volume of the mother's breast is such that the face can be pressed against it and the nostrils thus kept closed. Aspiration may be adequate in this case.

The swallowing process undergoes the greatest modifications. During normal deglutition, closure of the nasopharyngeal sphincter (by contact between the palate and the superior constrictor) enables the tongue to move the alimentary bolus towards the back of the mouth and down into the throat by exerting pressure against the lower surface of the velum.

When the palate is cleft, there is a gap in the roof of the mouth and the tongue must come to rest against the posterior wall of the pharynx. The isthmus of the fauces and the nasopharyngeal isthmus are missing, so the tongue enters the nasopharynx (the volume of the latter is simultaneously reduced by forward movement of the superior constrictor). There has been a good deal of controversy as to whether the tongue actually penetrates into the nasopharynx. This was clearly demonstrated in our studies of the swallowing process using videofluoroscopy (lateral views of the facial area) in collaboration with our colleagues from the Radiology Department, F. Brunelle and M. El Maleh. These images are totally different from those of normal infants (Fig. 10.6a and b). Bosma *et al.* (1965) noticed that the half-vela reposed on the base of the tongue when at rest, but drew away and apart during swallowing (Fig. 10.6c). He also remarked that the superior constrictor, in its attempt to re-establish a nasopharyngeal sphincter, could develop annular contractions seen as a transverse fold (Passavant's ridge).

The velar stumps are practically inert, and are therefore compressed by the tongue. There is a hinge-like structure that follows the line extending from the base of the skull (where the levator veli palatini inserts) to the half posterior nasal spine of the palatal shelf on the same side. Tongue pressure can make the muscle bundle found inside this line swing outward like a door, creating a bulge in the half-velum. This was pointed out by Bosma (Fig. 10.7).

As the muscle mass swings outward, it obstructs the choanae to a certain degree. This limits the reflux of liquids into the nasal fossae which, theoretically, should be greater than it is in actual fact. If reflux

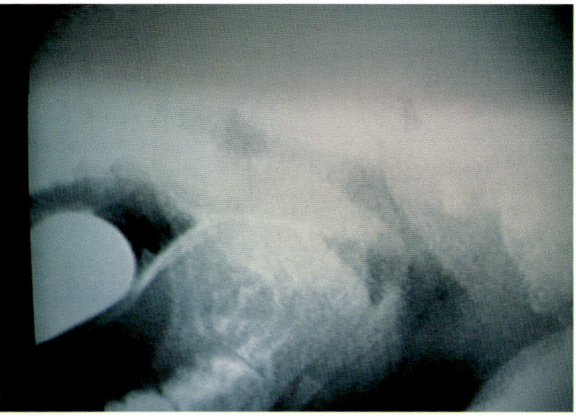

a

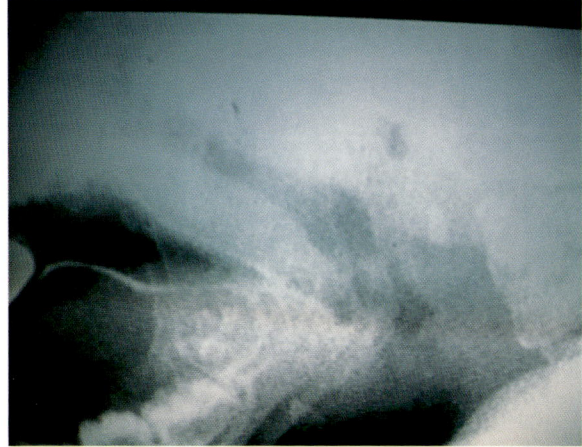

b

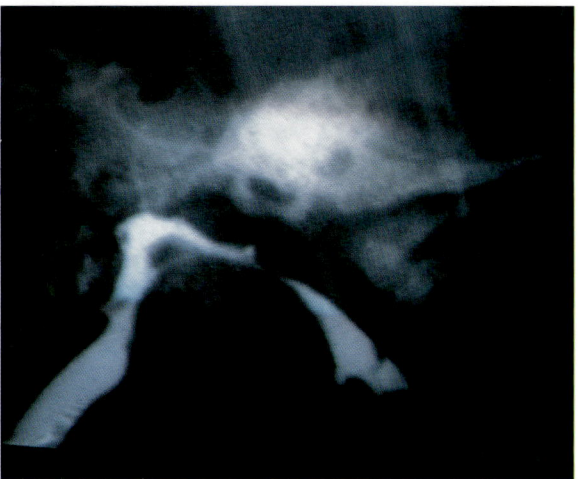

c

Fig. 10.6 *Swallowing disorders.*
a and b. Videofluoroscopic views of the swallowing process in normal children.
c. In cleft palate, the tongue is projected against the postero-superior wall of the pharynx. The two halves of the uvula are pushed upward and to the side.

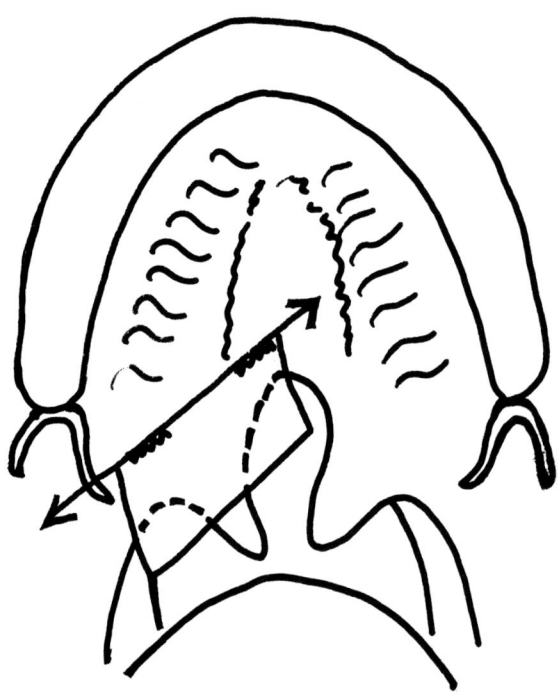

Fig. 10.7 *Passive movement of the half-velum, which swings outward like a door opening on its hinges.*

does occur, it does not generally produce serious consequences. Still, to avoid potential flooding of the nasal fossae, the infant should be held in a vertical position during bottle-feeding. In fact, the choanae are more easily obturated because of their reduced size, which is related to the elevation of the palatal shelves (under lingual pressure).

It must be remembered that the tongue pressure exerted towards the roof and the back of the oral cavity is responsible for widening the transverse diameter of the pharynx, a phenomenon evidenced by the angle of the pterygoid processes, which are set on a slant.

Below the nasopharynx, the physiology of the swallowing process remains normal and functions efficiently to move the alimentary bolus.

Normal infants show a characteristic manner of swallowing over the first months of life. During this process, known as infantile or primary deglutition, the tongue plays a major role due to its postero-inferior movement. During secondary deglutition, however, which usually appears at about 6 months of age, the swallowing reflex causes the base of the tongue to rise. This seems to be the type of swallowing necessary when the palate is cleft. It can clearly be detected on videofluoroscopy, even in very young infants (Fig. 10.8a and b).

It has already been seen that the palate is a vital trigger zone. Contact between food and the surface of the palate sets off the series of steps involved in the swallowing reflex: opening of the superior sphincter of the esophagus, esophageal peristalsis, and opening of the cardia.

Gastro-esophageal reflux is common in children afflicted with cleft palate, and could be linked to a

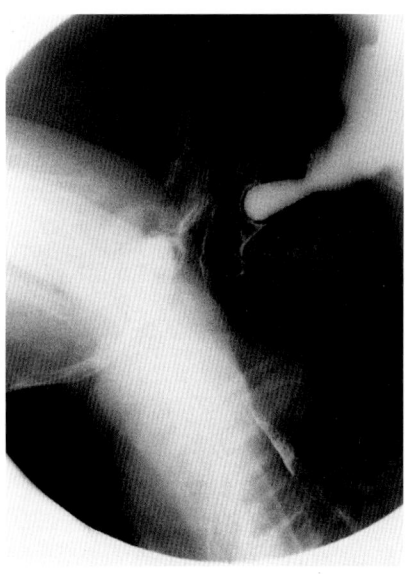

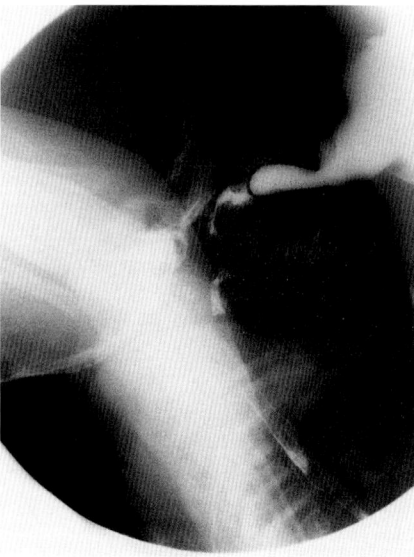

Fig. 10.8 *Secondary deglutition.*
a. Tongue at rest.
b. During deglutition, elevation of the tongue mass flexes the nipple.

a   *b*

reflex disorder secondary to the palatal anomaly. However, there are no reliable statistical studies on the subject to date. Whatever the case, early closure of the palatal cleft consistently produces favorable results. Associated with medical treatment, of course, it makes gastro-esophageal reflux disappear far more rapidly.

Respiratory disorders

Breathing is frequently oral among children with cleft palate. The choanae are small in size, and the nasopharynx is short in young infants and is congested with adenoid tissue. In its lower portion, the airway is not walled off by the palate due to the presence of the cleft but by the base of the tongue, which is itself positioned near the wall of the pharynx. This posterior position may be aggravated by retrognathia (primary or secondary). It can become a predominant factor of respiratory distress in the Robin syndrome, to which a separate section is devoted.

As a rule, there are no obvious respiratory problems connected with isolated cleft palate, but the dividing line between this anomaly and Robin syndrome is very hazy. What is commonly called 'minor' Robin syndrome may represent the transition between the two clinical types.

In the case of labio-palatal clefts, the passage towards the mouth cavity is wide open and oral breathing is usually adopted.

The Eustachian tube

The physiology of the Eustachian tube is impaired by the gap in the palate.

Normally, contraction of the levator veli palatini opens the pharyngeal orifice of the Eustachian tube thanks to a complex mechanism described previously: when the levator contracts, the mass of the torus raises the posterior portion of the tubal cartilage. The anterior wall of the tube then abuts the tensor veli palatini, which is also under tension. It is lowered by contraction of a slender strand of tensor fibers, which insert into it. These two simultaneous muscle actions open the pharyngeal orifice of the tube.

However, when the palate is cleft, the main muscle (levator veli palatini) has few or no contractions. The tube generally remains closed, which

results in an accumulation of secretions (hence the frequency of serous otitis).

If air pressure is not equalized on both sides of the eardrum, the transmission of sound waves is impaired (conductive deafness).

Speech disorders

Obviously, phonatory disorders cannot be perceived during the first weeks of life and are not the surgeon's prime concern. Nonetheless, the fact that phonatory mechanisms develop from birth provides an additional argument for early repair.

In a particularly pertinent article published in 1965, Bosma analyzed the production and quality of crying among very small infants with cleft palate, based on recordings and videofluoroscopy. It would seem that these infants expend a greater effort to produce sound. Furthermore, the sounds they do emit are characterized by a certain number of disturbances.

Phonetic disorders in unoperated cleft palate (M.-R. Mousset)

Immediately after birth and during the first months, the palatal gap does not affect early sound production. The unoperated infant can cry and vocalize like a normal baby, and glottal stops are common.

As of 6 months, however, significant differences begin to appear, the most striking of which concerns consonant production. For plosives, the impounding phase is impossible in the presence of a cleft because it supposes closure of the nasopharynx. Lack of pressure weakens the plosion, and blurs the characteristic sound of the consonant. Air escaping through the nose may produce an audible hiss and may be detected by placing a mirror or a more sophisticated device in front of the nostrils.

If there is no air pressure impounded behind the point of occlusion, the only effective constriction remains that of the laryngeal sphincter. This explains the continued occurrence of glottal stops.

For fricatives, impounding is also the phase affected by the cleft. The infant cannot articulate oral fricatives, and therefore resorts to a substitute consonant that involves oropharyngeal narrowing or restriction. Its production is often accompanied by hoarse laryngeal vibration (Fig. 10.9).

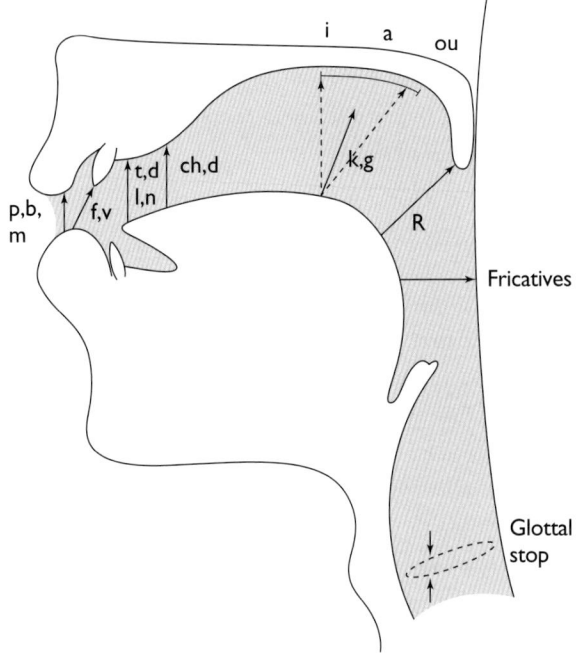

Fig. 10.9 Points of articulation corresponding to hoarse aspirates and glottal stops.

During the babbling stage, the infant cannot keep up with the progress of his or her peers. There is no syllabic vocalizing to stimulate parental response, so normal feed-back is compromised.

Primary palatal repair offers the logical solution to these problems; otherwise, babbling will remain monotonal, indistinct, undiversified and permanently distorted by hypernasal resonance interspersed only with glottal stops. Later on, in efforts to imitate what is heard and to be understood, the child tends to resort to the only manageable form of occlusion, i.e. the glottal stop. This becomes the major substitute for oral consonants.

From the first words onward, therefore, the child's language skills are based on abnormal patterns of speech. These grow increasingly difficult to correct as time goes by, a problem often encountered when children undergo surgery at the usual age of 18 months.

Infants operated on at an early age show far more satisfactory development. Parents often observe that veloplasty improves the quality of the voice, which they find higher in tone and more distinct. Vocalizing becomes more frequent and prolonged, and the tongue, which tended to remain in a posterior

position before the operation, shifts forward and constantly explores its new space. However, tongue activity does not yet participate in vocalization.

As of the age of 8 months, syllabic vocalizing is not uncommon, interspersed with clear plosives of a quality identical to that of normal infants.

Although a final prognosis cannot be established, the clarity of the plosives [p], [t] and [k] is in itself a good indication of velopharyngeal efficiency and of the normal acquisition of emergent language skills.

VELOPHARYNGEAL INCOMPETENCE

When the soft palate cannot fulfill its role in closing the nasopharynx, phonation is seriously affected. The analysis of resulting speech disorders calls for a detailed study.

Phonetic study

Even a moderate degree of velar insufficiency can be easily perceived by the ear during phonation. It is manifested by:

- Altered vowel quality
- Audible nasal air emission
- Indistinct consonant production
- Substitution mechanisms – the use of substitute consonants to replace phonemes that cannot be articulated.

Altered vowel quality
Vowel quality is affected when the nasal and oropharyngeal resonating cavities are no longer closed off from one another. Certain low frequencies are reinforced, while a number of characteristic high frequencies tend to disappear. The vowel [i], normally the most common and high-pitched of vowel sounds, is the most deeply affected by these changes. Only the open back vowel [a] generally remains recognizable, despite pronounced nasality.

Hypernasal resonance makes speech unintelligible. It also affects the esthetic aspect of the voice; a nasal tone or twang is usually considered displeasing to the ear.

Certain subjects attempt to counteract this defect by reducing nasal air escape. The laryngo-pharyngeal complex is strongly contracted to diminish airflow, and the resulting sound production takes on a nasal twang. The voice sounds shrill and unpleasant, and intonational patterns show little inflection. The scale of low frequencies and their harmonics is reduced. The strenuous effort expended to produce sound can be perceived by palpation of the larynx and can eventually lead to dysphonia.

Audible nasal air emission

Speech can be distorted by interference from audible nasal airflow. The hiss of nasal air escape can be heard most noticeably during the normally silent impounding phase of [p], [t] and [k]. These voiceless plosives require a build-up in air pressure behind the point of occlusion. Nasal emission also distorts the characteristic acoustic signal of the fricatives [s] and [f] with an additional sibilance, which makes them hard to recognize. It is most pronounced among subjects who make a considerable effort to articulate properly. A deviated septum or narrowing of the alar cartilage may contribute to making the sound of nasal air escape even louder. The condition is often accompanied by nasal and facial grimacing (knitted eyebrows, twitching of the nares, etc.).

The nasopharyngeal snort represents a further type of interference. It is louder in volume and arises deeper in the throat. Snorting is a sign of inadequate velopharyngeal closure forced open by the air pressure built up during phonation.

Indistinct consonant production

Any degree of nasal air escape lowers the oral air pressure necessary for proper articulation of consonants. This is particularly true of the plosives [p], [t] and [k]. For the fricatives [f] and [s], low pressure plus interference from audible nasal emission makes recognition difficult.

Substitution mechanisms

When nasal air escape is so extensive that pressure cannot be built up in the oral cavity, the subject attempts to produce intelligible speech by resorting to substitute points of occlusion and restriction. The points chosen are located before the velopharyngeal port of the access to the nasal cavity. Oral plosives ([p], [t] and [k]) are often replaced by the glottal stop, while pharyngeal or laryngeal fricatives

are substituted for the oral fricatives ([f], [s], [-sh-] or [ʃ]).

Once these gross substitution errors are acquired and integrated into speech patterns, they become habitual articulatory responses (learned compensatory patterns of misarticulation). They may subsist long after the subject has regained velopharyngeal competence thanks to pharyngoplasty, and can only be corrected by long-term speech therapy.

Classification

These various signs of velopharyngeal insufficiency do not all have the same significance. The nasal snort indicates that the velum is almost closed, perhaps over a mass of adenoid tissue. It is often corrected by appropriate therapy, particularly if the subject can hear the defect. The nasal hiss is far less easily eliminated. Most difficult of all is rhinolalia, particularly if accompanied by frequent use of the glottal stop.

Since 1935, the classification devised by S. Borel-Maisonny has been used to evaluate the competence of velopharyngeal functioning:

Ph 1: satisfactory velopharyngeal functioning.
Ph 2: velopharyngeal closure is not complete during phonation.
Ph 3: presence of gross substitution errors, glottal stops or hoarse pharyngeal fricatives, which indicate major velopharyngeal inadequacy.

Obviously, there are a number of intermediate degrees. For instance:

Ph 1/2: Velopharyngeal competence may vary according to the circumstances. The same child may articulate properly while speaking to the tester, then develop a slight nasal resonance when addressing parents or reciting a poem. Closure may be complete, but only over a short interval: the velum gives way towards the end of a sentence or during a series of connected syllables (as in 'papapa...'). Quite frequently in these borderline cases, the parents point out that the child tends to speak through the nose towards the end of the day or when tired.
Ph 2/1: Nasality predominates, but the nasopharynx can be closed with some effort during

breathing drills or in emphatic speech. Even in Ph 2 cases where the nasopharynx is never completely closed, there are many different levels of phonation. The nasal cavity differs from one person to the next. Individual resonance can vary as well. The degree of resonance is not necessarily determined by the amount of air emitted through the nose. Furthermore, certain individuals (thanks to motor skill, acute perception or successful therapy) manage to articulate with sufficient accuracy to make themselves understood. According to their level of intelligibility, a distinction can be made between Ph 2G (good) or Ph 2P (poor).

Ph 3:   Gross substitution errors reflect habituation to atypical motor patterns, which compensate for major velopharyngeal insufficiency. They correspond therefore to the category Ph 2/3. After pharyngoplasty and despite the re-establishment of velopharyngeal closure, these learned compensatory patterns may subsist for some time. As they are gradually eliminated by speech therapy, the individual progresses through temporary transitional phases classified as Ph 1/3 or sometimes Ph 1/2/3.

11. Surgical repair: the Malek procedure

ANESTHESIA

General anesthesia is always used. Since the patients are only a few months old, the anesthesiologist must be highly experienced. Discussion of anesthesiology techniques is not the purpose of this book, but the extraordinary progress made by our collaborators in this domain must be mentioned. They guarantee us pre-operative comfort and safety.

The use of pre-flexed tubes greatly simplifies the process of intubation and the installation of the operating area. The tubes must be set up in a strictly medial position so that the mouth gag manufactured according to our specifications can be properly installed. This instrument ensures patency of the tube, which can no longer be collapsed between the blade of the gag and the rim of the mandible.

During cleft palate surgery, hyperextension of the head prevents liquids from flowing into the larynx and trachea. This dispenses with the need for gauze in the pharynx, so there is nothing to hinder surgical maneuvres on the posterior border of the velum. The eyes are protected by an instillation of liquid and by taping the eyelids shut with strips of adhesive.

Unless there is some specific contraindication (associated cardiac malformations in particular), an anesthetic adrenaline solution of the Marcaine or Novocaine type is always used, which facilitates sub-periosteal dissection and minimizes blood loss. Thanks to this procedure, there is rarely enough hemorrhaging to justify transfusion. Nonetheless, as a precaution, a vein is always prepared when anesthesia begins and is available in case of need. It is not always easy to locate when the infant is chubby.

INSTALLATION

The same pattern is always followed. The infant is placed in the dorsal decubitus position. To provide easy access, the head is maintained in a hyperextended position by placing a rolled towel or similar support under the shoulders. The head rests on a rubber ring, which holds it stable.

The customary set-up for an otorhinolaryngology operation is respected, and the operator stands at the head of the table with the assistant on his right.

The mouth-gag manufactured to our design is similar to the widely used Dott–Gillies device, but we have incorporated a few improvements that adapt it to palatal surgery in very young infants.

Several small blades are sized to the mouths of infants only a few months old. The blades are notched at the tip of their right angles and there is a groove in the lower solid portion. This prevents any compression of the tube against the alveolar rim of the mandible or the base of the tongue. Since the tube is constantly in view, it is possible to keep track of the to and fro movement of condensation through its transparent wall. This confirms patency of the respiratory passages, and adds an extra safeguard to the already considerable security of multiple electronic measurements provided by modern anesthesiology equipment.

GENERAL PRINCIPLES

It has become our practice to perform early surgery on palatal clefts, in order to correct functional disorders as soon as it is feasible and permit virtually normal physiological development.

Previously, the most widely used technique for many years was that introduced by Veau, with which the name Wardill is associated in Anglo-Saxon countries. In this method, the two thick mucoperiosteum were used in their entirety to close the cleft in the hard palate. As will be seen, elevation of the fibro-mucosae produces major iatrogenic consequences in the case of complete labio-palatal clefts, and we came to the conclusion that it should be proscribed for isolated cleft palates as well. Indeed, orthodontists are well aware of how frequently dental occlusal disorders such as retrognathia and endognathia occur in such cases (Fig. 11.1). It is always possible to blame malformative hypoplasia of the maxilla. However, devascularization of the bone structure through detachment of the mucoperiosteum and secondary fibrotic scar tissue in the raw area left near the teeth after stripping the mucoperiosteum must necessarily contribute to the adverse effects. This is even more so when surgery is performed in the first months of life. We decided, therefore, to discontinue the practice of elevating the mucoperiosteum, a decision which may seem arbitrary since no valid statistics are available on the subject.

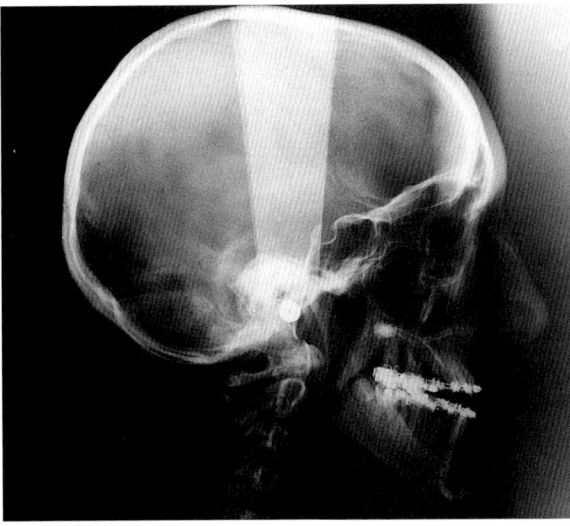

Fig. 11.1 Maxillary retrognathia in isolated cleft palate.

In cases of posterior palatal cleft, simple veloplasty is performed. For complete clefts involving the hard palate, the bony vault is closed on two layers to guarantee satisfactory healing. In this procedure only the thin mucosa from the margins of the cleft, which does not vector the essential blood supply is used. In our opinion, if the blood vessels and thick fibro-mucosa are left intact and if no area is stripped raw in the immediate vicinity of the teeth, the iatrogenic effects on maxillary and dental development are minimized.

Since a narrow pedicle is left intact in the anterior portion of the strip of thin mucosa dissected, our technique bears a resemblance to the procedure described by Von Langenbeck (1862). It is therefore called MVL (modified Von Langenbeck technique).

An analysis of both techniques follows.

VELOPLASTY

Incisions

The incisions include a transverse and a longitudinal segment.

A #12 blade is used to make the longitudinal incision along each margin of the cleft as far as the half-uvula. Ideally, it should follow the white dividing line between the red nasal and the more pinkish oral mucosa. The incision is extended as far as the apex of the cleft. At this point, it is possible either to trace an additional longitudinal incision, which meets the second transverse segment, or to leave a segment of oral mucosa intact between the two incisions. In this case, it is important to trace carefully the incisions on the borders of the cleft so that both sides meet in a perfect point without leaving a strip of mucosa, which might produce a fistula.

The transverse incision is curved. It begins laterally just beyond the posterior border of the alveolar ridge, and is oriented in a postero-anterior direction. It is then extended transversely right below the posterior margin of the palatal shelf, which it crosses before meeting the medial portion of the longitudinal incision at an angle. These two incisions therefore trace a small, triangular flap zone in the thin layer of fibro-mucosa (Fig. 11.2).

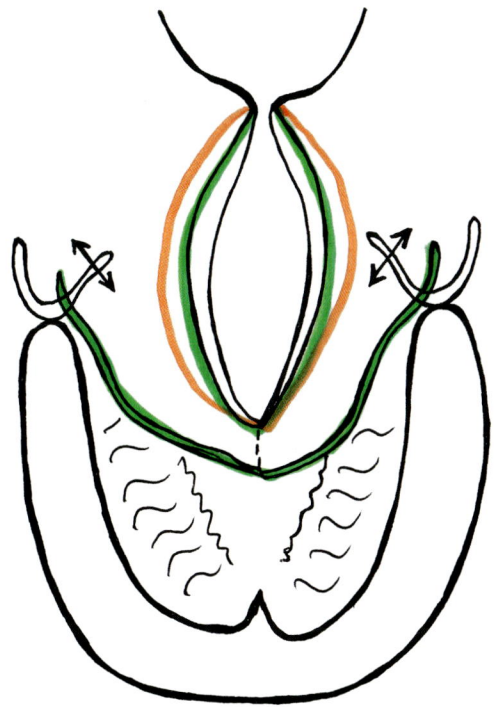

Green = Incision line
Orange = The line which indicates the change of colour
between oral and nasal mucosae

Fig. 11.2 *Pattern of incisions in posterior or simple cleft palate. The mucoperiosteum must be spared. Behind the maxillary tuberosities, the pterygoid hamuli are isolated and fractured.*

Undermining

On the outer side it is easy to locate the tendon of the tensor veli palatini, which winds round the hamulus of the medial ala of the pterygoid process. A Trélat elevator is used to fracture the hamulus so that this surface can be denuded as far as the base of the skull.

On the inner side, the elevator lifts the small triangular flap of the sub-periosteal layer. The half posterior nasal spine is denuded, as is the adjacent portion of the posterior border of the palatal shelf.

Between these two zones, the tissues are pushed back and carefully divided until detachment of the soft palate is complete. The division passes behind the posterior palatine neurovascular bundles, which must be left intact. Hemostasis may be necessary at this point.

The mucosa that lines the nasal side of the palatal shelves is easy to detach by displacing the velum towards the inside.

If a fissural muscle is present, its fibres are carefully sectioned without touching the nasal mucoperiosteum. Its tough tissue is needed to hold the suture fast. Any type of intra-velar dissection is deliberately avoided, since it produces fibrotic scarring. As will be explained, the argument of 'transverse reorientation of the muscle fibers' is refuted.

Suturing

Suturing is the next step. Thanks to extensive undermining, closure does not require undue traction in the vast majority of cases. Suturing is only unreliable during the very first days of life, when the cleft is broad and the velar stumps are still very tiny.

The first layer to be sutured is that of the nasal mucosa. Suturing, which begins at the very front, is done with 4/0 absorbable filament. The knots are tied inside the nose. Each stitch must take a bite of periosteum (which is clearly visible) to guarantee a firm hold. When the suture reaches the muscular portion of the velum, the needle should gather a small amount of mucosa and a larger bite of muscle fiber to prevent tearing when the knots are tightened (Fig. 11.3). At the base of the uvula, Donati or end-on mattress stitching is used to close the very fine mucosal layer. A length of suture left at the tip is held on a hemostat, and its weight exerts traction on the velum so that the symmetry of the second or oral layer will be retained during closure. The same end-on mattress stitches are continued as far as the anterior extremity of the flaps (Fig. 11.4).

Transverse approximation of the tissues produces spontaneous retraction. This is now possible thanks to extensive detachment of the nasal mucosa and medial rotation of the muscle fibers, which is necessary in order to unite the opposite portions at the midline.

A raw area of variable size remains near the free border of the palatal shelves. Despite the aforementioned retraction, the elasticity of the lateral mucosa permits an additional stitch to promote quick healing by approximating the lips of the transverse incision. Finally, an anchoring stitch fastens the oral layer to the roof of the vault near the apex of the small anterior triangular flaps. It should be tied moderately loosely to avoid endangering the blood supply to the flaps (Fig. 11.4).

Yellow = Bone
Brown = Muscle

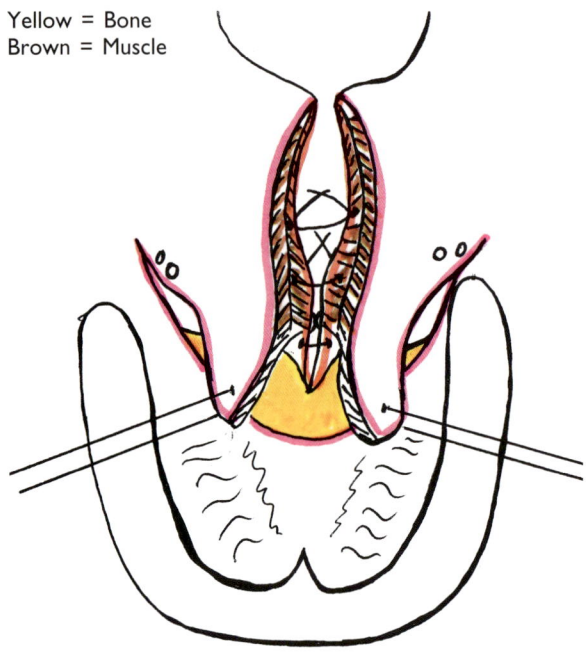

Fig. 11.3 Two small flaps, dissected, and reconstruction of the nasal muco-muscular layer from front to back. Notice the small bony surface that is denuded.

MODIFIED VON LANGENBECK TECHNIQUE (MVL)

This procedure is used when the cleft involves the hard palate to any degree. Despite extensive undermining of the nasal mucosa that covers the palatal shelves, it is difficult, if not impossible, to join the opposing borders directly. Suturing is not reliable and may result in residual fistulae. These can be avoided by using a second surface of oral mucosa to cover the nasal layer.

The major aim of this procedure is to leave the thick, heavily vascularized fibro-mucosa intact.

The only difference between the MVL technique and that of veloplasty concerns the transverse incision. In MVL, it continues forward along the furrow separating the thick and thin layers of fibro-mucosa and stops just beyond the anterior extremity of the cleft (Figs 11.5, 11.6a and b). It is relatively easy to undermine this narrow strip of flap, and the elevator is used to lift it inward.

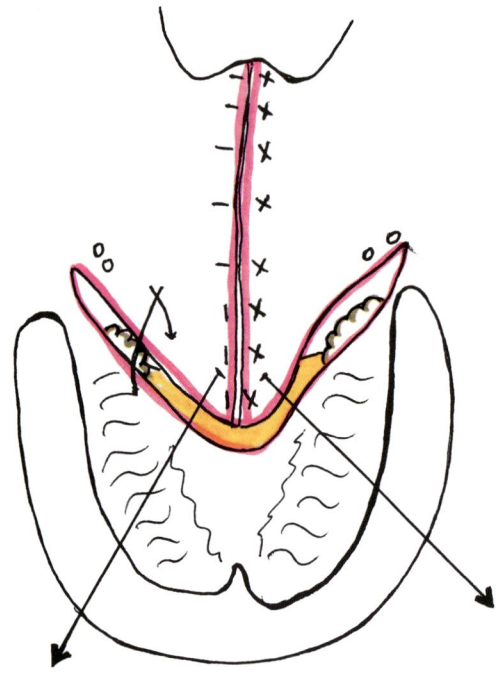

Fig. 11.4 Reconstruction of the oral layer proceeds anteriorly as of uvula, and is anchored to the nasal layer with transfixiating stitches. Spontaneous retraction of the soft palate requires no muscular dissection once the attachments of the palatal muscles have been sectioned on the posterior borders of the palatal shelves.

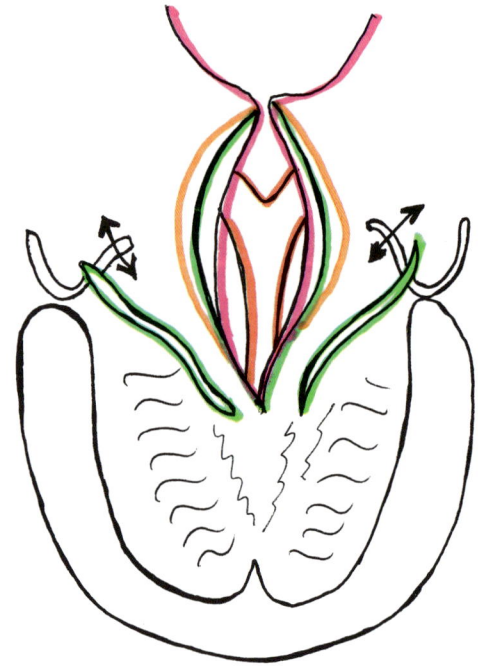

Fig. 11.5 When the cleft involves the bony vault, the transverse incisions can remain independent of one another to avoid leaving a zone with only the fragile nasal layer after suturing and spontaneous retraction of the soft palate. The procedure resembles the MVL technique.

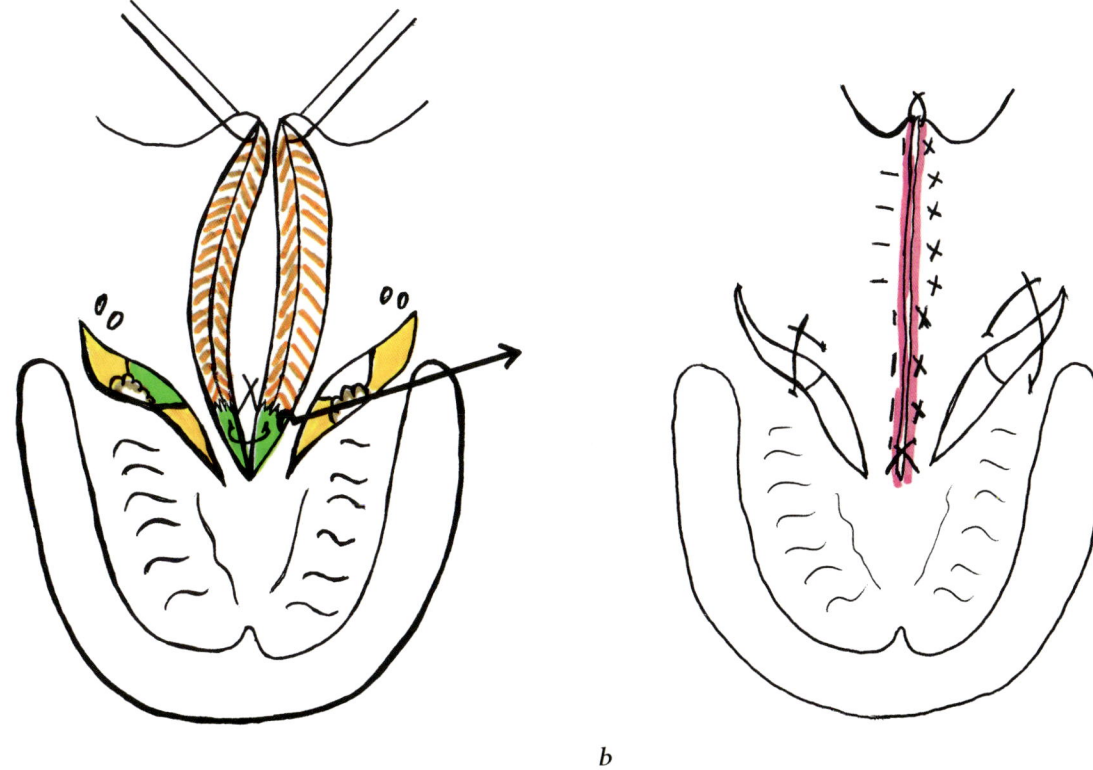

a *b*

Fig. 11.6 *Dissection (a) and suturing (b) in a minimal MVL procedure.*

Closure of the bony vault may present a problem. As already noted, despite its considerable mobility, nasal mucosa does not always permit direct suturing of one side to the other. In such cases, it becomes necessary to create a nasal layer using vomerine mucosa, a procedure practiced by Veau and later by Petit. A longitudinal incision is made in the lower edge of the vomerine mucosa, and it is sutured to the nasal mucosa on either side from front to back (Fig. 11.7). The first stitch is difficult and requires use of a Petit needle (small-sized Reverdin needle). The naso-vomerine suture continues until the tension appears to diminish, and at this point, direct suturing of the nasal mucosa can be performed (Figs 11.8 and 11.9).

Sectioning the fissural muscle calls for particularly careful attention in this procedure, since it is essential not to weaken either layer where the soft and hard palate meet.

The MVL technique is open to the same objections raised by Veau against the original version:

1. The soft palate is fastened in an anterior position and therefore cannot retract. However, long-term

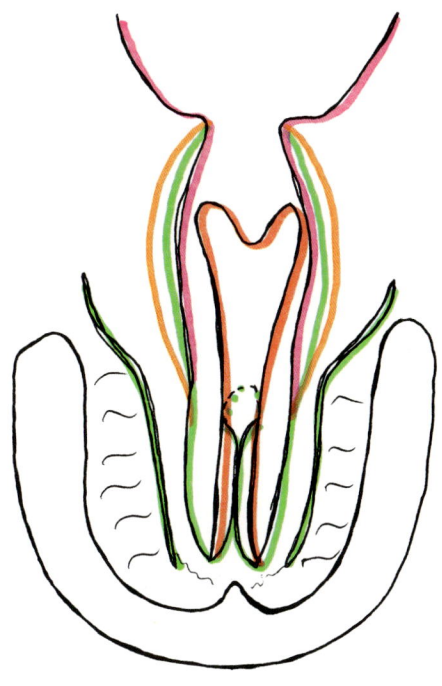

Fig. 11.7 *In bilateral cleft palate affecting the entire vault, the MVL technique is used. In the anterior portion, vomerine mucosa is used to create a nasal layer.*

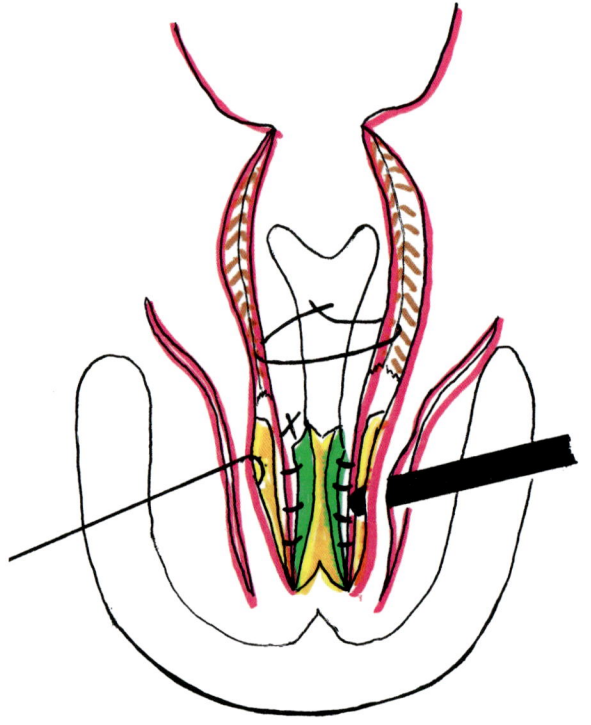

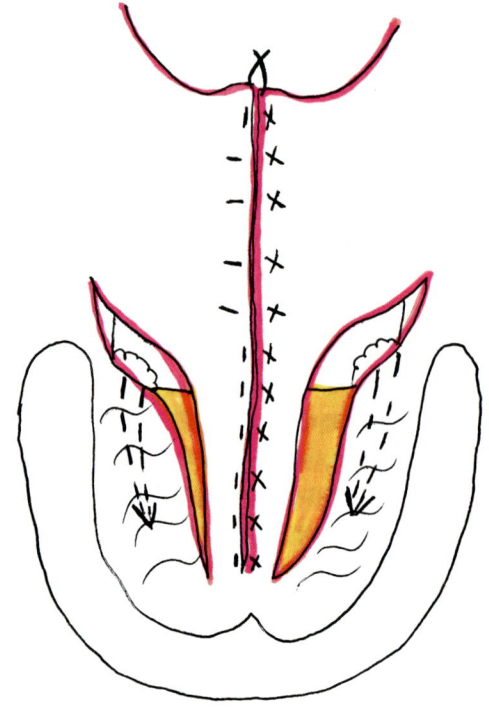

Fig. 11.8 *Dissection and suturing of palato-vomerine layers. This is feasible only in the anterior portion, and direct suturing of the muscles and nasal mucosa on the borders of the soft palate should begin as soon as possible. At the very front, the small portion of mucosa where the vomer and primary palate meet is resected to avoid a residual fistula.*

Fig. 11.9 *Post-operative view. No retraction is possible.*

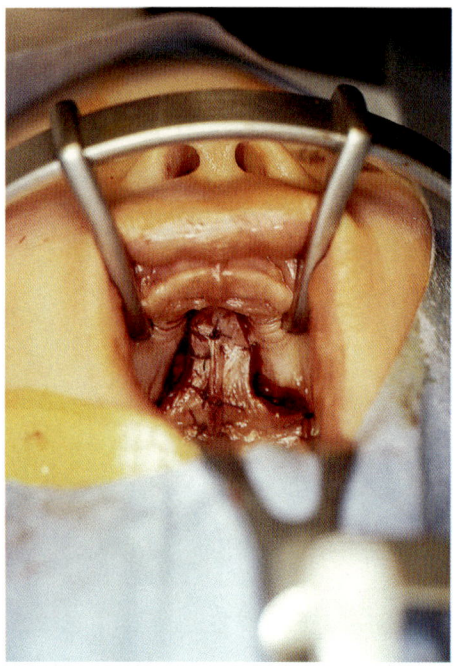

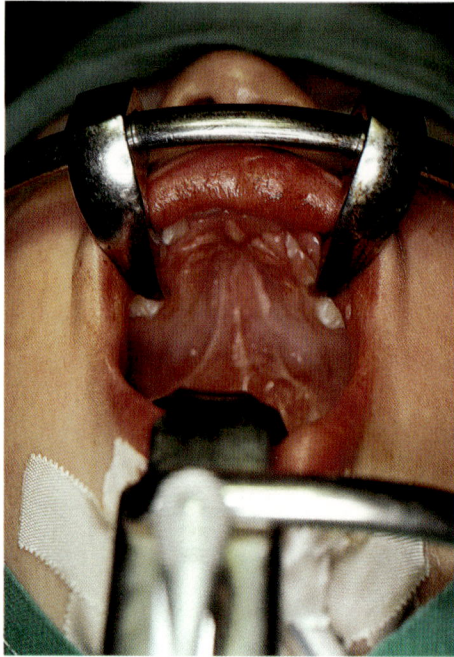

Fig. 11.10
a. *Post-operative view.*
b. *Scar after several months.*

a

b

speech results tend to refute the notion that the MVL procedure carries a greater risk of velopharyngeal insufficiency. In our experience (see below), results are similar to those of simple veloplasty.

2. The flaps or oral mucosa remain at a distance from the nasal layer, since anterior closure hinders upward as well as backward mobility. In Veau's opinion this was a major objection. In actual fact, healing proceeds quickly and easily in the roof of the mouth.

POST-OPERATIVE TREATMENT

This is identical to that for all cleft surgery:

- Short-term preventive antibiotic medication.
- Spoon-bottle feeding.
- Elbow restraints.

These measures can be discontinued once the stitches have been absorbed, which takes 3–4 weeks (Fig. 11.10a and b).

12. Surgical repair: other procedures

VEAU TECHNIQUE (STAPHYLORRAPHY)

This is the conventional or 'classic' technique, which has been used on hundreds of cases, whether of isolated cleft palate or of palatal closure in labio-palatal clefts. It is a simple, perfectly reliable procedure, which virtually never leaves residual fistulae.

As a rule, staphylorraphy is performed at about 18 months, before what was generally considered to be the age of emergent speech. An analysis of the phonetic results is appended (see page 152).

A vast number of procedures have been developed to prevent velar insufficiency by 'lengthening' the velum. Their routine use does not seem any more desirable or necessary than is extensive dissection of the velum to permit reorientation of the muscle fibers as recommended by Kriens (1969).

The recent evolution in therapeutic outcome, coupled with improvements in the field of anesthesia, has encouraged certain specialists to propose staphylorraphy at an earlier age; sometimes during the second semester of life.

Modern authors stress the drawbacks involved in elevating the mucoperiosteum, which is alleged to have an iatrogenic effect on maxillary growth. This attitude explains the popularity of the Schweckendiek method, which schedules veloplasty alone between the ages of 6 and 8 months, while the gap in the palatal vault is left open until a much later age. Elevation of the mucoperiosteum is reserved for secondary closure of the remaining cleft.

In our opinion, the 'classic' technique should no longer be used due to this iatrogenic risk. This exists even in cases of isolated cleft palate, which may present maxillary retrognathia at the end of the growth cycle. If elevation of the mucoperiosteum proves necessary, it should be postponed until maxillary growth is well under way.

Nonetheless, a working knowledge of this technique is an integral part of cleft palate background.

The operative site is infiltrated according to the customary procedure.

Incisions

Two incisions are involved. A straight, longitudinal incision divides the border and continues forward up to the apex of the cleft, which often extends into the bony vault. A curved incision starts behind the maxillary tuberosity, continues along the inside of the alveolar arch, and stops at the premaxilla (Fig. 12.1).

Undermining

Undermining of the mucoperiosteum is the next step. The tissues are generally quite easy to detach if this is the first time they have been elevated. The posterior palatine neurovascular bundle shows up very clearly, and is isolated near the posterior border of the shelves. Hemostasis should be thorough on the periphery of the flaps, since hemorrhaging can be abundant despite prior infiltration.

The hamulus of the inner ala of the pterygoid process is then located using a gentle diverging movement of the angulated forceps and Trélat hook. The latter is passed on the outer side of the hamulus, which is fractured by pushing the hook inward with gentle but steady pressure. The inner surface of the pterygoid ala is dissected, as is the posterior border of the shelves on either side of the pedicle.

All anterior insertions of the velar muscles are freed, particularly those fibers that may make up Veau's fissural muscle (Fig. 12.2).

In unilateral labio-palatal clefts, the vomerine mucosa is undermined (as is the nasal mucosa of the palatal shelf), as far as the site of hard palate repair previously effected during primary surgery, following the agenda of this 'classic' method.

In bilateral labio-palatal clefts or isolated cleft palate involving the bony vault, it may prove necessary to use vomerine mucosa to reinforce closure of the most anterior portion of the vault. A longitudinal incision is made in the vomerine mucosa from the lower border to the premaxilla to permit undermining of both surfaces of the bone (Fig. 12.2).

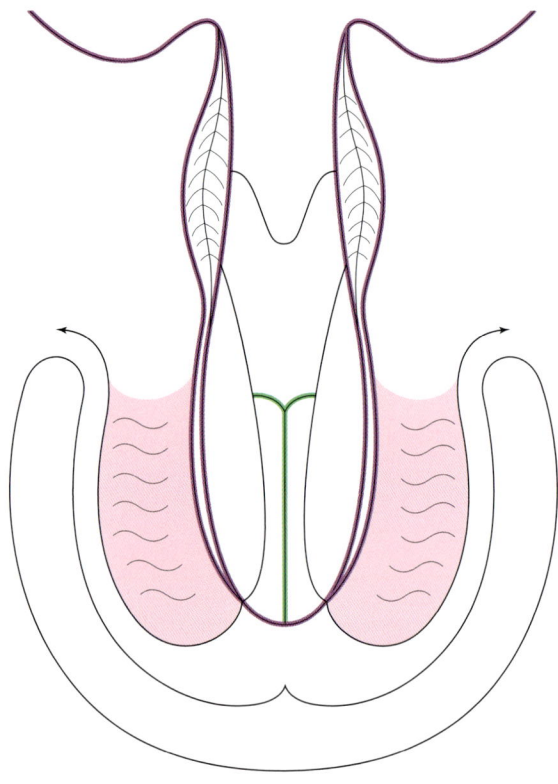

Fig. 12.1 *Pattern of incisions along the borders of the cleft and on the periphery of the mucoperiosteum. In the bilateral form, a longitudinal incision is made in the lower border of the vomerine mucosa.*

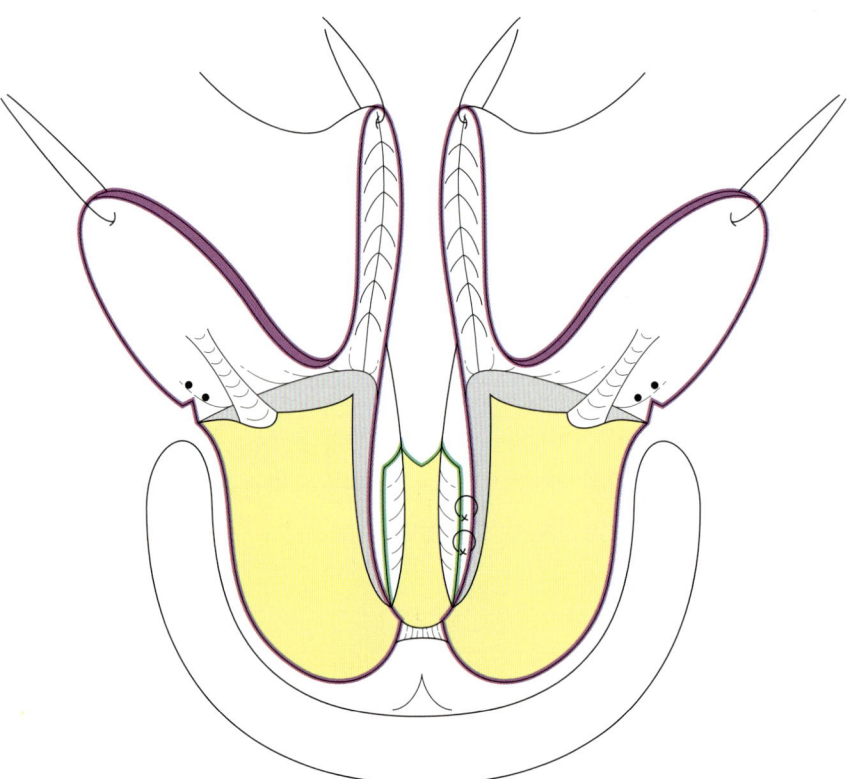

Fig. 12.2 *Elevated flaps and fracture of the pterygoid hamuli. A vomero-nasal suture creates a nasal layer in the anterior portion of the bony vault. Notice the freshening necessary at the primary palate.*

Suturing

Suturing begins with the nasal layer, and proceeds from front to back. Whenever required, the vomerine and lateral nasal mucosae should be sutured together first. The initial stitch is rather tricky and may require use of a fine Petit (Reverdin) needle, which is introduced into the corresponding nostril so that the knot can be tied inside the nose. Only two or three stitches are placed on the naso-vomerine layer, followed by direct suturing of the two sides of palatal mucosa. Each suture takes a larger bite of muscle than of nasal mucosa.

On reaching the uvula, Donati stitches are used. As of the summit of the uvula (suspended by the traction stitch at its tip held on a Halsted forceps), the oral layer is closed with the same Donati stitching. A stitch or two fastens the palate snugly to the nasal layer on the midline.

LENGTHENING THE SOFT PALATE

Velar incompetence is a pathological speech disorder, which represents the most detrimental functional repercussion of cleft palate (see Chapter 10). This defect manifests itself when the nasopharyngeal orifice fails to achieve complete occlusion during the production of plosive consonants, evidenced by the audible emission of nasal air.

The physio-pathological explanation for this phenomenon is highly complex, and varies from one case to another. Naso-endoscopy has clearly demonstrated the activation of the nasopharyngeal sphincter. However, the most common explanation nowadays is that the soft palate presents a deficit in length, which prevents it from establishing contact with the wall of the pharynx. This concurs with the diagnosis of a short velum. A congenital length deficit related to some embryological anomaly is correctly incriminated. Thus, plastic surgeons, whatever the specific technique used, have consistently endeavored to lengthen the short, soft palate in the course of primary repair.

Simple Z-plasty based on nasal mucosa does not seem particularly promising. As in all Z-plasties, inversion of the flaps can only obtain additional length at the expense of width. It so happens that the greatest tension created during correction is

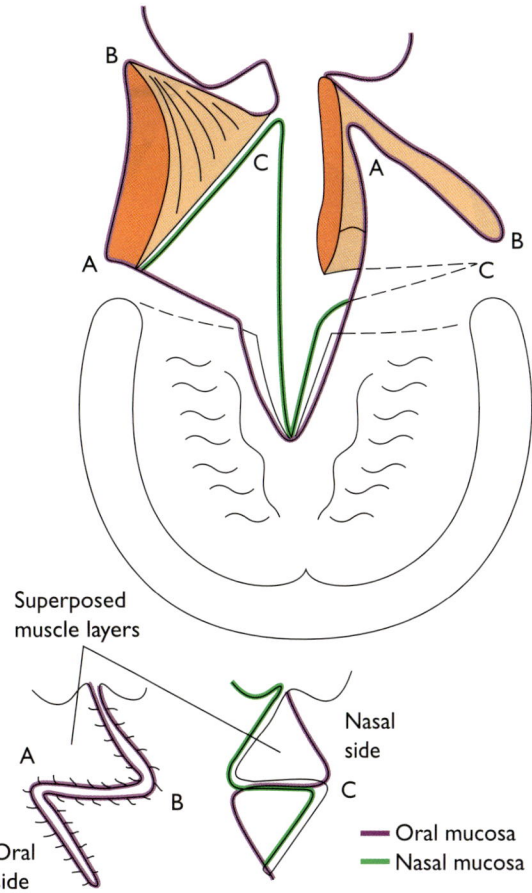

Fig. 12.3 *Furlow technique of double opposing Z-plasty.*

produced precisely in that zone where the tissues should be able to lend extra width (the posterior borders of the palatal shelves). Any increase in this tension may well lead to a rupture of the nasal layer, and this can prove disastrous unless the Veau procedure, which involves elevation of the mucoperiosteum, has been employed. In addition, after healing the scar tissues show a tendency to retract. The muscles are drawn forward again towards the posterior borders of the shelves, thus cancelling out the initial gain in length obtained.

The Furlow technique (1986), which offers a different version of the Z-plasty, has won a certain following in the USA (Fig. 12.3) (see below).

Retrodisplacement of the velar muscles and primarily of the levator veli palatini based on intravelar dissection of the muscle fibers, which are directly sutured end to end so as to reconstruct a 'muscle sling' (automatically located in a posterior position due to the loss of anterior muscle attachments), represents one of the solutions proposed to prevent velar inadequacy (Kriens, 1969).

Unlike many other specialists throughout the world, we have not chosen to apply this procedure. By definition, it implies extensive dissection of the muscles, which strikes us as a source of fibrosis and hence of velar sclerosis. Recent studies reporting the phonetic results of this technique show no clearly significant improvements.

As concerns primary pharyngoplasty (Stark and Dehaan, 1960) and, more specifically, repositioning obtained thanks to a pharyngeal flap, we have always found that this procedure amounts to too much, too soon. This is a difficult technique to apply at a very early age, when the cavum is still clogged with adenoid tissue (see Chapter 13).

Early surgery – early veloplasty, to be more precise – appears to provide the best safeguard against velar incompetence. By reconstructing the muscle structures of the soft palate at a stage when the bones are still easily remoulded, veloplasty reduces the dimensions of the cavum, which has been enlarged by the cleft, and favors the development of normal strength and function in muscles hitherto underdeveloped through lack of use.

FURLOW TECHNIQUE

According to Furlow, who described it in 1986, this technique offers two advantages:

1. It lengthens the soft palate without using the mucoperiosteum (a factor favorable to satisfactory growth).
2. It permits a better muscular suture, which does not impair velar contraction.

The procedure is endorsed by Peter Randall, who has become its principal advocate.

The technique is based on a large Z- or rather double Z-plasty (known as the Furlow double opposing Z-plasty). The design of the mucosal incisions traced in the oral and nasal layers is reversed. The levator muscle fibers, which remain continuous with the oral layer on one side and with the nasal layer on the other, are detached from the palatal shelves. Closure of the hard palate should remain on the midline. The two isolated muscle layers are overlapped and due to the tension created, they shift into a more posterior position, which benefits the lengthening achieved by the plasty. Because of this lengthening, the technique is recommended in the treatment of velar inadequacy over and above the other techniques of pharyngoplasty.

The theoretical concept may arouse enthusiasm, but it overlooks what has been learned from long experience of Z-plasties: a gain in length can only be obtained at the expense of width. Also, the tissues of the velopharynx are not extensile. If, as Furlow suggests, the incisions should be continued as far as the pterygoid hamuli, then lateral undermining must be quite extensive. It follows that the levator palatini undergoes considerable displacement, which is not in the order of normal physiology and must have some effect on local functions. Anterior suturing of the two large mucosal flaps presents a risk due to the transverse tension thus created.

The report on 22 cases presented by Furlow is somewhat limited, and the cephalometric studies were still pending at the time of writing. Speech results were excellent, with only 10 per cent of moderate velopharyngeal incompetency. Hearing was satisfactory in 70 per cent of the cases.

Our main objection to this technique concerns its unphysiological aspects.

13. Pharyngoplasty

GENERAL PRINCIPLES

Pharyngoplasty is an operation designed to reduce the distance between the velum and the posterior wall of the pharynx so that efficient occlusion of the rhinopharynx can be obtained. This is a prerequisite for satisfactory phonation.

The procedure is often mistakenly construed as a means of lengthening the soft palate, based on the notion that oropharyngeal valving is defective when the velum is too short. In reality, pharyngoplasty involves retrodisplacement of the velum as a whole, which can only be obtained by severing all its anterior attachments. This is usually accomplished by elevating the fibro-mucosae on the oral side and sectioning the nasal mucosa at the posterior border of the bony palatal shelves. Retrodisplacement of the soft palate necessarily leaves raw surfaces denuded of mucosa behind the incisor teeth on the oral side and behind the palatal shelves in the area of the nose. These surfaces heal rapidly, but show a marked tendency to retract. This is likely to pull the palatal tissue forward again, which means that all or most of the recession originally gained may be lost.

This explains why a muco-muscular flap must be elevated from the superior constrictor to anchor the soft palate in its posterior position. This procedure (described by Rosenthal, 1924) maintains the retrodisplacement. It also reduces the transverse diameter of the nasopharynx, an effect which combines with velar recession to permit far more efficient active occlusion of the velopharyngeal sphincter (this sphincteric action reinforces the valving mechanism).

There has been a considerable amount of debate over which direction to choose for the orientation of the pharyngeal flap and where to place its pedicle. A single flap is generally used. It can be incised with a superior pedicle, and is then applied to the freshened upper surface of the velum. This is the method we have adopted, as it seems to offer more advantages than an inferiorly-based flap applied to the oral or lower surface of the velum. Since the soft palate is elevated during closure, it does not seem logical to anchor it from below. This argument may be purely theoretical, however, because in the vast majority of cases an adhesion of fibrous scar tissue develops linking the area where the flap was lifted to its base (for superior pedicles). Therefore, theory notwithstanding, the velum is undeniably anchored from below. Moreover, the theory does not take into account the dynamics of the system, which brings the superior constrictor forward into contact with the soft palate.

If a superior flap procedure is used the flap pedicle is located on the level of the anterior tubercle of the atlas, which is easily palpated in the posterior wall of the pharynx. This is the point of contact revealed on profile X-ray views of adults when the subject holds the phoneme [i].

The well-known Hynes technique (Hynes, 1950) relies on bilateral palato-pharyngeal muscle flaps with their attached mucosa. The flaps are swung toward the midline, overlapped and inserted into an incision in the mucosa of the posterior pharyngeal wall above the anterior arch of the atlas. The end result is a sort

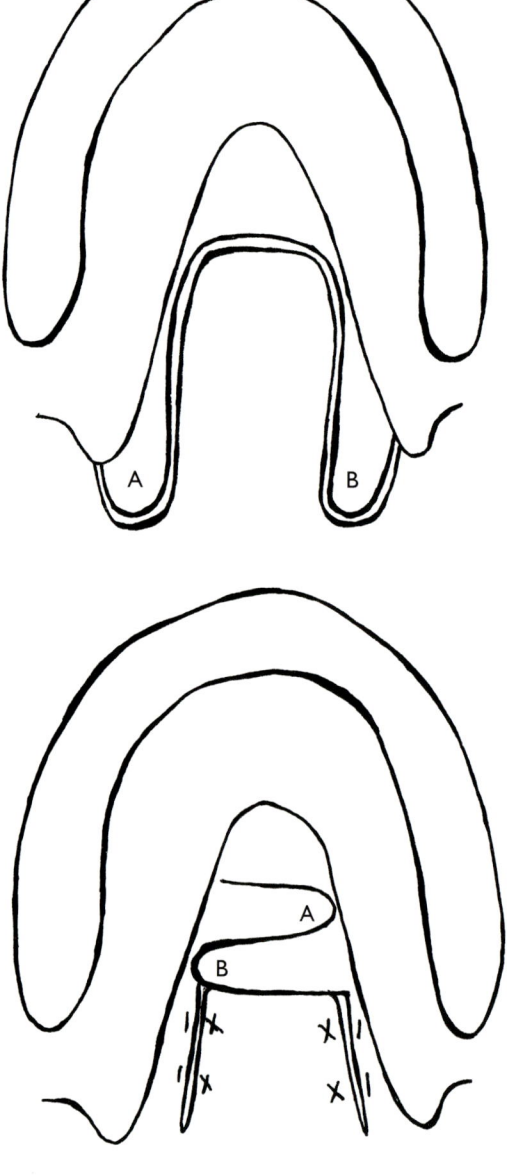

Fig. 13.1 *Incisions for the Hynes technique.*
A and B. Flaps at posterior pillars.

retains its anterior attachment to the palatal shelf. This produces a permanent separation between the oro- and nasopharynx, which does not strike us as being satisfactory from a physiological standpoint (Fig. 13.2). In our opinion, the flap has no active role to play. Once the healing process is completed, it can very well be sectioned as is sometimes done in the case of rhinolalia (speech impaired by nasal tract obstruction).

Rather than resort to a flap, another school of thought advocates covering the raw area with nasal mucosa to eliminate any risk of having the velar structures shift forward again.

Cronin (1957) advises sectioning the nasal mucosa much further forward (Fig. 13.3).

Millard (1963) described a flap with a pedicle

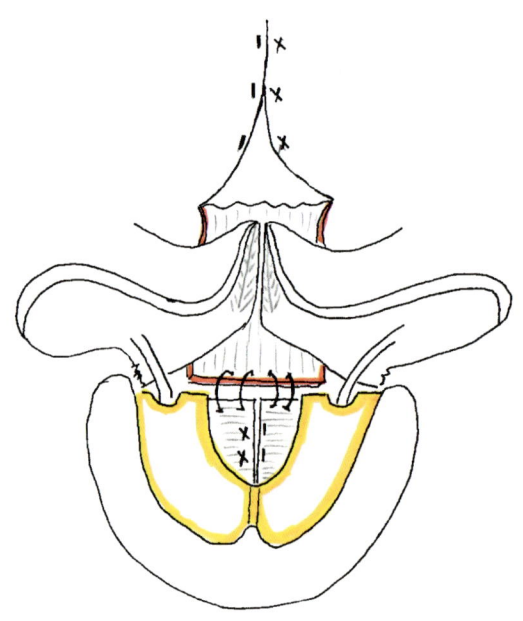

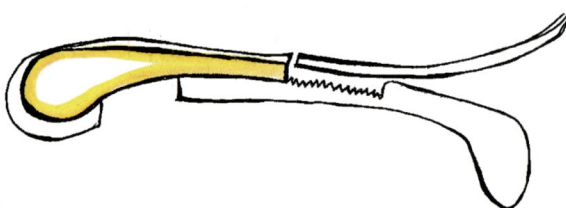

Fig. 13.2 *San Venero-Rosselli procedure. A large, superior pharyngeal flap is sutured anteriorly to the nasal mucosa.*

of super Passavant's ridge. However, we find the procedure over-complicated and poorly suited to small infants (Fig. 13.1).

Some surgeons use the 'sandwich' procedure, whereby the flap is interleaved between the two halves of the velum, which is incised lengthwise.

Lastly, a certain number, like San Venero-Rosselli (1955), anchor the extremity of a flap dissected from the superior constrictor to the nasal mucosa, which

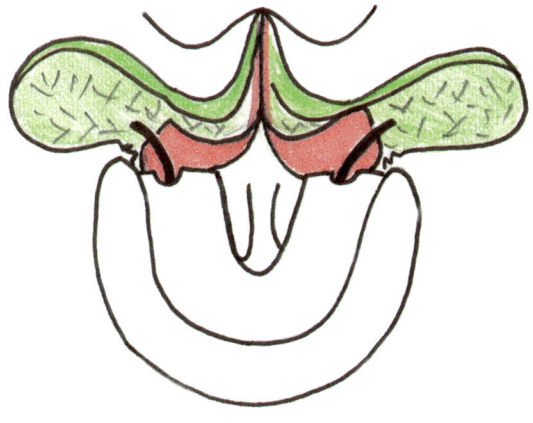

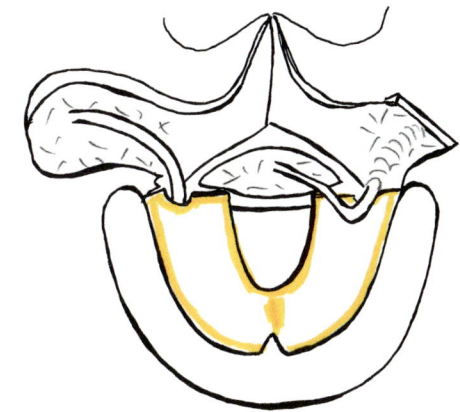

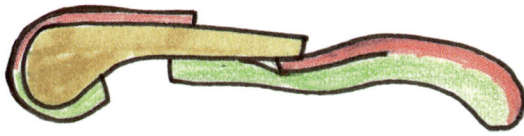

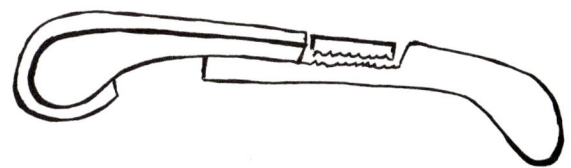

Fig. 13.3 Cronin operation using the nasal mucosa to cover the raw area.

Fig. 13.4 Principles of Millard (1963)–Edgerton (1965) technique, with island flap of mucoperiosteum.

elevated from one of the fibro-mucosae, which could be inserted between the two edges of the sectioned mucosa (Fig. 13.4). Flaps of cheek mucosa have also been suggested.

In the Furlow procedure, endorsed by Randall, a particularly large Z-plasty is performed using flaps of different thicknesses, which are inverted so that closure does not leave a raw area.

As far as we are concerned, the reliable pharyngeal flap with its bonus effect of narrowing the pharyngeal port offers such significant advantages that it supersedes all other techniques.

Pharyngoplasty is usually performed at 5–6 years of age. There are several arguments in favor of this choice:

1. The true degree of speech impairment can be evaluated by this age, since the child is old enough to respond to testing. The patient has usually undergone enough speech therapy so that surgery can be reserved for only those cases in which retrodis-

placement of the soft palate is indeed a necessity.
2. As a rule, the nasopharynx is no longer congested with adenoid tissue at this age.
3. Improved speech production becomes particularly important by the time the child reaches the age for primary school.

It goes without saying that pharyngoplasty can be performed at any age, even on elderly patients. However, in such cases it is extremely difficult to eradicate defective speech patterns because they are deeply ingrained.

Problems of pharyngoplasty

The major drawback of pharyngoplasty is the inevitable need to elevate the fibro-mucosae (Petit *et al.*, 1956). There are a number of repercussions, particularly on the growth process of the upper maxilla. However, it has been clearly established that maxillary growth decreases considerably as of 6–8 years of age.

In the long-term follow-up on the outcome of the 'primary palate' procedure, we have not observed a correlation between pharyngoplasty and poor dental results. However, we must admit to our lack of enthusiasm for elevating the fibro-mucosae although, unfortunately, we have found no other method of obtaining retrodisplacement of the soft palate that better meets our demands. This is a domain where additional research may perhaps lead to future technical improvements.

If an oro-nasal fistula exists after primary surgery, it is often difficult to determine whether speech defects are to be attributed to a short palate or to the residual opening. In these cases, speech therapists provide valuable assistance. A study is devoted to this subject in Chapter 23.

To avoid repercussions on dental development while the raw surfaces heal, we customarily fit a retainer plate after pharyngoplasty. This also serves to protect the sutures.

A study of the general aspects of pharyngoplasty would not be complete without discussing the problem of the tonsils and adenoids. There is often a considerable mass of tonsillar and adenoidal tissue at the age when surgery is usually performed and, in addition to the latent danger of infection, the flap used in pharyngoplasty creates an obstruction that seriously complicates their subsequent removal. Furthermore, bulky tonsils may hinder retrodisplacement of the soft palate or block the air flow by obstructing the cavum, which has already been reduced in volume by the retrodisplacement and the presence of the flap.

It is therefore preferable to remove the tonsils and adenoids a few months before pharyngoplasty. The parents may wonder why this decision has been made, because they have been repeatedly told that the adenoids should not be removed in cases of cleft palate since this might create or aggravate velar insufficiency. However, once velar inadequacy is confirmed, the parents are in a position to understand that these precautions are no longer justified and that the adenoids can represent a source of problems if not treated with radical measures.

It is advisable to perform tonsillectomy by dissection under general anesthesia with intubation. It is important to leave the tonsillar pillars absolutely intact, since their muscle structure has a vital physi-

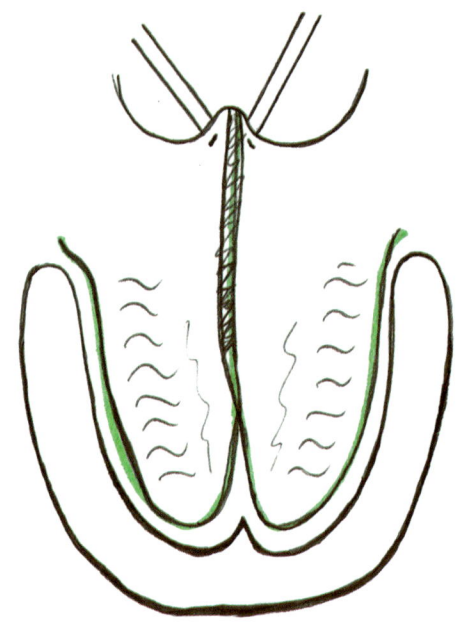

Fig. 13.5 Our technique (Petit). Two flaps of mucoperiosteum are dissected and the velum is re-opened on the midline.

ological role to play.

PETIT TECHNIQUE

Installation of the patient is identical to that for cleft palate repair. A rolled towel or similar support is placed under the shoulders to obtain hyperextension of the neck.

The fibro-mucosae and soft palate are infiltrated with a solution of marcaine and adrenaline. Two traction sutures are used to suspend the uvula, and thus the soft palate can be divided down the middle. The incision should not go beyond the posterior borders of the bony palatal shelves (Fig. 13.5).

Incisions

The fibro-mucosae are elevated. We routinely make a peripheral incision, which passes a few millimetres inside the teeth. The midline incision, however, depends on the nature of the congenital cleft.

When the soft palate is cleft and the hard palate intact, the midline incision is made immediately. There is no risk of leaving an anterior gap when the velum is set back. It may be advisable to spare a small amount of medial tissue, which can serve as a support for the suspension of the two fibro-mucosal flaps from the bony roof of the vault during the final stage of the operation. However, this strip of tissue often comes off spontaneously since it has little hold on the underlying bone. If a significant amount of medial tissue has been spared, it must be freshened by scraping it with the blade of the scalpel to avoid the development of a horizontal slough lined with the mucosa left in place.

When the initial lesion involves a cleft in the hard palate (bilateral cleft palate or uni-/bilateral labio-maxillo-palatal cleft), elevation of the fibro-mucosae implies a risk of leaving a gap in the nasal plane. The risk is all the greater because this anterior hole is located in such a position that it cannot be covered by the fibro-mucosae once retrodisplacement has been obtained. In this context, it is wise to begin undermining the fibro-mucosae laterally in order to locate the lateral border of the ipsilateral palatal shelf. The midline incision can then be made with utmost caution in plain sight to avoid rupturing the nasal plane.

In the case of isolated cleft palate with significant involvement of the bone structure, we use the MVL (modified Von Langenbeck, 1862) technique to guarantee risk-free closure of the vault. This procedure calls for two narrow flaps dissected from the palatal mucosa. To carry out pharyngoplasty with retrodisplacement, the two fibro-mucosae must be elevated. During undermining, the blood vessels that irrigate these slender flaps anteriorly are sectioned. This does not fundamentally compromise blood supply to the flaps. However, if the sutures gather too large an amount of mucosa on either side (in the event that Blair–Donati stitches are used), necrosis may affect a portion of this inner mucosa and result in a fistula. This pitfall must not be underestimated; closure of these fistulae is extremely difficult. It is better to resect most of this mucosa and suture the two well-vascularized fibro-mucosae together.

Undermining

The next step concerns lateral undermining of the soft palate. The posterior palatal pedicle is isolated. The posterior borders of the shelves are freed from their muscle attachments, and the pterygoid hamuli are fractured if this has not already been done during

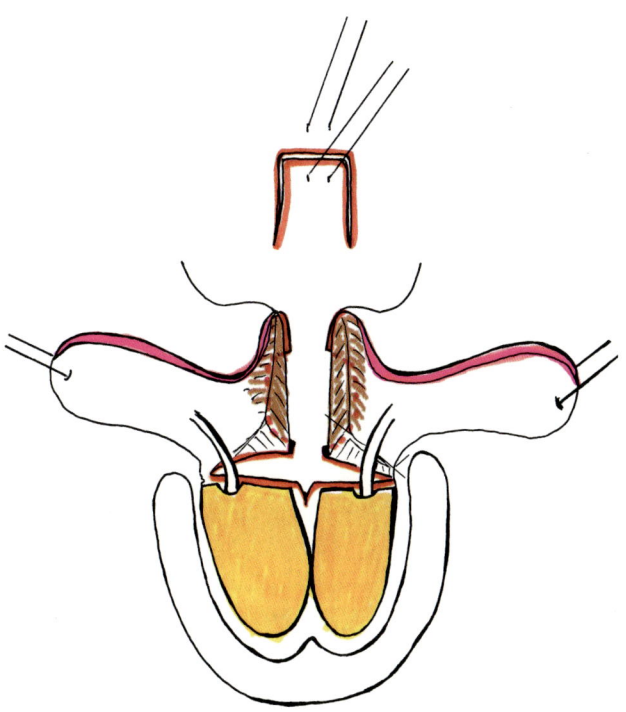

Fig. 13.6 *Petit technique: transverse section of the nasal mucosa and dissection of a superior muco-muscular flap from the pharyngeal wall based at the protuberance of the anterior tubercle of the atlas. The nasal surface of the velum is freshened.*

earlier primary surgery. The orifice of the Eustachian tube is located on either side, and the nasal mucosa is sectioned with the blade held at a right angle. This can cause hemorrhaging, and should be performed with cutting diathermy.

The palatal pedicles alone now provide an anterior attachment for the soft palate. These should be sufficiently dissected to permit retrodisplacement without creating undue tension. It may be necessary to depress the bone structure to the rear slightly if it impinges on the pedicles at the posterior border of the palatal shelves.

The upper surface of the velum is freshened. A strip of nasal mucosa is resected on either side to permit application of the raw side of the pharyngeal flap, which is incised during the following phase (Fig. 13.6).

The protuberance of the anterior tubercle of the atlas is easy to locate with the tip of the index finger. Before infiltration, a shallow vertical incision is made on either side to mark off the width of the flap. It should measure about 1 cm across, or slightly more if the cavum is particularly broad. The tissues are infiltrated. Next, to serve as suspension, two heavy transverse sutures that bite through the entire thickness of the muscle are placed on either side of what is to become the lower border of the flap, about 2 cm from the tubercle of the atlas. Once these stitches are pulled taut, a transverse incision is made all the way through the superior constrictor along the desired length (about 1 cm). A long-handled scalpel is then used for the two vertical incisions. As the flap is elevated, it exposes the white, shiny surface of the prevertebral aponeurosis.

Suturing

The zone where the flap was elevated can now be closed with reasonably heavy absorbable suture material (3/0). Suturing begins at the base of the flap

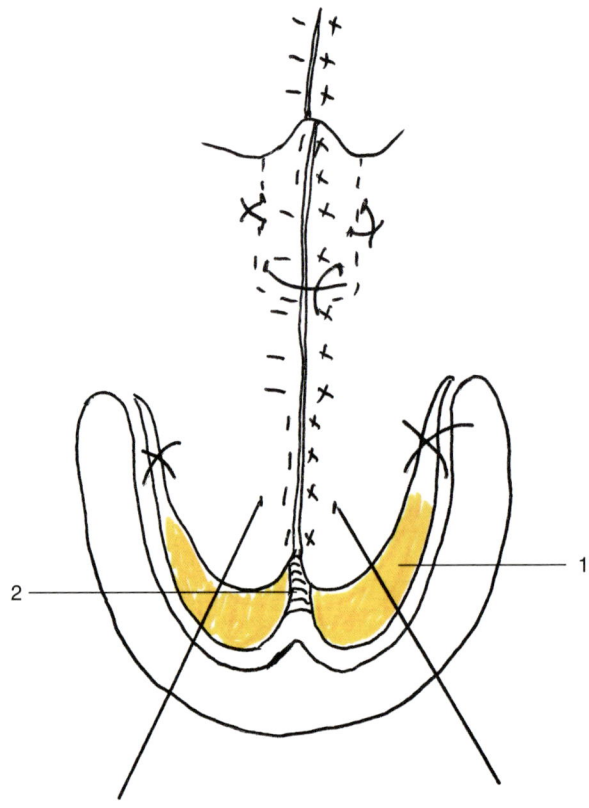

Fig. 13.8 *Petit technique, at the end of surgery. This shows the denuded zones behind the arch and the anchoring stitch after freshening of the mucosa on the midline.*

1. *Low area corresponding to the first back*
2. *The mucosa must be exised here*

using Donati stitches, and continues to its lower end. The crimp of tissue produced by approximating the edges of this quadrangular zone can be disregarded.

Retrodisplacement of the soft palate is held fast by stitches that apply the flap to the upper surface of the velum and that are heavy enough to prevent tearing of the adjacent tissues (Fig. 13.7). These are U-shaped stitches, which are set in place (one or two on each side of the flap and one at its end) but left untied until the final stages of the operation, after reconstruction of the palate.

Medial suturing of the palate begins at the base of the uvula, first the nasal, then the oral layer. It continues with mattress stitching of the velum, followed by suturing of the fibro-mucosae.

Once the heavy sutures that anchor the flap are tied and the retrodisplacement securely fixed, the

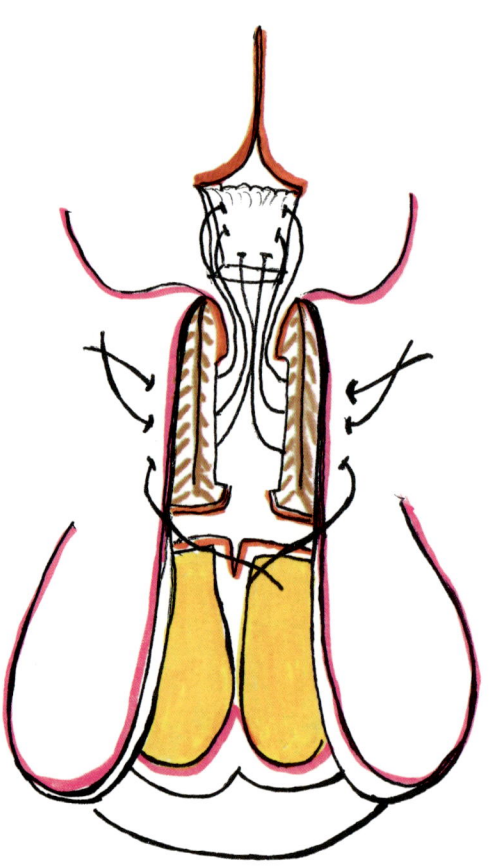

Fig. 13.7 *Placement of stitches on the velum and flap that anchor the retrodisplacement. The zone where the flap was elevated is sutured.*

fibro-mucosae are applied over the bony portion with a few stitches that grab the tissue left on the midline and along the sides (Fig. 13.8).

Post-operative care

Local post-operative care is minimal. The patient has a sore throat for 2 days at most. If the patient is unable to swallow fluids, the drip is left in place with an antibiotic and sedative supplement. Oral feeding can be resumed as soon as possible (liquid or puréed). Healing is very rapid, but it is better to restrict solids for a month or so until the stitches are no longer apparent.

Retrodisplacement of the soft palate frequently causes fairly loud snoring, which gradually lessens and finally ceases after a few months. Certain special-ists have debated whether this deliberate retrodis-placement might result in chronic respiratory and cardiovascular disorders. However, the techniques they used were probably different from ours. So far, despite the considerable number of operations performed by Petit and his assistants or by myself, there have not been any such disorders after pharyn-goplasty using our procedure.

The phonetic results cannot be validly assessed until the soft palate has resumed its proper function, which takes a few months. A certain improvement may be noted in the days following surgery, but local edema makes it hard to tell whether active closure is satisfactory or not. The parents should therefore be informed of the necessary delay before the results can be evaluated.

14. Speech results

When we opted for early primary veloplasty at the age of 3 months in complete labio-maxillo-palatal clefts, we also radically modified the timetable of palatal closure in isolated cleft palate. Although elevation of the mucoperiosteum presents less of a problem in the latter form, the risks involved cannot be totally disregarded since there have been many cases of subsequent maxillary hypoplasia with undesirable repercussions on dentition and facial appearance.

The advantages of early cleft palate repair seemed particularly obvious from a functional point of view. If virtually normal anatomy of the muscle structures is re-established, this promotes the satisfactory development of muscles which, for the most part, were underdeveloped from the start because they were used so little in the sucking/swallowing process.

Early repair at a stage when the bone structures are easily remodeled helps to reduce the transverse dimensions of the nasopharynx, which was originally widened by pressure from the tongue. Effective 'closure of the nasopharynx' promises satisfactory velopharyngeal competency, even if the velum is short. Moreover, it should also restore the normal functions of the Eustachian tube. Above all, early closure of the cleft fosters better conditions for phonetic development, as was stressed in Chapter 10 (M.-R. Mousset).

Our modified technique was applied as of the late 1970s. Subsequently, it was encouraging to find a number of articles appearing in favor of early repair (Kaplan, 1981; Dorf and Curtin, 1982). The results of this program cannot be quantified as yet, but they are very clear-cut: speech is more precocious among these children, and parental feed-back functions successfully.

Phonation 1	Normal velopharyngeal competence
Phonation 1/2	Slight and occasional nasal escape
Phonation 2	Permanent nasal escape: velopharyngeal incompetence
Phonation 2/1	Nasal escape is predominant, but the nasopharynx can be closed in some instances (effort, emphatic speech)
Phonation 3	Major nasal escape with compensatory speech patterns such as glottal stops or hoarse pharyngeal fricatives

Fig. 14.1 The Borel–Maisonny scale.

Compared with infants who underwent surgery at a much later age, the differences are very striking.

Insofar as velar insufficiency is concerned, the results have always been evaluated on a strictly clinical basis thanks to repeated testing and assessment on the part of therapists. As soon as the child was capable of co-operating, a program of speech therapy was set up as required.

The results concerning nasal air escape were rated on the Borel–Maisonny scale (Fig. 14.1).

STATISTICAL STUDY

At the 1993 International Congress on cleft palate and related cranio-facial anomalies in Broadbeach (Australia), the first statistical study presented was based on 345 of our patients who underwent surgery using the PP2 technique (early primary veloplasty between 3 and 6 months of age) with complete closure (Malek *et al*, 1993). The statistics covered patients operated on over a 10-year period (1979–89) and who had been submitted to a sufficient number of testing sessions to guarantee a reliable evaluation of speech patterns. This series included 20 children classified as Robin syndrome (see Chapter 15).

To reflect phonetic evolution during the growth cycle, the focus was placed on two different age brackets: 136 case studies were retained.

At age 4:   Of 111 children

$$\left.\begin{array}{l} \text{Ph 1} \quad = 53 \\ \text{Ph 1/2} = 31 \end{array}\right\} = 76\% \text{ competency}$$

$$\left.\begin{array}{l} \text{Ph 2/1} = 13 \\ \text{Ph 2} \quad = 12 \\ \text{Ph 2/3} = 2 \end{array}\right\} \begin{array}{l} = 24\% \text{ marginal cases or} \\ \text{incompetency} \end{array}$$

At ages 5–8:   Of 80 children tested, 55 had been examined at age 4.

Of the 25 not seen at age 4:

$$\left.\begin{array}{l} \text{Ph 1} \quad = 13 \\ \text{Ph 1/2} = 5 \end{array}\right\} \begin{array}{l} 72\% \text{ with good spontaneous} \\ \text{speech patterns} \end{array}$$

$$\left.\begin{array}{l} \text{Ph 2/1} = 3 \\ \text{Ph 2} \quad = 3 \\ \text{Ph 3} \quad = 1 \end{array}\right\} \begin{array}{l} 28\% \text{ of marginal cases or} \\ \text{incompetency, who were} \\ \text{oriented towards speech} \\ \text{therapy followed by} \\ \text{pharyngoplasty} \end{array}$$

Of the 55 already seen age age 4:

Ph 1   = 32   (8 had undergone
                   pharyngoplasty)

Ph 1/2 = 14   (1 pharyngoplasty)

$$\left.\begin{array}{l} \text{Ph 2/1} = 7 \\ \text{Ph 2} \quad = 2 \\ \text{Ph 3} \quad = 0 \end{array}\right\} \begin{array}{l} \text{(9 were oriented towards} \\ \text{pharyngoplasty)} \end{array}$$

According to these statistics, among our oldest patients (111 children born between 1979 and 1986) 18 (16.2 per cent) underwent pharyngoplasty. This figure may sound high, but it reflects the more demanding standards now applied. Formerly, some degree of nasal air emission was deemed acceptable if it did not compromise intelligibility. Nowadays, we are determined to eliminate nasal air escape altogether.

Lastly, 10 children presented with hearing disorders (40 per cent loss). This statistic must be compared with those of classical surgery.

COMPARISON WITH SPEECH DEVELOPMENT FOLLOWING LATE SURGICAL CORRECTION

At 6 months, an infant with cleft palate develops the same mandibular activity as normal children in this age group and vocalizes or babbles in syllabic sequences combining consonant and vowel repetition.

However, although the infant exercises the pharyngeal muscles, the cleft palate prevents closure of the nasopharynx. The infant cannot build up enough pressure to produce plosive consonants of the [p], [t], [k] type, and the only consonant sounds that can be pronounced are the nasals such as [m] or [n]. The babbling is slow, monotonous and indistinct, and is characterized by hypernasal resonance interspersed with glottal stops.

Such vocal emissions do not stimulate parental feed-back. The parents are not encouraged to respond, and do not recognize consistent – let alone meaningful – sounds.

Later on, in efforts to imitate language and make him- or herself understood, the infant tends to resort to the only point of occlusion possible which is the glottal stop. The latter develops into a compensatory speech pattern substituted for plosive consonants.

The child's emergent language skills are therefore acquired according to abnormal neuromotor patterns, which may subsist long after the soft palate has been reconstructed.

Statistics on staphylorraphies performed at 18 months (P. Oger, 1976)

Of 657 cases:

$$\left.\begin{array}{l} \text{Ph 1} \quad = 268 \\ \text{Ph 1/2} \quad = 140 \end{array}\right\} \begin{array}{l} = 408 \text{ or} \\ 62.1\% \end{array}$$

$$\left.\begin{array}{l} \left.\begin{array}{l} \text{Ph 1/2/3} = 11 \\ \text{Ph 2G} \quad = 106 \\ \text{Ph 2M} \quad = 51 \end{array}\right\} = 168 \\ \left.\begin{array}{l} \text{Ph 2/3} \quad = 24 \\ \text{Ph 3} \quad = 33 \\ \text{Ph 0} \quad = 24 \end{array}\right\} = 81 \end{array}\right\} \begin{array}{l} = 249 \text{ or} \\ 37.9\% \end{array}$$

15. Pierre Robin syndrome

This chapter was prepared with the collaboration of Patrice Oger.

Pierre Robin syndrome deserves a chapter of its own within a work devoted to labio-palatal malformations.

Robin described the association of respiratory and digestive disorders linked to micrognathia. A great number of problems are involved with this syndrome:

1. Definition and fixing the limits of what is covered by Robin syndrome, details of which remain hazy and controversial (particularly as to the presence or absence of cleft palate).
2. Clinical description – confusion exists between those symptoms specific to the syndrome and those secondary to its development or which concern associated malformations.
3. Interpretation of the etiology of the physio-pathological disorders it involves – purely mechanical causes according to some; neuro-functional immaturity of the aero-digestive system to others.
4. Therapeutic outlook, which varies from one school to another.

HISTORICAL OVERVIEW AND PROBLEMS OF DEFINITION

This pathology is a fairly recent finding. It is customarily attributed to Pierre Robin, who reported it in 1923; hence the widely recognized diagnostic eponym.

Robin, a Parisian stomatologist, coined the term glossoptosis, which refers to the tendency of the tongue to fall back into the air passages. In his opinion, this anomalous position was linked to a defect in mandibular growth (micrognathia). Micrognathia itself could be either primary (congenital hypoplasia) or secondary to a wide range of causes. As the base of the tongue shifts backward and downward, it presses against the posterior pharyngeal wall. This produces narrowing and, at times, obstruction of the airway at a point situated above the larynx.

It is interesting that Robin did not insist on the presence of cleft palate, although he had observed it in his seminal case. In later publications, and particularly in his work on glossoptosis, it was not even mentioned. In an article published in the US in 1934, Robin quoted a study by Eley et al. (1930), which included a patient with cleft palate. He saw this malformation as a simple aggravating factor. Thus, according to Robin, the major feature of this disorder was mandibular hypoplasia.

It is also intriguing to remark, in passing, that Veau did not make a single allusion to this pathology in his book on palatal clefts (1938).

Only around the time of World War II, and above all during the 1960s and 1970s, did publications on Robin syndrome begin to appear in significant numbers. The development of pediatrics and of neonatal intensive care units led to a complete inventory of pathological obstructions of the upper airway in newborns. Progress in therapeutics helped to reduce the high rate of mortality in serious cases.

Cleft palate came to be considered a major factor in the description of the syndrome. Cases of Robin syndrome without cleft palate consistently involve a mandibular pathology which justifies their inclusion, according to certain authors. Such non-cleft cases are uncommon.

In an attempt to more clearly delineate the symptomatology, North American specialists first adopted the term Robin 'anomalad'. It was used to designate a non-specific symptom complex of diverse etiology, resulting in respiratory and swallowing disorders. Over the years, Robin 'sequence' came to be preferred to 'anomalad'. This term clearly indicates that a large number of secondary clinical signs can be traced to an initial factor, which many recognized as micrognathia, thus confirming Robin's original hypothesis. Although the theory is debatable, the term Robin sequence does contribute to a more accurate understanding of the pathology, and it has gained acceptance world-wide.

For facial cleft surgeons, Robin syndrome is defined by a triad of clinical criteria:

• Retrognathia
• Severe respiratory and/or digestive disorders in early infancy
• Cleft palate.

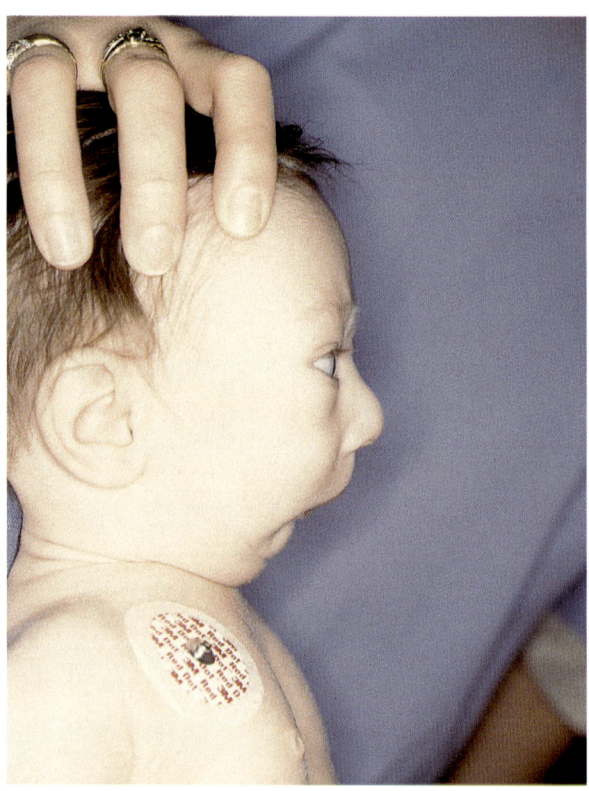

Fig. 15.1 *Characteristic profile of an infant with pronounced retrognathia.*

CLINICAL FORMS

The prenatal diagnosis of suspected retrognathia is often established due to family antecedents. It is sometimes combined with oligoamniosis. The diagnosis is generally made in the maternity ward, at birth or shortly thereafter.

Presentation

These infants present with a characteristic facial appearance, where the underdeveloped chin immediately suggests the presence of a cleft palate (Fig. 15.1).

The cleft may take different forms, and may involve only the velum. It can be V- or U-shaped, in which case its considerable width and extremely frail stumps are particularly typical. The form is often bilateral, since it extends considerably into the bony vault (Fig. 15.2).

The tongue tends to be small and retropositioned, with its tip pointing upward. In the floor of the mouth on either side of the midline a transverse protrusion can be observed, which corresponds to a

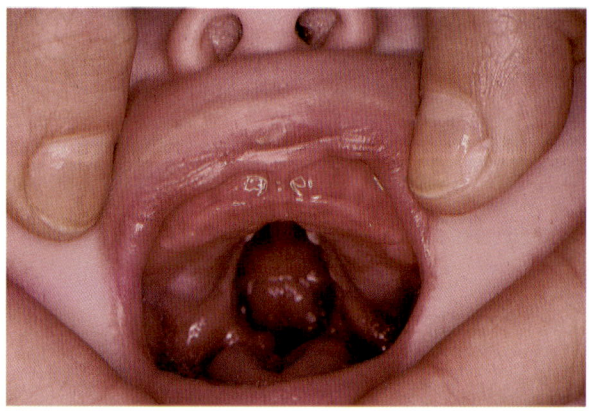

Fig. 15.2 *Cleft palate, bilateral V-shaped form.*

pronounced sublingual ridge (Fig. 15.3).

Respiratory distress may be more or less severe, and is characterized by inspiratory dyspnea with suprasternal, epigastric and even sternal depressions, which can be pronounced because the ribcage is not very sturdy at this age (Fig. 15.4). A state of acute asphyxia may set in, accompanied by cyanosis of the extremities, and

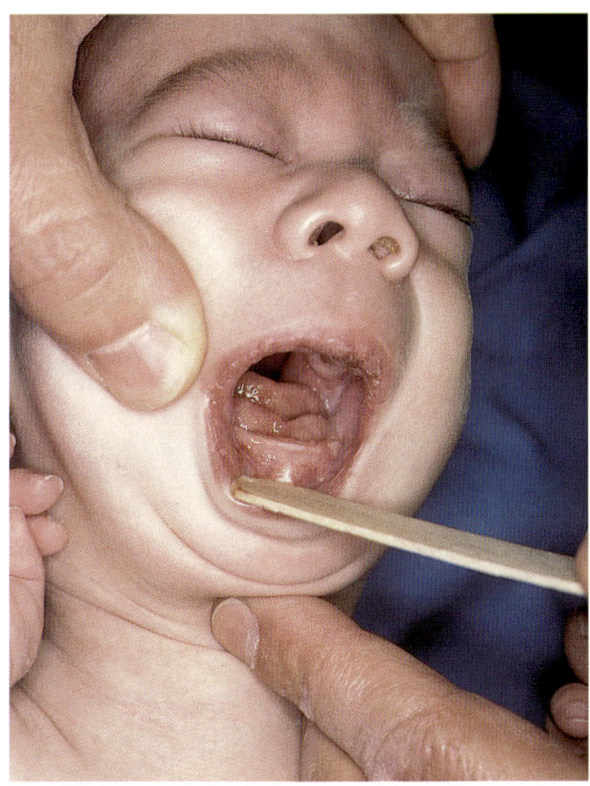

Fig. 15.3 Small tongue rotated backward, protruding sublingual ridge.

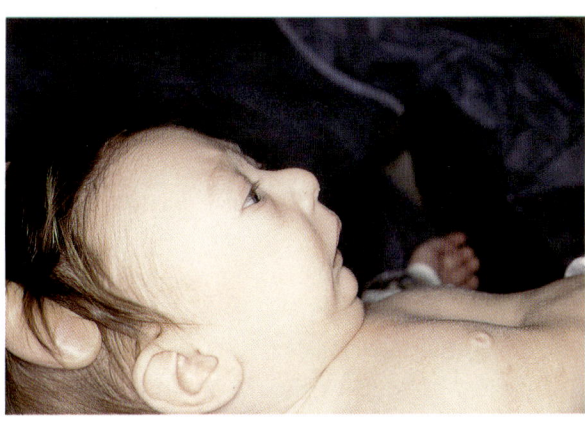

Fig. 15.4 Sternal depression during inspiration is often very pronounced.

emergency measures may be required to secure the airways. If at all feasible, the infant should be admitted to a neonatal intensive care unit for examination by a surgeon specialized in the treatment of clefts.

The situation may be less life-threatening, and immediate prone positioning is sometimes sufficient to relieve breathing difficulties. However, acute distress may occur at any moment.

In this context, feeding problems take on particular prominence. The infant is unable to suckle, whether breast or bottle (dyspnea may be prompted or aggravated in the process). Milk intake is often insignificant, and the infant becomes exhausted by vain efforts. Weight loss soon arouses concern, and leads to nasogastric feeding. Repeated insertion of a nasogastric tube becomes an arduous process. On the other hand, if kept in place the tube triggers hypersecretion of the mucous membranes, which may increase the breathing problems.

Assessment

During the first days after admission to the surgical ward or pediatric intensive care unit, a complete check-up is performed.

Respiratory problems

Above all, an evaluation of respiratory compromise is performed.

Blood gas monitoring is the most important continuous test:

- It provides data on the level of oxygen (Sat O_2). The reading decreases during crying or feeding attempts.
- It is essential to ascertain the quantity of CO_2 in the blood stream if a valid prognosis of the adequacy of ventilation is to be established.
- The amount of alkali reserve is also a useful item of information, since it is proportional to acidosis in the blood, caused in turn by hypercarbia.

Polysomnography is performed if possible, but this is not of major importance. However, it may help to determine the particulars of surgical treatment.

Episodes of apnea of peripheral origin are recorded, which reflect airway obstruction due to glossoptosis. Their frequency may indicate a risk of subacute hypoxia.

Intermittent apnea of central origin would uphold the theories of those who attribute a neurological source to the disorder. The fact is that episodes of this type of apnea occur in all newborn infants. Their only significance might be their unusual frequency. Still, this is not a consistent phenomenon among the majority of young patients, and obstructive apnea is far more common.

Feeding problems

The assessment of feeding problems is next on the agenda. In most cases, breast feeding is impossible. Attempts at bottle feeding must be conducted with caution, under conditions that will be discussed in a later section. They generally obtain poor results.

Intake may be impossible because feeding aggravates respiratory distress and may induce syncope of the neurovagal type, which is a cause for serious concern. Alternatively, if intake is inadequate, the frequency of feeding must be increased, and recourse to nasogastric feeding then becomes imperative.

The risk of food going down the wrong way must be taken into account, but does not occur with any significant frequency.

The possibility of an additional digestive disorder, particularly a gastro-esophageal reflux must be subject to routine investigation. It may well be responsible for syncope, and requires curative or preventive treatment.

Associated abnormalities

The detection of associated malformations is essential to the prognosis.

It is important to evaluate the neurological condition of the newborn infant. The clinical examination should be supported by a transglabellar ultrasound examination, or even by a CT scan, which may reveal anomalies of the encephalon, the corpus callosum or the ventricles. The infant's tonicity varies according to its weight and respiratory condition. Reflexes are not easy to test in these cases.

Examination of the cardiovascular system may show a murmur, which suggests a malformation of the aurico-ventricular ostium or an abnormal communication between the right and left sides of the heart. Arrhythmia is often observed. Here, too, ultrasound is indicated, as are X-rays of the cardiac image and an electrocardiogram.

An eye examination is difficult in the first days of life, but the ophthalmologist is called for consultation because there may be specific associated malformations.

Finally, the general check-up and orthopedic examination furnish results that may vary from case to case. A blood count may detect anomalies in the cell color ratio linked to hypoxia. A rather paradoxical anemia may show up as well.

A prognosis can be formulated and a program of treatment implemented after the first few days of hospitalization.

Severe forms

There are severe forms of Robin syndrome which are life-threatening emergencies, and these include respiratory and digestive forms.

Respiratory forms

Respiratory forms may begin with a dramatic incident of acute asphyxia, or gradually set in with a state of precarious oxygenation. For various reasons, there is a constant risk of aggravated hypoxia or of developing a subacute condition. Prolonged hypoxia presents a risk for the brain (it may produce cortical degeneration) and/or for the heart. Combined with hypercarbia, hypoxia leads to elevated pulmonary-vascular resistance, and eventually to right-sided heart failure or cor pulmonale.

Rising pH levels cause renal compensation, with an accumulation of bicarbonates. This reading is a more reliable sign of subacute hypoxia than blood gas rates. O_2/CO_2 levels can be misleading, as they vary over a period of time proportionally to changes in breathing.

Freeing the airways is an emergency procedure that will restore normal metabolic balance provided it is carried out immediately.

Digestive forms

Digestive forms are often accompanied by respiratory risk during bottle-feeding.

Feeding presents tremendous difficulties, with weight loss leading to the constant need for nasogastric tube feeding, which does little to improve the problems of sucking and swallowing and contributes to the irritation of the aero-digestive passages by causing hypersecretion.

When treatment of these severe forms proves difficult or doubtful, surgery must be considered. Currently, however, the techniques can only provide temporary relief.

Mild forms

In less severe forms, appropriate nursing care, keeping the infant in ventral decubitus, and more frequent, lighter feeds backed up by intermittent nasogastric feeding will help get through the first days and even the first weeks more calmly, while avoiding possible complications.

It is advisable to keep the infant in hospital, because there is the constant risk of the respiratory condition worsening due to intercurrent phenomena such as secondary pulmonary infection.

Appropriate methods of treatment are most controversial where these forms are concerned. This is particularly true of the decision as to if and when primary surgery (especially velar repair) should be undertaken.

Associated forms

These often come under the heading of well-defined syndromes involving lesions that must be clearly differentiated from possible complications of the standard forms outlined above.

From personal experience, syndromic forms are rare. They seem to figure far more frequently in statistics published elsewhere, particularly in Anglo-Saxon studies. There is no known explanation for this rather baffling difference.

The most well-known syndromes include the following.

The Stickler syndrome is characterized by its association with the Robin sequence. It is typified by ocular disorders and, in particular, severe myopia. This condition can be treated and blindness forestalled, providing the diagnosis is made early on. Additional ocular disorders may also be detected. There is no need to provide an exhaustive list here because they concern the ophthalmologist, who is routinely consulted in cases of Robin syndrome. However, retinal detachment is very important and should be mentioned.

Skeletal defects, with hypermobility of the ligaments and spondylo-epiphyseal dysplasia visible on X-ray, may also occur.

The Di George syndrome is far less common. It involves aplasia of the thymus and parathyroid glands and may be combined with a Robin-type symptom complex.

Cardiac anomalies are common. The diagnosis must be rapid, based on immediate auscultation, an electrocardiogram and, later if need be, a digitalized angiography or catheterization. It is essential to make the distinction between these disorders and those caused by pulmonary hypertension or cor pulmonale linked to recurrent hypoxia due to glossoptosis.

The velocardiofacial syndrome (VCFS), isolated by Schprintzen *et al.* (1978), seems to occur frequently, at least in North America. It is reportedly linked to a defective chromosome 22.

A vast number of additional congenital abnormalities could be added to the list. Despite what certain authors contend, these are not directly related to Robin syndrome, but can probably be attributed to a teratogenic incident some time during the embryonic period.

INTERPRETATION OF PATHOLOGICAL DISORDERS

The interpretation of pathological disorders linked to Robin syndrome or 'sequence' remains hazy and controversial. It is nonetheless essential to the establishment of a coherent and efficient program of treatment.

An important question hinges on whether the *primum movens*, or primary cause, is pathognomic or not. In other words, is there an initial phenomenon of pathological anatomy which gives rise to a chain or cascade of secondary anomalies?

The roles of micrognathia, functional dysmaturity of the nervous system and, lastly, of cleft palate will be studied in turn.

Micrognathia (mandibular hypoplasia)

Robins's initial hypothesis linked these disorders in their entirety to mandibular hypoplasia. In his opinion, hypoplasia causes the tongue as a whole (including its floor) to shift backward towards the spinal column, thus creating a low obstruction of the upper airway at the level of the oropharynx. Furthermore, as the tongue moves backward it falls downward into the throat and under its pressure, the epiglottis becomes horizontal. This phenomenon compounds oropharyngeal obstruction with reduced

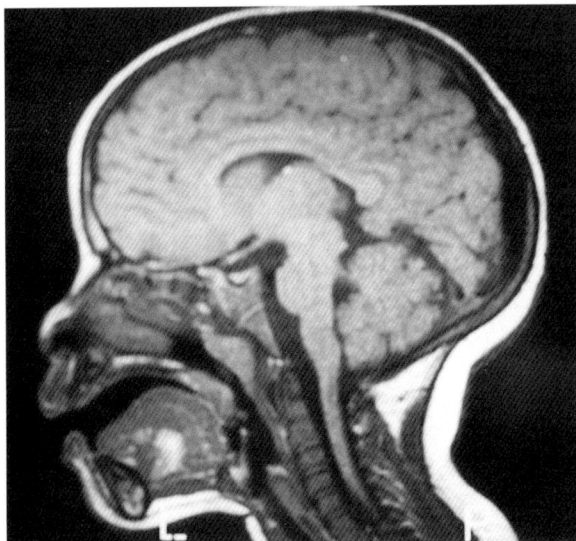

a

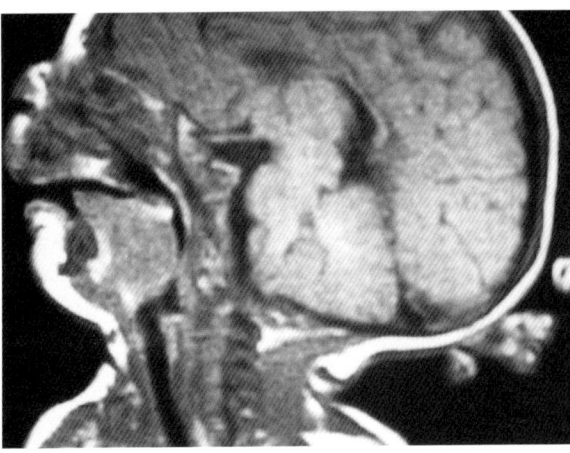

b

Fig. 15.5 *MRI profile view of face.*
a. Normal image. Closed faucial isthmus rests on the base of the tongue, with the epiglottis in a vertical position.
b. Robin syndrome. The tongue is rotated backward, with the base touching the posterior wall of the pharynx.

access to the laryngeal orifice.

To describe these phenomena, Robin coined the term glossoptosis, which was to gain world-wide recognition.

Robin's work (1928) set forth a number of concepts worth retaining:

1. The essential idea that tongue retraction produces low obstruction of the airways has been confirmed by endoscopy and video-fluoroscopy, as well as by MRI profile images (Figs 15.5a and b). However, these examinations do not reveal retrodisplacement of the hyoid bone towards the spinal column. The base of the tongue itself swings backward and bulges, hernia-like, towards the pharynx above the hyoid bone.

2. Robin also had an interesting theory on sucking disorders. He believed that milk intake is difficult for affected infants because they cannot close the front of their mouth properly. (At the time, Robin was not aware that a palatal cleft produces the same effect: intra-oral pressure cannot be lowered unless the cavity is sealed tight, and sealing cannot be obtained if there is constant oro-nasal communication.) Infants are therefore unable to compress the nipple of breast or bottle at the proper level to extract milk and draw it inward.

3. Robin explained digestive problems as being due to constant aerophagia and insalivation resulting in flatulence, and disorders of the Eustachian tube as being due to defective reflexes of the aero-digestive junction.

If mandibular hypoplasia is accepted as the primary cause, it might also explain how and why cleft palate occurs. During embryogenesis, the tongue may not descend as it normally should in the course of facial development when the neck flexes upward. Forced backward, it remains positioned between the palatal shelves as they grow, and obstructs their fusion on the midline. The obturating presence of the tongue would therefore explain the U-shaped palatal cleft.

If such were the case, mandibular abnormality would indeed be the primary factor that triggers a cascade of secondary anomalies.

In itself, micrognathia can be ascribed to a variety of causes:

- Positional deformity, linked to protracted downward flexion of the neck towards the fetal thorax due to intrauterine constriction (oligohydramnios, crowding from multiple embryos, uterine abnormality).
- Genetic, as encountered in certain syndromes. Schprintzen pointed out typical antegonial notching in the horizontal ramus of the mandible, which is a constant in Stickler syndrome.
- Neuromuscular, such as muscle tone disorders or myotonia; lack of 'mandibular exercise', i.e.

intrauterine mandibular movements which promote normal growth.

- Lastly, tissue disorders, which affect bone tissue (Larsen syndrome, politeal pterygium syndrome).

Neurological origin

Many practitioners, pediatricians or surgeons attribute the disorders of Robin syndrome to a neurological cause. This interpretation favors a dysfunction of the aero-digestive tract produced, theoretically, by a congenital abnormality or by dysmaturity of the central nervous system control seated in the brain stem. The etiology of Robin syndrome might thus be traced to a disorder of the central nervous system.

Certain specialists carry the theory even further (Couly *et al.*, 1988), and link this neurological anomaly to a 'dysneurulation of the rhomben-cephalon'. Neurulation is a stage of development that takes place between the 20th and 50th days of embryonic life. During this period, the neural tube is formed and cells from the neural crests migrate towards the periphery. These neural crests make up the different structures of the head and neck.

Robin syndrome could be the result of a neurochristopathy (disorder of cell migration), which might explain subsequent malformations (cleft palate and associated defects). Micrognathia itself might reflect a fetal sucking disorder.

Be that as it may, these rather esoteric definitions are of little assistance in understanding the clinical signs that are observed. Nor have we found, in our experience, that they explain the rapid and complete reversal of these same signs after veloplasty.

The evidence listed below is used to support the neurological theory but it is not wholly conclusive:

- Postmortems of victims of sudden infant death syndrome (mistakenly linked to Robin syndrome) purportedly revealed a reduced number of motor neurons in the brain stem (Ollsson, cited in Couly *et al.*, 1988).
- Tests such as polysomnography do indeed show incidents of central apnea alongside obstructive apnea but, as stated earlier, these episodes occur among all newborns. Could they be more frequent or longer lasting? Our observations do not confirm such findings.

- EMGs of muscles in the vicinity do not reveal peripheral symptoms, but this does not furnish sufficient grounds to permit a distinction between reflex and initial central disorders.
- Studies of auditory-evoked potentials furnish little relevant data.

All in all, the hypothesis of a neurological origin for Robin syndrome is unsubstantiated, to say the least.

In our opinion, the major flaw of this theory resides in the fact that it inevitably inspires a program of palliative treatment over a long period of time, to the exclusion of direct corrective action. While awaiting a spontaneous improvement in the aero-digestive functions (through maturation), the infant is subjected in the meantime to constant nasogastric feeding, which can last several months. Tracheostomy is performed to guard against acute or subacute obstructive respiratory problems, but this does have side-effects in very young infants.

Cleft palate

Cleft palate could, in itself, explain the entire range of symptoms, and it represents a third interpretation of Robin syndrome.

Memo on the consequences of cleft palate

In the physio-pathological study of isolated cleft palate, it has already been seen that sucking and swallowing disorders are caused by the existence of the cleft. During the swallowing process, the tongue is forced to enter the nasopharynx in order to move

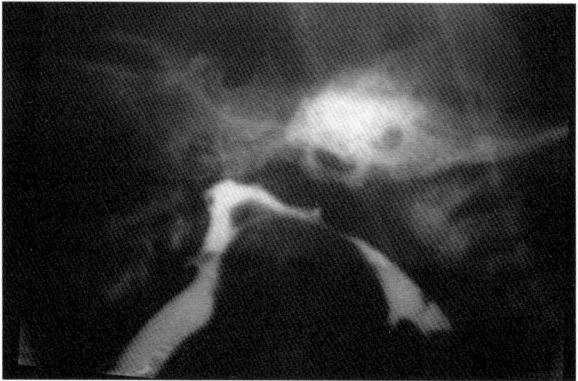

Fig. 15.6 During deglutition, the tongue penetrates the nasopharynx and pushes the stumps of the cleft velum to the side.

the bolus of food towards the esophagus. In so doing, it makes contact with the posterior wall of the pharynx. This backward tongue pressure is largely responsible for widening the pharynx (a well-known phenomenon demonstrated by the divergence of the pterygoid processes) (Fig. 15.6).

Backward displacement of the tongue also explains the receding jaw. This retrognathia is often observed in cases of isolated cleft palate; hence the term 'Robin-like syndrome', which adds to the difficulties of clear-cut delineation.

The choanae are undersized due to tongue pressure on the posterior margin of the palatal shelves. Breathing is largely oral.

This tongue position and functional disorder disrupt the first phase of swallowing, and may lead to additional problems further down the digestive tract since the reflexes are affected. The existence of gastro-esophageal reflux (GER) in particular is probably a result of asynchronous functioning of the esophageal sphincters.

It is even more enlightening to observe what happens during the breathing process in both isolated cleft palate and Robin-like syndrome, when the laryngo-tracheal system has to descend. The tongue remains in its posterior position, but only moderately, and breathing space is adequate so signs of dyspnea do not usually appear except in cases of superinfection.

How can cleft palate be distinguished from severe Robin syndrome?

It would seem logical to conclude that it is only a question of degree due to an anatomical difference.

The role of micrognathia, whether primary or secondary to cleft palate, brings us back to the first of the physio-pathological interpretations. Whatever the degree, the entire range fits into this framework and the notion of 'Robin-like syndrome' is easy to justify.

The magnitude of the palatal cleft is also a factor (broad clefts may have more severe repositioning of the tongue). A specific phenomenon may occur in what are known as horseshoe or U-shaped clefts. The retracted tongue is often small in size with its tip pointing upward, and it may become impacted between the velar stumps within the nasopharynx, catching on the upper borders of the cleft and thus producing an alarming episode of acute asphyxia. This is easy to understand in U-shaped clefts, but, practi-cally speaking, certain V-shaped forms involve a similar risk of asphyxia.

The series of symptoms observed in severe forms of Robin syndrome, other than those connected with airway obstruction, could be explained by cleft palate alone. This remark will be developed in detail in the following chapter. However, at present it seems logical to presume that, if the anatomy of the aero-digestive junction (which is recognized as a major reflexogenic zone) is abnormal, then the reflexes associated with it will automatically be affected. The reasons for sucking/swallowing disorders have already been examined, including 'wrong way' degluti-tion and GER, which are no doubt of reflex origin; the lesion at the junction of the aero-digestive systems modifies the succession of contractions further down the line. GER itself may cause spells of vagal syncope. Problems of cardiac rhythm (again of the vagal type) can also be attributed to a reflex origin.

Moreover, the associated malformations that seem to compound the problem are only related to it by coincidences of the embryopathic calendar.

A major question seems relevant here: Why are no tell-tale signs of Robin syndrome observed in complete uni- or bilateral labio-palatal clefts, however severe? After all, cleft palate does produce the same consequences on retropositioning of the tongue, at least during phases of sucking/swallowing activity.

This question can only be answered by hypotheses:

1. It may be that retrognathia plays a predominant role here as well. It does not intervene to the same degree in labio-maxillo-palatal clefts. The causes and the mechanisms responsible for non-fusion of the facial growth buds vary according to the different stages of the embryonic timetable.
2. Isolated cleft palate occurs during a later phase of embryonic development, at a period when micrognathia is more likely to appear.
3. It might also be thought that the tongue has more space towards the front of the oral cavity, due to widening of the cleft between the anterior maxillary segments.

Whatever the case, this remains a thorny question in a discussion intended to demonstrate the decisive role of cleft palate.

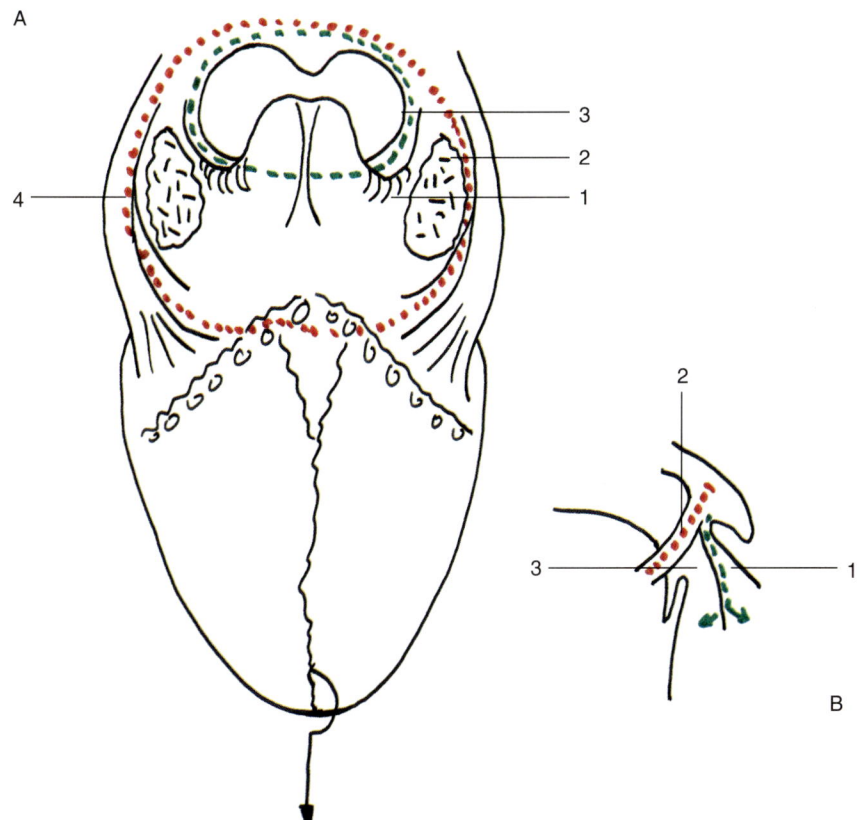

Fig. 15.7 Oropharyngeal isthmuses: red, isthmus of the fauces; green, pharyngo-nasal isthmus.

A. Base of the tongue, seen from above.

1. Lateral fold between tongue and epiglottis
2. Tonsil
3. Fold between pharynx and epiglottis. Posterior tonsillar pillar
4. Anterior tonsillar pillar

B. Location of isthmuses on profile view.

1. Posterior tonsillar pillar
2. Anterior tonsillar pillar
3. Tonsil area

Our working hypothesis

Our suggestion is based essentially on the third physio-pathological interpretation: that cleft palate is the main cause.

As soon as our technique for closing the cleft at a very early age had been perfected, we asked the following question: Could veloplasty shift the tongue forward, particularly during the breathing process when the digestive system is at rest? If this were the case, adequate breathing space should be established. In addition to restoring the tongue to its proper place, palatal closure should also re-establish satisfactory physiological conditions at the aero-digestive junction, thus achieving a return to nasal breathing, efficient sucking and normal swallowing. As the reflex disorders were corrected, the chain of problems involving the rest of the tract should disappear as well.

In order to justify this hypothesis, at least from a theoretical point of view, a closer study of the factors linked to glossoptosis and more specifically of the isthmus of the fauces and the pharyngo-nasal isthmus, their definitions and respective roles must be made (Fig. 15.7).

The isthmus of the fauces represents the posterior opening of the oral cavity. It is normally bounded:

- Laterally, by the anterior pillars of the fauces or palato-glossal arches.
- Superiorly, by the under surface of the soft palate. Its anterior portion (palatine aponeurosis) is relatively fixed. Inclined on a backward and downward slant, it continues the lower surface of the bony palatal vault (this zone forms a concave arch that is in fact capable of a slight up and down movement, but only at its very center). The posterior portion of the normal soft palate shows greater mobility, moving like a door with its hinges along the transverse line where it joins the anterior portion. Seen in longitudinal section, the soft palate thus resembles a valve.
- Inferiorly, by the tongue – or to be more specific, by a surface that corresponds to the base of the tongue, flanked by the epiglottis behind it. The latter follows the movements of the hyoid bone, and is also subject to pressure exerted by the base of the tongue. This causes the angle of its slant to range from vertical to horizontal.

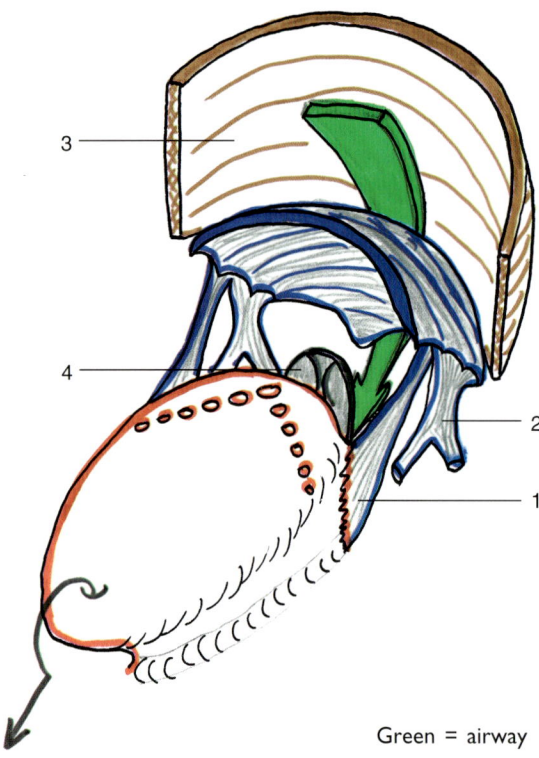

3

4

2

1

Green = airway

Fig. 15.8 '*Parachute*' *mechanism, which keeps airway free. Harnesses are represented by the anterior and posterior pillars (palatoglossi and palatopharyngei).*

1. *Pilaris anterior*
2. *Posterior pillar*
3. *Constrictor superior*
4. *Epiglottis*

The pharyngo-nasal isthmus is situated behind the isthmus of the fauces. It is formed by the soft palate and the posterior pillars of the fauces, which correspond to the arch of the underlying palato-pharyngeal muscles.

For a normal individual in a state of rest, i.e. breathing, the faucial isthmus is virtually closed (Fig. 15.8). The soft palate fits over the base of the tongue like a parachute, drawn at the same time forward and downward by its harness, represented here by the velar arches. As described above, the arches or pillars are formed by the palatoglossus for the anterior pillars and by the palato-pharyngeus for the posterior. The latter muscles, which are far more developed than the former, are thought to play the predominant role. They are placed in a state of passive tension when the pharyngo-laryngeal system descends during

inspiration and expiration. As a result, the soft palate is lowered, shifting the base of the tongue forward, and the posterior pillars are drawn closer together. The epiglottis then becomes vertical and its upper edge nears the uvula, which frees the laryngeal passageway (Fig. 15.9).

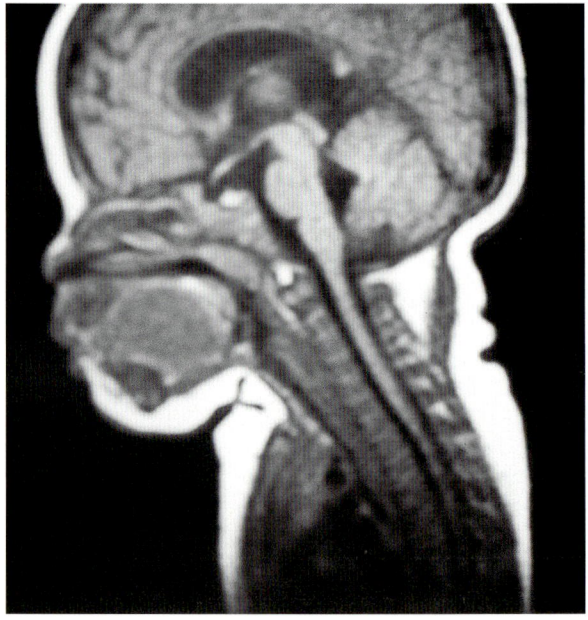

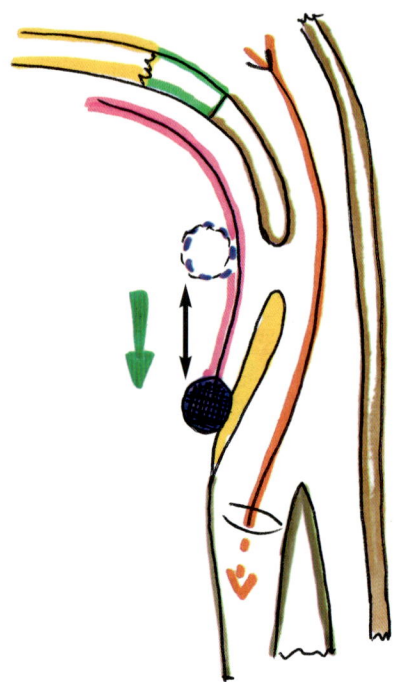

Fig. 15.9 In a normal infant, the patency of the airway is maintained when the base of the tongue is blocked by the 'parachute' under tension during descent of the airway.

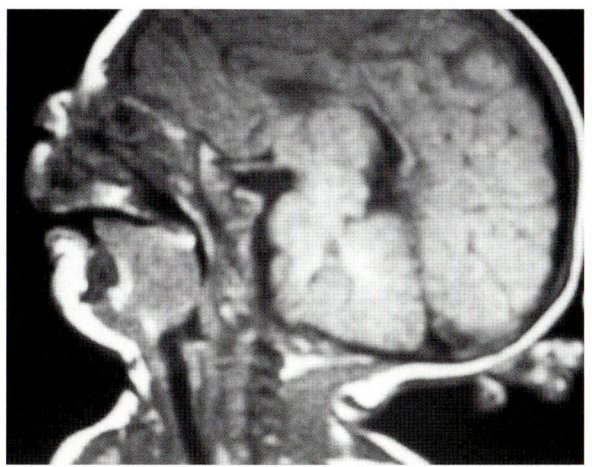

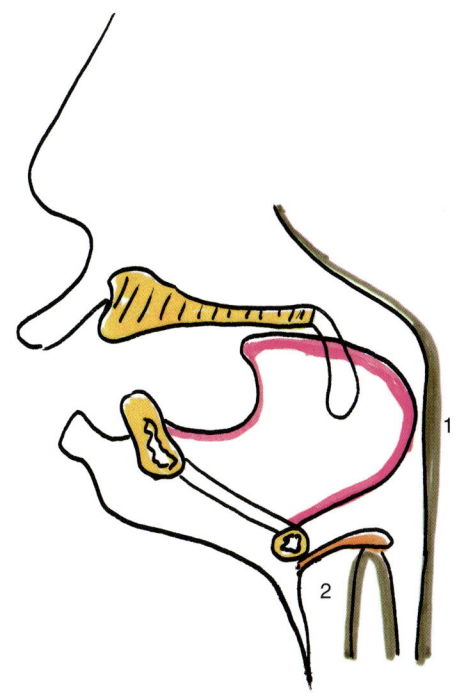

Fig. 15.10 *In Robin syndrome, the narrow base of the tongue favors its backward rotation since the parachute mechanism is missing. Notice the bend in the airway at the laryngeal vestibule. Areas marked 1 and 2 are described in the text.*

During the process, all these elements – the velum in particular – are at some distance from the posterior wall of the pharynx, with the pharyngeal constrictors at rest. The hyoid bone is in a low position (this bone is known to move in only two directions; up during swallowing and down during breathing).

Therefore, the airway is always patent, whatever the position of the subject. In dorsal decubitus in particu-

lar, the weight of the tongue has no effect. Its base is maintained by the velum, which functions as a type of cradle or sling. The image of the parachute seems particularly appropriate here. Keeping the airway clear depends on a certain amount of motor activity, which calls into play those muscles that determine the position of the hyoid bone and those that lower the soft palate. In the latter case, the action is mainly passive resistance to retrodisplacement of the tongue.

However, when there is an anomaly of the faucial and pharyngo-nasal isthmuses, air flow may be compromised by the disappearance of the parachute mechanism, which allows the base of the tongue to retract.

This tongue retraction is more likely to occur when the insertion of the lingual muscle mass in the floor of the mouth is comparatively narrow, as demonstrated by lateral X-rays or MRI (Fig. 15.10).

The base of the tongue therefore approaches the posterior wall of the pharynx (1 in Fig. 15.10). The floor of the tongue does not shift backward, as Robin contended; rather, the base of the tongue rotates around the hyoid bone, which represents a fixed point, as stated earlier (Bosma *et al.*, 1965) (Fig. 15.11). The epiglottis (2 in Fig. 15.10) becomes horizontal and further constricts the airway. Lateral X-rays show that the passage is bent almost at a right angle above the thyroid.

This type of airway constriction can be aggravated to

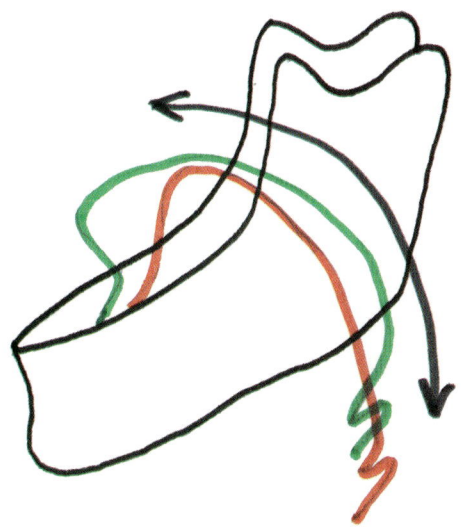

Fig. 15.11 *Rotation and lowering of the tongue according to Bosma et al. 1965.*

the point of complete obstruction by a phenomenon familiar to physicists. Bernouilli's theorem comes to mind, but it would be more accurate to refer to Venturi's phenomenon, which is more relevant to the movement of gases. This phenomenon produces a centripetal attraction on the walls of a flexible duct when gas passes through a narrowed portion of the tube. The diameter of the elastic tube is reduced even further in the process. Thus a vicious circle sets in and, in this context, gradually aggravates respiratory compromise.

In our opinion, this discussion gives a clear explanation of the phenomena involved in what Pierre Robin called glossoptosis.

As Robin observed, position has no effect on normal subjects. However, it can significantly modify the degree of obstruction in pathological cases. Indeed, ventral decubitus (which brings the weight of the tongue into play) and, above all, opening the mouth do cause the base of the tongue to shift forward to some extent. This explains the benefits of a prone position. Related hyperextension of the head also advances the jaw and, therefore, the tongue.

We have come to believe that, in cases where retrognathia is not too severe, veloplasty offers the ideal solution to the problems of infants with Robin syndrome and guarantees rapid recovery. It restores the normal anatomy and physiology of the faucial and pharyngo-nasal isthmuses and re-establishes the aptly named parachute mechanism. This is the hypothesis on which our experimental program was based, and it has produced very favorable results (see Statistics, below).

In cases where retrognathia is extremely severe, correction by simple veloplasty will take time. Nonetheless, cleft palate repair can greatly improve the situation, particularly regarding the reflex phenomena described earlier.

Contrary to certain preconceived ideas, veloplasty in no way aggravates the obstruction. The initial blockage is located below the palate and is removed by velar repair, which restores the possibility of nasal breathing customary to young infants.

Needless to say, during the first days of life before veloplasty can be performed, these infants may require neonatal intensive care.

TREATMENT – RESULTS

Treatment involves two totally distinct aspects:

1. Treatment of a potential acute phase before any etiological measures are undertaken.
2. Treatment during a secondary phase, when corrective procedures intervene.

The first days of life

Respiratory problems

At times, treatment is required for true asphyxia, which does not respond to simple face-down positioning.

Remembering that the obstruction is located low in the oropharynx, simple probe will not solve the problem but will afford only temporary relief. The Guesdel tube or Mayo cannula, improved and adapted for use in small infants, can, thanks to its form and volume, shift the base of the tongue forward and restore a certain amount of airflow. However, nasopharyngeal tubes must be of considerable length in order to reach beyond the obstruction deep in the throat, and are not easily tolerated. They irritate the membranes, cause mucus hypersecretion and impair swallowing. The lesions they leave may become a long-term source of constriction.

Endotracheal intubation is effective, of course, but has disadvantages. First, initial placement is difficult. Visualizing the glottis is complicated by the right-angled bend in the pharyngo-laryngeal vestibule and by the horizontal epiglottis, which forms a screen. Anesthesiologists have described a great many helpful tricks of the trade, particularly in view of the fact that drugs of the curare type are proscribed until their successful use is guaranteed. These include intubation in a prone position, by nasal tube or 'blind' (guided by airflow), or after placement of a lighted stylet visible beneath the skin. Fibroscopic intubation represents an advance, but calls for equipment specially adapted to the size and age of tiny infants and requires a good deal of experience. Secondly, although the endotracheal tube is useful in cases of acute distress, it cannot be left in place over a long period – certainly not for the length of time generally necessary for the initial symptoms to show significant improvement.

It seems that one valid solution to the problems of intubation lies in the use of a laryngeal mask. The mechanism of this device meets the specific needs of the problem; the mask lifts the base of the tongue and thrusts it forward. Again, however, the device cannot be left in place for more than a few hours at a time, since it also obstructs the digestive passages. However, as a pre-operative measure it offers a worthwhile alternative if intubation fails.

If the foregoing maneuvers are not successful and the blood gas reading is poor, tracheostomy becomes inevitable. This is a difficult procedure when the infant presents acute obstruction and cannot be anesthetized under satisfactory conditions. In these circumstances, the laryngeal mask is of great assistance.

In actual practice, acute asphyxia is fortunately far less common than obstructive dyspnea, which usually responds to simple prone positioning and minor procedures like intubation, keeping the infant under close observation.

Once the oxygen level is satisfactory, round-the-clock surveillance and nursing care should suffice to get the infant through the waiting period.

During this interval, which might be termed the early secondary phase, a number of specialists advocate certain operative measures intended to correct glossoptosis and prevent an acute episode, provided the patient's general condition permits.

The oldest procedure is the Douglas–Routledge operation (or glossopexy), which consists of attaching the tip of the tongue to the lower lip. Simple suturing of the denuded raw surfaces has been replaced by the use of two flaps of mucosa – the first gingival and the second lingual – which are sutured to one another (Fig. 15.12). This is a relatively simple technique (except for the problems of intubation for the anesthesiologist), but its results do not meet with unanimous approval. Although the operation does frequently improve airflow, the flaps show a tendency to spontaneously pull apart, and often the only effect is on the lip, which is drawn backward, while the forward shift of the base of the tongue remains a matter of theory rather than reality. The promising results reported sporadically are not necessarily produced by the operation itself, but by spontaneous improvement that would have occurred regardless.

Certain other techniques have fortunately been disregarded – for instance, the Kirschner wire, which advanced the lingual mass by skewering the tongue to the mandible, or the use of weights and pulleys to exert continuous forward traction of the tongue.

The latest technique proposed by a group of Canadian specialists (Delorme *et al.*, 1989) is based on disinsertion of the floor of the mouth. One might well wonder how this could affect glossoptosis. The authors speak of a retraction of the components of the floor of the mouth, which they see as responsible for tongue recession, and include references to the work of one of our former collaborators, Epois (1983), who did raise the subject in her study on our reasons for velar repair in labio-palatal clefts (Chapter 7). The Canadian findings are based on a limited number of cases (Caouette-Laberge *et al.*, 1994). Considering this technique, it is possible to imagine that increasing the volume of the anterior portion of the oral cavity (by supposedly lowering the floor of the mouth in relation to the mandibular arch) might make the tongue less likely to rotate behind the hyoid bone. However, this remains a matter of pure conjecture.

In our opinion, this entire range of procedures can be set aside in favor of early primary veloplasty.

It is true that velar repair cannot always be performed in the first weeks of life. The cleft is still wide and the velar stumps are very fragile due to lack of contraction. Although ideally the operation should be performed as soon as possible, in practice there is a certain waiting period to be respected.

This interval can be made more comfortable for

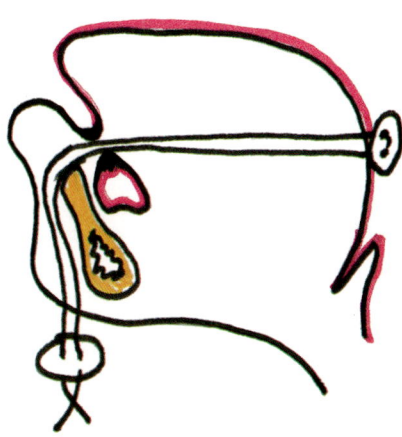

Fig. 15.12 Principles of the Douglas–Routledge procedure.

all concerned if the infant's mouth is fitted with a palatal plate. Theoretically, if the appliance provides sufficient coverage of the velum, it should prevent the tongue from becoming impacted in the cleft (cases with a wide horse-shoe or U-shaped cleft and small tongue). By keeping the tongue from entering the cleft (broad and bilateral forms), the plate helps to reduce its width. In addition, it should encourage the tongue to move forward by facilitating compression of the nipple and anterior suction. Although the benefits of a plate remain somewhat hypothetical and its placement presents a problem in frail infants who have difficulty breathing, the treatment should be attempted, if only to reassure the parents.

During this waiting period, it is essential to keep the infant under constant surveillance in hospital. Blood gases in particular must be monitored routinely for signs of long-term hypoxia, which can cause permanent brain damage and cardiovascular complications. If this is the case (and *only* in this case, in our opinion), then tracheostomy is the best solution, bearing in mind that it is only a temporary stop-gap. The major objective is still veloplasty at the earliest possible date.

Digestive problems

In severe forms, digestive problems are associated with respiratory disorders, and in fact often predominate.

The sucking/swallowing problems specific to these patients have already been discussed. Feeding is difficult, time-consuming and exhausting for the infant, whose milk intake is far from adequate. The situation may be relieved by following the guidelines set up by Robin himself (orthostatic feeding), and by increasing the frequency of feeding.

Nasogastric feeding often proves necessary, but should not become a matter of course. It must not stop attempts at normal feeding, which help develop the sucking/swallowing process.

Gastro-esophageal reflux frequently occurs, probably of reflex rather than central origin. It can cause pain and faintness (vagal type). Suitable positioning and pharmaceutical treatment must be applied automatically, backed up whenever possible by the assistance of a pediatric gastro-enterologist. Needless to say, it is not easy to maintain the infant in a position both prone and on an incline, which may hinder breathing by reducing the effect of gravity on the lingual mass.

After several weeks

Following several weeks of treatment and surveillance in a specialized neonatal intensive care unit, the infant's condition generally improves. As far as breathing goes, this is due primarily to the prone position. A weight gain also permits nasogastric feeding to become less frequent or be discontinued.

However, these patients remain tiny and frail. Their state of health is precarious, especially if there are associated malformations. The gastro-esophageal reflux, which is often severe, predisposes them to swallowing the wrong way and to fainting spells. The danger of superinfection, a subsequent relapse of major respiratory problems, is always present.

The decision must be made to combat glossoptosis or, at least, to deal with the low obstruction, which compromises breathing space.

Possible options

These infants are kept in hospital so that more or less acute incidents can be dealt with. Two different approaches can be adopted here; 'wait and see' and surgical.

Those practitioners who believe that dysmaturity is the main cause of Robin syndrome disorders strongly advise both tracheostomy (if it has not already been performed in a postnatal emergency) and nasogastric feeding. To support their opinion, they put forth polysomnographic data that stresses the frequency of central apnea. Their standpoint does seem to be corroborated by the spontaneous improvement that generally occurs over a certain length of time, although substantial improvement may take 6 months or more. In any event, this approach rules out any surgical action to correct glossoptosis.

However, since the pathological anatomy remains unchanged during this period, there is a constant risk of acute episodes. Thus, tracheostomy must be maintained for quite some time, which is most undesirable considering its drawbacks. This 'wait and see' approach may also have harmful effects on functional development (speech, hearing, digestive processes).

A common surgical alternative is the Douglas–Routledge operation, which is advocated by many surgeons during the secondary phase. This temporary attachment of the tongue to the lip is maintained until the infant is several months old and seems to have survived the crisis of glossoptosis-related incidents. The method is not problem-free however.

Once again, it is emphasized that the disorders (both mechanical and reflex) related to the palatal cleft and to the dysfunction of the aero-digestive junction continue to exist.

An original approach is proposed because we feel that reconstruction of the faucial isthmus is an absolute necessity and must be accomplished as soon as possible. Veloplasty shifts the tongue forward, restores the anatomy to normal and does away with all the pathological reflex or mechanical factors. It can generally be performed after a few weeks of life since the cleft tends to narrow, with or without a plate. The velar stumps acquire a certain volume due to muscle contraction, however inefficient, and are better adapted to surgical closure.

The operation requires the collaboration of a skilled anesthesiologist capable of practicing successful endotracheal intubation. The technique of primary veloplasty is identical to that described for correction of isolated cleft palate (see Chapter 11). The mouth-gag manufactured to our specification is equipped with a very small blade adapted to the mouth size of tiny infants. It can be handled without flattening the endotracheal tube against the alveolar rim of the mandible.

Ever since we perfected a veloplasty technique based on the Von Langenbeck procedure using narrow longitudinal flaps, which spare the thick portion of vault mucosa, it has been possible to close any type of palatal cleft in a single operation. Our technique has a very high success rate and leaves no residual fistulae.

Statistics for primary veloplasty on Robin syndrome

These statistics were compiled in collaboration with Patrice Oger.

From 1978 to 1997, we treated 80 cases of Robin syndrome, two of which did not involve cleft palate. Seventy-one presented with the triad described early in this chapter: micrognathia, cleft palate and clinical signs of severe respiratory and/or digestive disorders.

Gender has no bearing here.

Associated malformations were detected in only 20 per cent of our cases, a low figure compared with the data found in literature (40–75 per cent).

Thus, 78 cases of Robin syndrome were surgically treated over a period of 20 years. Early primary veloplasty was performed on 63 infants, and only fifteen were operated on at a relatively late date.

Thirty-six were classified as critical or serious. These were the cases that threw the most light on the effects of early velar repair. We have retained their relevant data to stave off the usual critical reaction: specialists are often accused of relating only satisfactory results, which can often be explained by the fact that they concern pseudo-Robin syndrome cases no different basically from 'run of the mill' palatal clefts. This is definitely not the case for the remaining 27 children in the group; however, their results are not included.

Virtually all these infants underwent nasogastric feeding, and 20 received major respiratory treatment prior to veloplasty such as nasopharyngeal intubation, 7; endotracheal intubation, 8.

In the majority of cases a *status quo* was obtained after several weeks, which enabled the infants to undergo surgery in a better state of health. Nonetheless, there were still grounds for concern.

Two pre-operative tracheostomies were performed. The circumstances will be discussed presently.

Thirteen infants presented severe gastro-esophageal reflux.

True primary veloplasty was performed in 36 cases:

26 underwent modified Von Langenbeck technique.
10 underwent simple veloplasty.

A plate was fitted in 31.5 per cent of cases.
Operations were performed at the following ages:

First month: 1
Second month: 2
Third month: 14
Fourth month: 9
Fifth month 5
Sixth month 6

A total of 36 infants underwent surgery before the

seventh month, and improvement was spectacular in the majority of cases.

The dates of release accurately reflect the improvements obtained and the end of the 'at risk' period, since the infants were on normal feeds when discharged to their parents:

17 patients were released during the week following surgery, including 11 before the fifth day

14 were discharged during the second week

 5 stayed longer

The average date of release was 12 days.

Seven infants continued to present respiratory problems for a few days after surgery. Only two cases suffered from serious longer-lasting sequelae, but they too eventually recovered.

Tracheostomy proved necessary in five cases, an enlightening figure in our point of view.

There were two pre-operative tracheostomies. These may have resulted from arbitrary decisions on the part of residents called in from other departments in an emergency, who thought this was the appropriate procedure for Robin syndrome with respiratory distress and cannot be faulted for recommending it.

It is significant that these particular patients underwent veloplasty in the days that followed (anesthesia was simplified by the presence of the tracheostomy tube). These tubes were soon removed (about 3 months later), since conditions at the aerodigestive junction were back to normal.

Three post-operative tracheostomies were performed: one on the seventeenth day after surgery, because blood gas readings aroused concern; another 6 months after veloplasty, related to pulmonary infection in an infant presenting with severe malformation and hypotonia; and the third, for general failure to thrive in the third month after surgery.

We have no cause to regret these tracheostomies, which were prescribed in a state of emergency and must certainly have helped rather than harmed the patients with the exception of one case of complications directly linked to the tracheostomy itself, which involved a pneumothorax and neurological troubles subsequent to post-anesthetic cardiac arrest.

It is worth mentioning that, in one case where tracheostomy was performed prior to velar repair, decannulation took place after only 3 months – far earlier than is customary. This confirms the beneficial effects of veloplasty.

The degree of retrognathia was not measured. Only a few clinical estimates were available in the files, which lacked information on this aspect of the problem despite its relevance. In six cases, it was noted that retrognathia had disappeared within 2 years.

Speech development among these infants deserves a study of its own, but the field has yet to be researched. We did notice in the follow-up on this series that five pharyngoplasties were performed before the age of 10 years. As things stand, however, it is impossible to affirm whether these short vela are more likely to present phonetic difficulties or whether primary veloplasty has a favorable effect on this particular aspect of the problem.

CONCLUSION

In conclusion, we remain firmly convinced that cleft palate plays an essential role in the disorders related to the Robin sequence. Consequently, the option of primary veloplasty always deserves consideration.

Needless to say, this operation does not enter into the emergency treatment of respiratory disorders, which are the domain of neonatal intensive care units. However, once the crucial period of acute accidents is past, and regardless of the therapeutic measures previously applied, veloplasty is the most logical and effective treatment.

It seems illogical, therefore, to leave a cleft palate untreated under the pretense that the young patients are too weak and immature for anything but long-term tracheostomy. Indeed, except in the case of multiple malformations, all or most of the symptoms they present are linked to the cleft, which is aggravated by the degree of retrognathia.

The operation itself is a demanding procedure, due to the usual width of the cleft and to the problems of anesthesia involved. Nonetheless, within the context of a pediatric hospital, well staffed with specialists in the various related fields, primary veloplasty stands out as the most appropriate technique.

IV COMPLETE CLEFTS

16. The normal maxillary skeleton

BASIC ANATOMY

The study of embryology reveals that the maxilla, which might appear to be one single solid bone, is in fact made up of several parts.

On either side, there is a sizeable segment that anatomists call the maxilla or superior maxillary bone. It is irregular in shape and consists of a central portion articulated towards the rear with the fragile pterygoid process of the sphenoid bone and the palatine bone. This entire portion is hollowed by the maxillary sinus. The superior maxillary bone makes up the greater part of the orbital floor, and presents three extensions:

1. The malar process which, along with the malar bone, forms the prominence of the cheek bone.
2. The processus frontalis or frontal process, which is situated between the orifice of the nasal fossa towards the inside and the inner side of the orbit towards the outside (Fig. 16.1).
3. The third element, located on a deep level, is the palatal shelf, a horizontal plate which is joined to its contralateral as well as to the vomer. The latter forms a vertical plate perpendicular to the midline.

Seen from below, the maxilla presents (at the outer limit of the bone) the alveolar ridge or dental arch, which is the seat of the dental buds and surrounds the palatal shelf within the oral cavity.

In the anterior central portion, on either side of the midline, is the premaxilla (also known as the

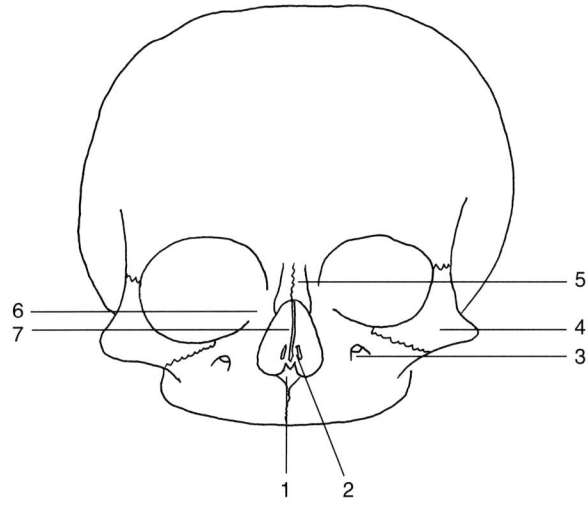

Fig. 16.1 Maxilla in the very young infant.

1. *Anterior nasal spine*
2. *Jacobson's cartilage*
3. *Infraorbital foramen*
4. *Malar bone*
5. *Nasal bones*
6. *Frontal process*
7. *Septal cartilage*

premaxillary segment or intermaxillary bone). The premaxilla is rather poorly described in literature although, as Veau has pointed out, it is of major importance in the study of labio-palatal clefts. This paired bone is derived from the two inner nasal processes located on either side. It presents an alveolar protuberance, which contains the buds of the incisor teeth, and a posterior extension or palatine

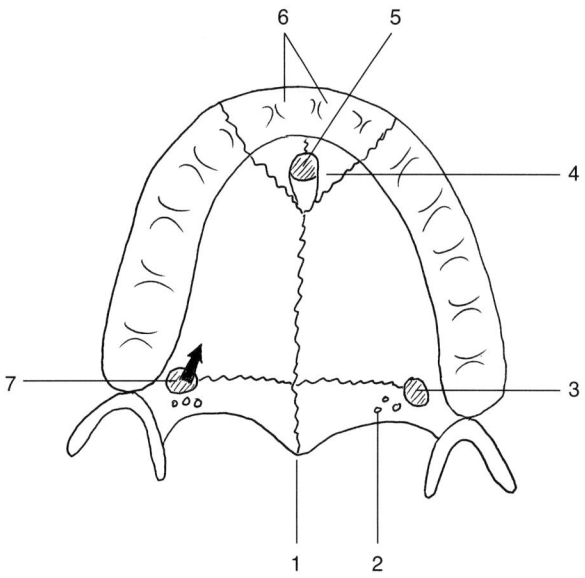

Fig. 16.2 *Bony palatal vault seen from below.*

1. *Posterior nasal spine*
2. *Lesser palatine foramina*
3. *Major palatine foramen*
4. *Primary palate*
5. *Anterior palatine foramen*
6. *Premaxillary bone*
7. *Posterior bundle*

process of the premaxilla, which fits between the anterior extremities of the palatal shelves. This extension forms the primary palate as opposed to the secondary palate, which is composed of the palatal shelves (cf. Embryology) (Fig. 16.2).

The nasopalatine nerves and blood vessels run between the two premaxillary bones in what are at first two separate canals. These merge further downward and open into the mouth through a funnel-shaped common opening called the incisive or anterior palatine foramen.

Anteriorly, the upper borders of the two small premaxillary bones rise to form the anterior nasal spine, a pyramidal structure into which all the superficial facial muscles are inserted. It is therefore the major fixed point for the facial muscle layer. This upper border, which is hollowed into a sulcus, articulates along its entire length with the lower border of the septal cartilage. The connection is completed by a pincer-shaped configuration made up of the two

Jacobson's small cartilages (cf. anatomy of the septum).

Ossification of the maxilla involves two centers: an anterior ossification center, which corresponds to the premaxilla, and a second posterior center, which plays a more important role. The corresponding suture lines are usually still evident in the skulls of infants (notably those separating the incisive portion from the remainder of the maxilla).

The congenital cleft is not related to a defect in the process of ossification; the gap occurs before ossification takes place. We have already seen that, depending on which theory of embryology is retained, it results from defective fusion between the facial processes or from the failure of the mesenchyme to penetrate these processes. It is thought that the premaxillary bone gives rise to most of the bone corresponding to the nostril sill rather than the frontal process, which does not, in fact, contribute to its formation.

The bony palatal vault, which is derived from the maxillary processes, is continued towards the rear by the palatal shelves of the palatine bone. The posterior border of the latter unites with its contralateral to form the posterior nasal spine. Between the palatine bone and the palatal shelf of the maxilla, near the alveolar ridge, lies the orifice of the posterior palatine canal or major palatine foramen. The arteries and greater palatine nerves emerge through this and course towards the hard palate. The arteries and lesser posterior palatine nerves that supply the soft palate emerge through the lesser palatine foramina, which are found in the palatine bone (Fig. 16.2).

The premaxillary bones and the vomer form a supporting structure or veritable beam of bone, which is broad towards the rear and narrower towards the front. Oriented in a postero-anterior direction and set on a superior–inferior and postero-anterior slant, it supports the middle level of the facial skeleton and participates in its growth. Abnormalities that affect this beam structure determine several of the deformities which are most typical of complete clefts.

In the normal skeleton, dentition is arranged according to the following pattern:

•   The premaxilla produces the four incisor teeth.
•   The alveolar arch of the maxilla gives rise to the rest of the teeth.

In the presence of a cleft, there is always a central incisor tooth. However, the lateral incisor is sometimes missing. In most cases it has split into an anterior or mesial tooth, which is usually malpositioned, and a distal incisor positioned posteriorly in the maxillary segment, often in a palatal location.

This phenomenon has led to the idea that the congenital cleft is responsible for the division of the lateral incisor bud and that the premaxillary bone segment is therefore cleft as well. In fact this theory has not been substantiated, since the skulls examined show no sign of a fragment of premaxillary bone on the outer border of the bony cleft.

BASIC CONCEPTS OF FACIAL GROWTH

Before introducing the study of complete clefts, a few basic reminders about postnatal growth of the facial structures might provide a useful supplement to the chapter on embryology of the face and contribute to a better understanding of the lesions involved.

Facial skeletal elements are known as 'membranous' bones. Unlike long bones, which have cartilaginous growth plates, facial bones do not have well-defined growth centers. Their growth is determined by the mechanical forces that act upon them. These forces are generated by muscle actions exerted on a permanent basis. Indeed, even in the absence of obvious contraction of the muscle fibers there is a low-level muscle activity or tonus which is never interrupted.

Balanced muscle forces, which are usually distributed among a system of counteracting antagonists, are essential to the harmony of skeletal growth. The size and shape of bone units are genetically determined, but only to a certain extent. They also depend on the effects of muscle balance, which is established at a very early stage of development.

New facial bone is generated by the periosteum, which covers the skeletal elements. Conversely, bone tissue can degenerate if the mechanical forces diminish. Thus, notwithstanding the intrinsic quality of the periosteum, a distinction is made between zones of bone apposition and those of bone resorption in terms of the intensity of muscle forces at work.

Volumetric growth of bone occurs when zones of apposition (which are on the surface) predominate

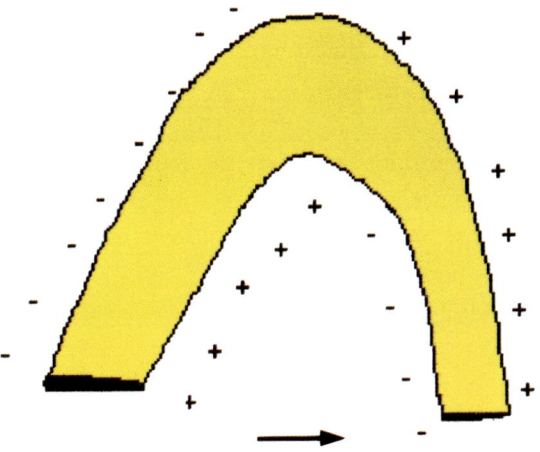

Fig. 16.3 *Apposition–resorption mechanism in bone growth. Arrow indicates virtual displacement of bone in space.*

over deeper-lying zones of resorption (Enlow, 1975) (Fig. 16.3). Superficial forces are essentially produced by the facial muscle layer. On a deeper level, the muscle forces are exerted by the tongue, which plays a major role in the morphogenesis of the face (Oblak, 1975a; Delaire, 1976). Thus, during the first 6 years of life at least, the facial bone structure has a peripheral surface that undergoes the phenomenon of apposition, and a deep-lying resorptive surface.

The palatal shelves are believed to have a nasal surface of resorption and an oral surface of apposition.

It is clear that the presence of a congenital cleft alters these mechanical factors; indeed, neither the muscle insertions nor the mechanical forces produced correspond to those found in a normal subject. The problem can be described as a state of imbalance. The growth process is disrupted from the earliest stages of fetal development. As Wallace (1968) observed, the pathology of each stage of prenatal life is influenced by the physiology of that same period, just as it in turn affects the pathology of the period that follows.

The principle of apposition–resorption growth in itself helps in understanding deformities of the bone structure due to the existence of a cleft. These deformities can be misleading in that they suggest there has been displacement of the bony segments. The problem is compounded by a gap in the maxillary arch that causes unusual mobility of the bone segments. In fact, only very thin laminae of malleable, fragile bone tissue attach the bone segments to the rest of the facial structure and the base of the skull. This abnormal mobility can be held responsible for the true displacements.

In the case of complete clefts, therefore, it can prove very difficult to tell the difference between those anomalies that represent authentic deformities and those that are caused by displacement of the various bone segments.

Concerning the program of treatment, the first step is to re-establish virtually normal muscle insertions at the earliest possible date. The goal is to recreate a state of muscular balance between the antagonistic actions of the facial muscle layer and the tongue. This is the foundation of our present method, which we call early primary palate repair.

It is obvious that our method is based on a theory which would be open to debate were it not substantiated by irrefutable evidence, but the long-term results of our experience at the end of the growth cycle should suffice to demonstrate whether we are on the right track or not.

The potential iatrogenic effects that surgery can have on the growth process must always be taken into account.

The surgical procedure seeks to modify surface muscle forces by correcting the insertions of the superficial muscles of the face. The lingual pressure exerted on the inner walls will also vary due to changes in the volume of the oral cavity and closure of the palatal cleft, which reconstructs the faucial isthmus. However, there may be undesirable side-effects. The tension created when the borders of the cleft are drawn together to close the gap is sometimes so great that it produces prejudicial consequences, and this situation may be aggravated by post-operative edema. Fibrotic scar tissue may also be detrimental to future growth. Lastly, development can be impaired by vascular disorders of the tissue caused by damage when the flaps were raised.

Needless to say, cleft surgery calls for a great deal of caution and skill. The same caution should be exercised in interpreting the long-term results.

17. The nature and consequences of bone lesions

Lesions of the lip and of the palate have already been described.

In complete clefts, these lesions are combined with those that affect the bone structures, i.e. deformities of the skeleton and cartilages and displacement of the bone structures. Indeed, the separate segments of the cleft maxilla are extremely malleable in the early stages of development, and they are also mobile due to the weakness of their attachments to the other facial structures.

These two types of lesion are related to muscular anomalies. The bone insertions of the superficial facial muscles are modified, and the muscle bundles are oriented in new directions, which results in actions altogether different from their normal behavior (Fig. 17.1). At the same time, the pressures exerted on the bony segments and also by the tongue on the deep-lying structures are altered due to the presence of a wide gap in the roof of the oral cavity (Fig. 17.2).

Both categories of anomaly can be partially corrected by cleft repair. It seems logical, therefore, that correction should be attempted at a stage when they can still be reversed (i.e. during the first months of life). The muscle insertions must be re-established in a pattern which approaches that of 'normal anatomy'; however, in most cases the initial bone lesions subsist unchanged.

Surgery does not automatically reverse the anomalous muscle forces responsible for the problems. Also, the operation itself can produce consequences which are likely to aggravate these lesions. What is known as the 'iatrogenic' effect of surgery may be of a purely mechanical nature, created

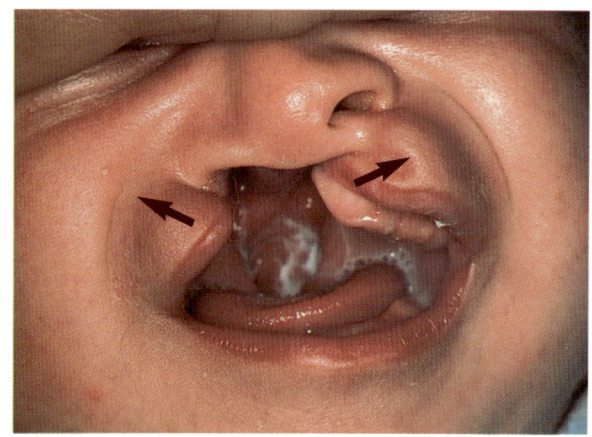

Fig. 17.1 *Diverging forces appear in superficial muscles due to the presence of a cleft.*

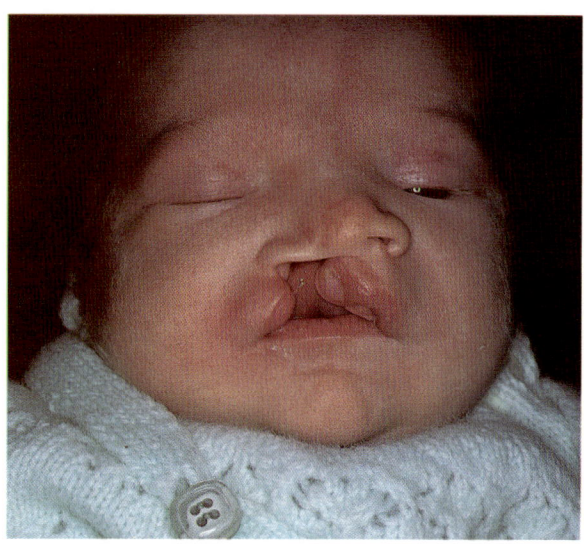

Fig. 17.2 *Tongue penetrates into the cleft.*

by the new forces it generates. This may also be compounded by the detrimental side-effects of disorders in the vascular supply to bone structures due to extensive subperiosteal undermining, or of an unsatisfactory healing process which leaves retractile or non-extensile fibrotic scar tissue.

Bone growth can therefore be affected by a multitude of causes, among which congenital hypoplasia (often over-hastily incriminated) is not always the major factor.

These bone lesions include an altogether new but consistent phenomenon linked to the existence of a cleft. This is the abnormal periosteal junction observed on the borders of the cleft.

THE PERIOSTEAL JUNCTION

A complete cleft implies the existence of a gap in the bone structure. Since the bone is lined by the periosteum, an abnormal junction is automatically established both on the level of the superficial periosteum and on that of the periosteum that covers the deep lying structures.

Therefore, in the alveolar region there is continuity between the superficial periosteal layer and the deep periosteum of the retro-alveolar or palatal zone (Fig. 17.3).

At the piriform aperture in unilateral clefts, on the outer or small segment there is another abnormal junction between the superficial periosteum and that which lines the inner surface of the frontal process of the maxilla above and below the inferior nasal concha (thus meeting the mucoperiosteum on the upper or nasal surface of the palatal shelf). On the large or major segment, the superficial alveolar periosteum unites at its upper level with the perichondrium that lines the septal cartilage, and below with the periosteum of the free surface of the premaxilla.

At the piriform aperture in bilateral clefts, the abnormal connection with the perichondrium and with the vomerine periosteum is established on both sides of the premaxilla. On the small segments, the periosteal junction is identical to that described in unilateral forms.

Behind the alveolar ridges, the abnormal periosteal junction varies according to the anatomical

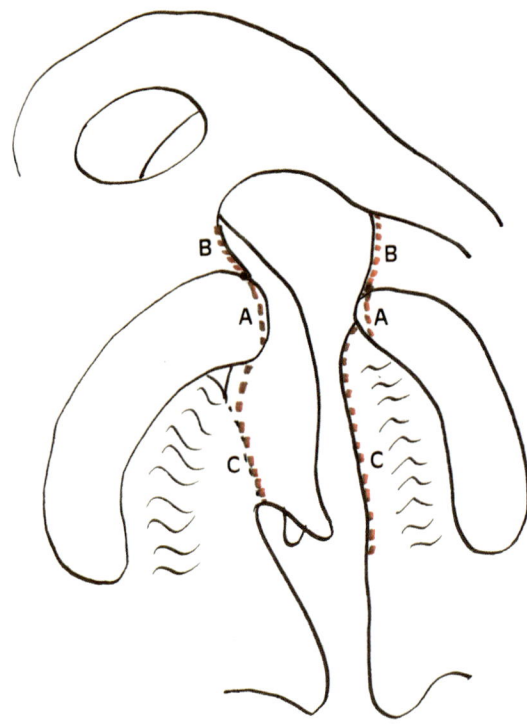

Fig. 17.3 *Periosteal junction on borders of the cleft. These are established along two lines, which converge towards the anterior portion of the mouth corresponding to the alveolar region (A), nostril sill (B) and palatal cleft (C).*

form of the palatal cleft. In unilateral cleft palate, it is located at the juncture between the vomer and the palatal shelf on the major segment and, on the minor segment, between the superficial and buccal surfaces of the palatal shelf along its entire length. In bilateral cleft palate combined with a labio-maxillary cleft, there is only a partial periosteal junction with the vomer.

Muscle insertions

Due to both the division of the facial muscle layer and the periosteal configuration, abnormal muscle insertions are developed. Since the muscles remain attached to the underlying periosteum, each of the muscle bundles finds itself anchored to the periosteal junction described above. Thus, the facial muscles have lost their normal midline insertions on the anterior nasal spine on the cleft side, and have found new insertions on the frontal process of the

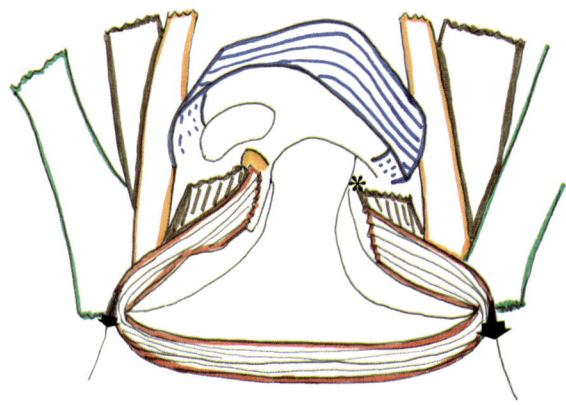

Fig. 17.4 *Gap in the facial muscles leads to a new insertion on the frontal process of the maxilla.*

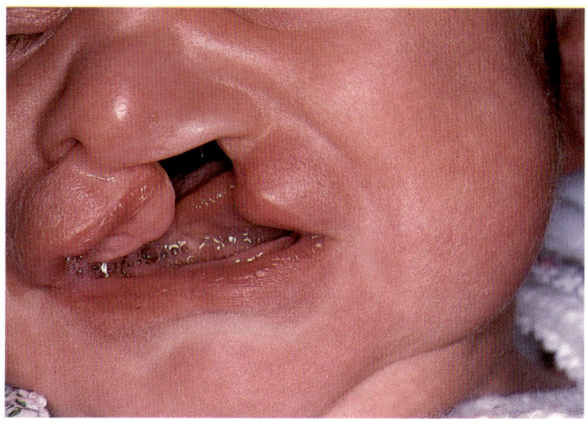

Fig. 17.5 *The two segments are spread apart; the lateral soft tissues are lowered due to muscle action.*

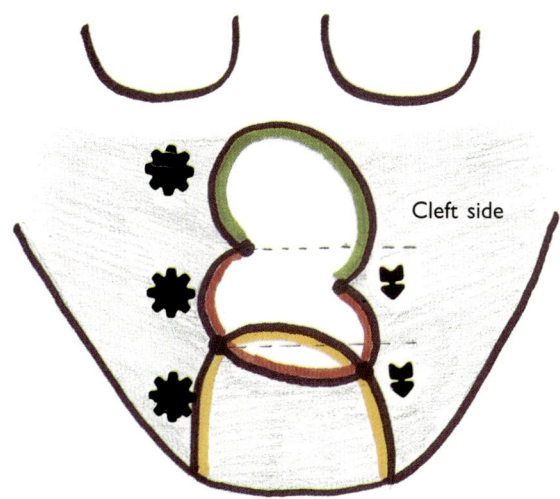

Fig. 17.6 *Delaire's diagram of the muscle loops shows how the muscles are lowered by the loss of their insertions on the anterior nasal spine.*

maxilla. In unilateral clefts, however, the muscles on the level of the major segment retain their midline insertions on the non-cleft side (Fig. 17.4).

As these two muscle bundles contract in opposite directions, they cause the anterior portions of the bone segments to diverge (Fig. 17.5). They also lower the small segment due to the predominant action of those muscles that depress the corner of the mouth (Fig. 17.6).

Lastly, on the outer border, the abnormal insertions on the frontal process anchor the deep fibers of the muscles while their superficial fibers create an eversion of those structures that form the outer base of the alar wing.

Misalignment of the borders

Malalignment of the borders in an antero-posterior direction can be linked to two factors:

1. Forward growth of the vomer (in a postero-anterior direction) can be considerable since it is no longer held in check by labial pressure when the lip is cleft.
2. Pressure exerted by the superficial muscle layer on the small segment, which is the more mobile, forces it backward into the oral cavity (Figs 17.7, 17.8).

In all labio-palatal clefts, surgery seeks to eliminate the gap.

It is obvious that the pathological periosteal junction must be corrected in order to re-establish a virtually normal anatomy. After surgery, the superficial periosteum of the two segments should form a continuous layer. The same holds true for the deep periosteum. Moreover, due to the bone misalignment, it is essential to section the periosteum vertically at its abnormal junction on the small segment(s) facing the ascending ramus of the maxilla (Fig. 17.9). This will permit proper realignment of the cutaneo-muscular structures so that they can be sutured to one another.

Lastly, in the frontal plane, bone misalignment notwithstanding, the periosteum must be sectioned to allow correct reinsertion of the facial muscle layer on the nasal spine.

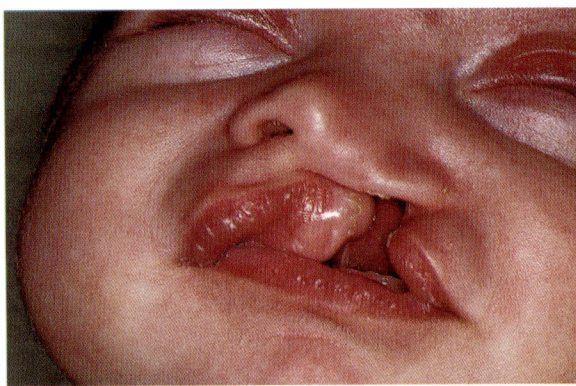

Fig. 17.7 *Misalignment of borders.*

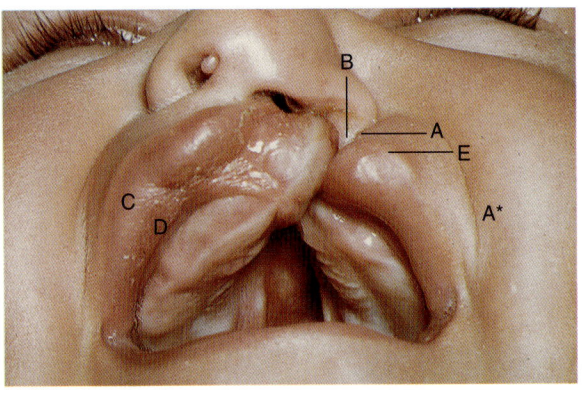

Fig. 17.8 *Narrow complete labio-palatal cleft from below.*

A). Furrow extending nasogenian fold (A*).

B). Cutaneous surface of outer border corresponding to pilous zone of nasal vestibule, visible due to eversion of outer alar base.

C). Dry zone of vermilion.

D). Moist zone of vermilion.

E). End of ridge above skin—vermilion line.

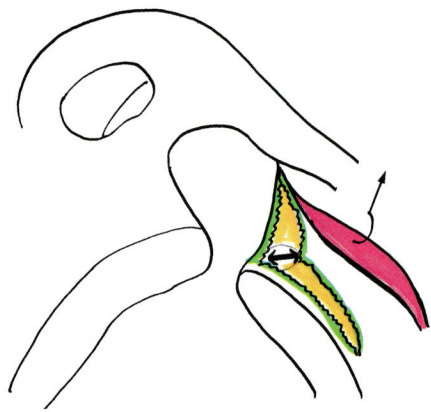

Fig. 17.9 *A periosteal incision is necessary to correct misalignment of the borders.*

Surgical correction

From the above, it can be seen that labial correction (and particularly muscle repair) requires a compulsory subperiosteal approach, although certain specialists deem this pointless, not to say harmful.

Simple 'drawing the curtain' closures, which do nothing to correct the periosteum, should therefore be proscribed. This form of closure presents another serious drawback; if secondary surgery is later performed on the bone segments to obtain complete closure of the cleft, the entire lip must be re-opened. This step is usually totally unproductive as far as the lip itself is concerned.

There are no grounds for the argument that primary repair involving the periosteum of this inter-alveolar zone jeopardizes maxillary growth.

Our experience, based on a large number of cases, proves that complete closure of the cleft, whatever its site, has no harmful repercussions on the growth process. On the contrary, it fosters normal growth by correcting abnormal structures and configurations.

UNILATERAL CLEFTS

Medial margin

The large or major segment includes the premaxilla, the alveolar rim and the palatal shelf as well as the vomer and the components of the nasal septum. Deformities of the large segment may date from the fetal period and be produced by the abnormal position of the tongue, which remains high between the palatal shelves. They can be further accentuated by the lack of muscle balance. The inner border is subject to unilateral traction from the superficial facial muscles, which insert into the anterior nasal spine, and also to pressure from the tongue, which exerts an oblique force upward and outward towards the normal side as it penetrates the cleft.

Thus, the anterior portion of the greater segment of the maxilla is shifted towards the non-cleft side and undergoes a more or less pronounced rotation, which lifts it above the normal horizontal plane. The transverse axis of the premaxilla is tilted on a slant, while the anterior nasal spine tends to intrude into the nostril opening on the non-cleft side. It is lateralized compared with the normal sagittal plane (Fig. 17.10).

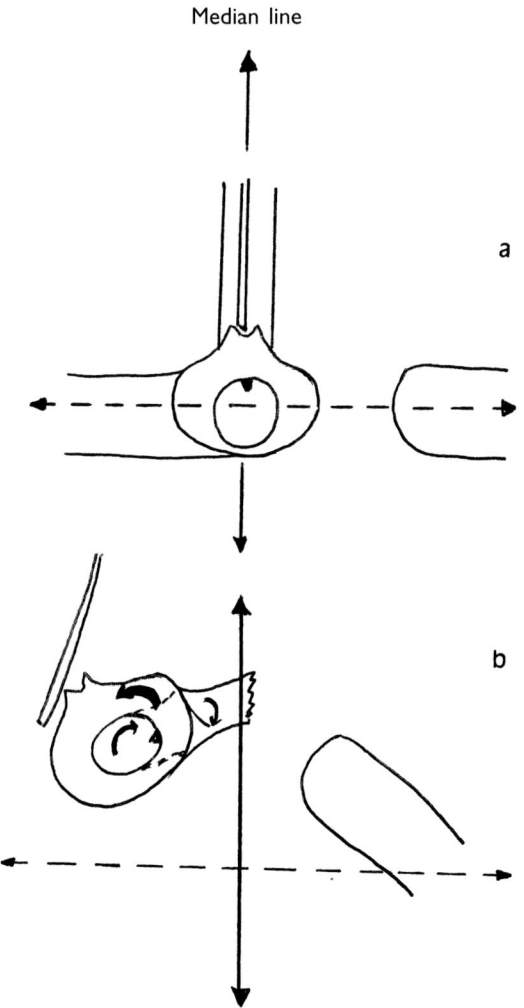

Median line

a

b

Fig. 17.10 Displacement of bony structures on borders of a complete cleft and, in particular, of premaxillary bone: a. Theoretical aspect. The dot represents the superior pole of the palatal extension of the premaxillary bones; the septum is lodged in the groove of the nasal spine. b. Elevation and outward displacement of outer border. There is a torque effect on the intermaxillary bones, whose posterior portion is rotated in the same direction as the vomer. Note possible dislocation of lower end of the septum.

The palatal shelf, which is attached to the large segment, follows the rotation of the alveolar rim and is exposed to pressure from the tongue. It therefore slants upward and inward and articulates with the vomer, which presents a certain number of deformities.

The septal cartilage, which is normally attached to the nasal spine and to the premaxillary bone, tends to slip out of the latter's upper groove. Under the

effects of growth, it comes to rest against the nasal spine on the non-cleft side.

The tongue also exerts pressure on the lateral aspect of the vomer which faces the cleft. This rotates the vomer in the opposite direction from the alveolar rim. A torque effect is thus created, which produces a fold in the bony septum. This fold, which bulges into a more or less rounded prominence towards the cleft, is known as Poutriquet's ridge or crest, although the precise origin of the term has not been clearly identified (Fig. 17.11). During surgery, once the septal mucoperiosteum is denuded, Poutriquet's ridge is often found to correspond to the junction between the vomer and the perpendicular plate of the ethmoid bone (Fig. 17.12).

Thus, there occurs a double rotation in opposite directions of the vomer and the premaxillary bone on the level of the palatine process of the premaxilla. This creates an un-named groove, which is often very deeply indented (Fig. 17.12b). At the upper edge of the premaxillary bone (which undergoes the greatest amount of torque), there is a second furrow corresponding to its line of contact with the lateral aspect of the septal cartilage which faces the cleft. Since the perichondrium of the cartilage and the periosteum of the bone into which it continues both penetrate deep

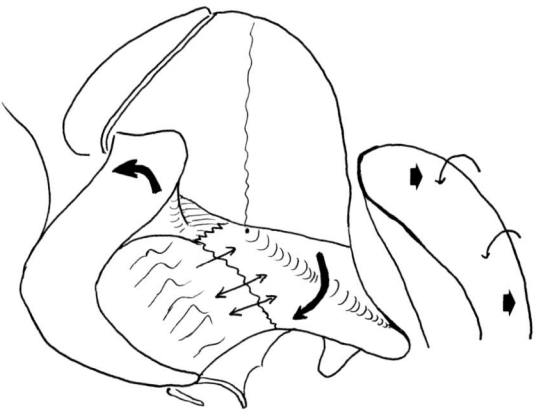

Fig. 17.11 Greater segment viewed laterally and from below (lesser segment artificially moved to the side). Under pressure of the tongue, the lateral aspect of the vomer is located in the extension of the palatal shelf, producing Poutriquet's ridge or crest and, anteriorly, a furrow at the point where the premaxillary bones are twisted. When the septal cartilage is dislocated, a furrow appears in the continuation of Poutriquet's ridge.

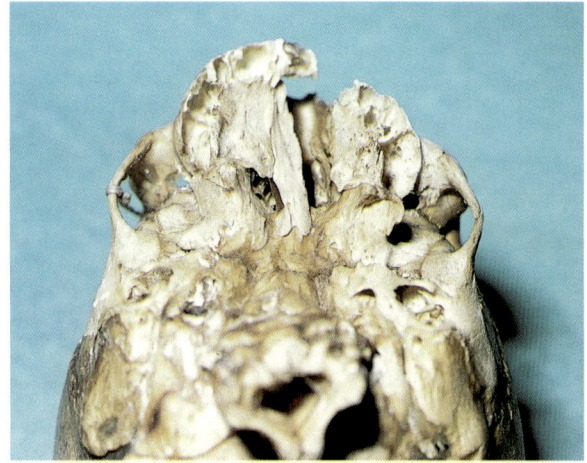

a

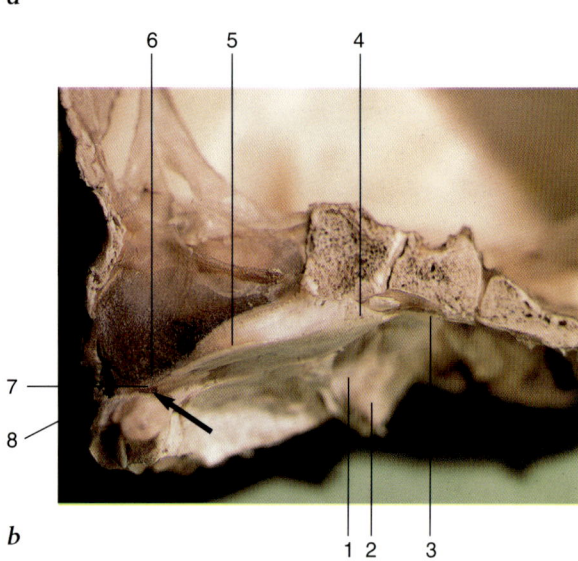

b

6   5   4

7 —

8 —

1 2   3

Fig. 17.12 *(a and b) Skeletal lesions in the neonate (Veau's collection).*

a   Poutiquet's crest is sometimes very sharp.

b

1. *Palatine bone*
2. *Pterygoid process*
3. *Sphenoid bone*
4. *The alae of the vomer*
5. *Poutriquet's crest*
6. *Un-named furrow*
7. *Second furrow*
8. *Anterior nasal spine*

within the furrow, this can make undermining difficult during cheiloplasty.

Behind this furrow, rotation of the vomer swings its lateral aspect into the same plane as the palatal shelf of the greater segment so that Poutriquet's ridge

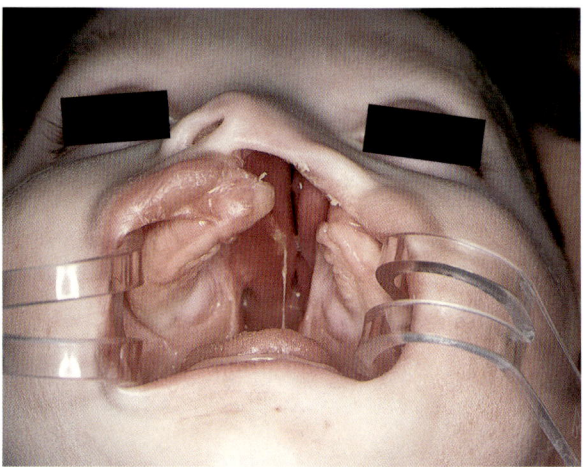

Fig. 17.13 *Difference in color between oral and nasal mucosae.*

seems to form the inner limit of the cleft itself. The palatal shelf looks unusually broad. The dividing line between the vomerine and oral mucosae can only be identified by their different colors (a brighter red for the nasal or vomerian mucosa compared with the paler oral mucosa) (Fig. 17.13).

Lastly, due to the labial cleft the upper lip no longer exerts restraining pressure on the premaxilla, which advances under the influence of postero-anterior vomerine growth. This accentuates the impression of displacement as the large segment rotates. Unchecked forward growth of the vomer aggravates the horizontal misalignment of the anterior extremities of the two segments produced by the displacements described above (Fig. 17.14a and b).

Lateral border

The outer border also presents a certain number of characteristic deformities.

The small or lesser segment of the maxilla is subject to pressure from the facial muscle layer, which has lost its midline insertions on this side but retains its effect on the deep-lying bone structures due to the integrity of the other facial sphincters. The anterior portion of this segment tends to tilt towards the theoretical midline of the face, and is deformed into the shape of an inverted letter *J*.

The tongue is believed to limit this movement. Prior to treatment, tongue pressure causes the

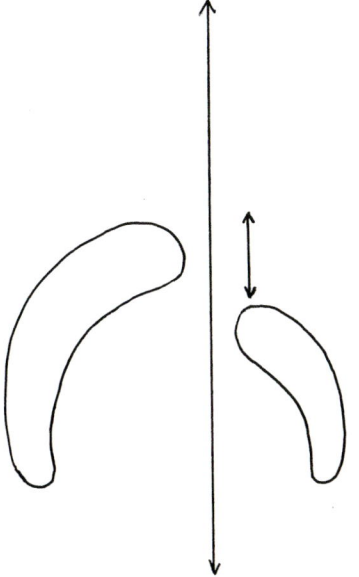

a

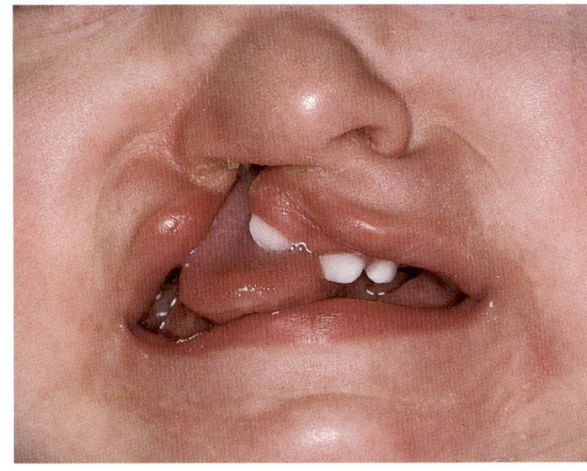

Fig. 17.15 *Role of tongue in moulding anterior infragnathia.*

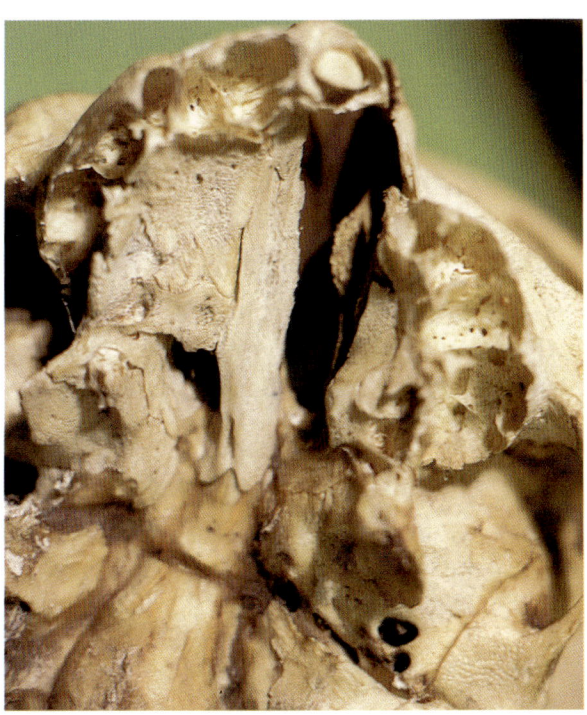

b

Fig. 17.14 *(a and b) Misalignment of bony borders: diagram and skeleton.*

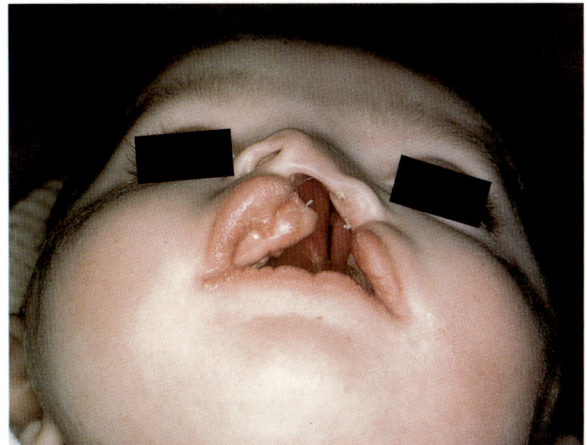

Fig. 17.16 *Edge of inferior concha protruding into cleft.*

horizontal plane of the lesser segment to rotate in the opposite direction to that of the greater segment. This rotation can be combined with inferior positioning or lowering of the anterior portion of the small segment, which curves upward when the tongue intrudes between the segments (Fig. 17.15).

The palatal shelf on the same side follows this rotation so that it slants upward and inward. Its free border is situated on a level with Poutriquet's ridge in the most typical forms.

Because of the muscular forces in play, the outer border of the cleft is likely to be located on a lower level than the inner border. Owing to the periosteal junction described earlier, the facial muscles retain their insertions at the nostril sill. They tend to lower the small segment when the mouth is opened, which places them under passive tension.

CT scans or coronal X-ray views reveal that the inferior nasal concha is also in an abnormally low position. When the mouth is open it is easy to identify its lower border, which sometimes protrudes into the cleft (Fig. 17.16).

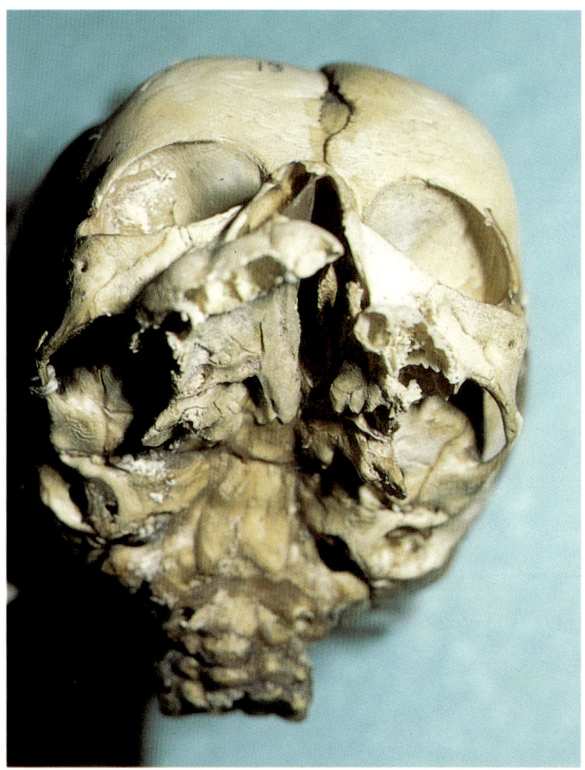

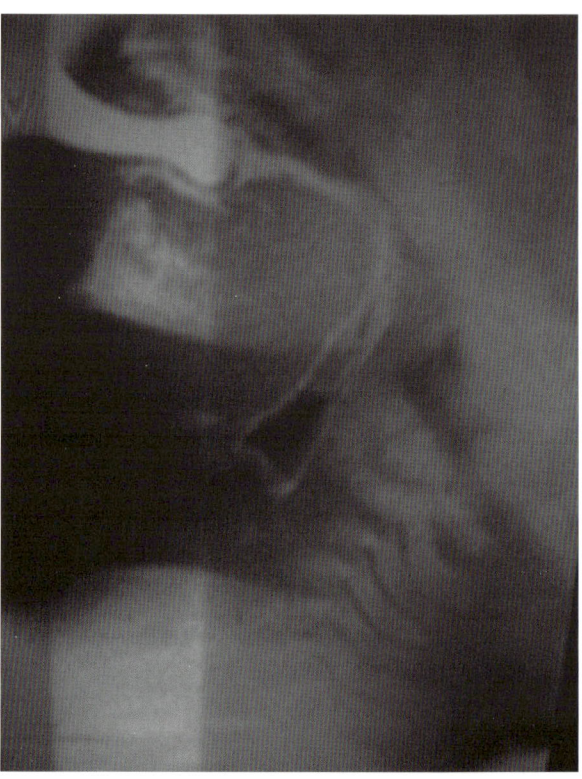

Fig. 17.17 *Distortion and flattening of face on the cleft side.*

Fig. 17.18 *Videofluoroscopic profile view of the swallowing process shows posterior pressure of the tongue in the nasopharynx.*

The bony borders present a variable degree of antero-posterior misalignment, which shows up clearly on profile views. This factor contributes to the nasal deformities that we will study later on. This misalignment distorts the shape of the entire face, which appears to be flattened on the cleft side (Fig. 17.17).

Deep structures

The pharynx is enlarged due to the gap in the palatal muscles and, above all, pressure from the tongue. During deglutition, the tongue shifts to the back of the oral cavity to help advance the alimentary bolus towards the esophagus. In the presence of a cleft, the base of the tongue must establish contact with the wall of the pharynx rather than with the palate, since the two separate halves of the palate serve little purpose in the process (as videofluoroscopy during the swallowing process has clearly demonstrated) (Fig. 17.18).

When we speak of a widened or enlarged pharynx, we are referring to an enlargement of its skeletal walls. The increased distance between the tuberosities and the divergence of the pterygoid processes constitute a well known anatomical fact (Brophy and Izard's law, quoted by a number of authorities including Veau, Rosenthal, Calnan, Subtelny, Wardill, Peyton, Psaume and Delaire). With the assistance of colleagues from the Radiology Department, the author's team measured the distance between the pterygoid hamular processes and, in collaboration with Brunelle (1985), established a pterygo-maxillary index (Fig. 17.19a and b). This index is based on the ratio between two distances: that measured between the pterygoid hamuli, and the intermandibulary distance measured from one vertical mandibular ramus to the other on the same cross-section (for instance, between the most prominent portions or between two given points located at the center of the vertical ramus). This ratio has proved to be remarkably constant among healthy subjects (about 0.35), but it increases to almost 0.50 in cases of cleft palate (Fig. 17.20a and b). Thanks to this index, measured before and after surgery, we have shown that the enlarged pharynx can be corrected by

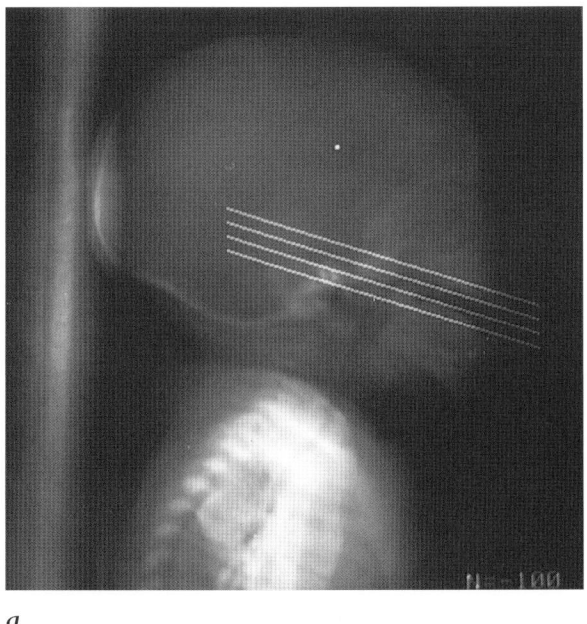

a

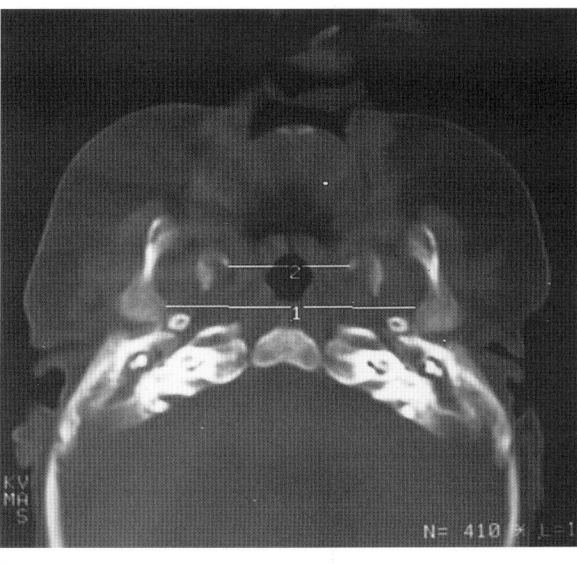

b

Fig. 17.19 *(a and b) CT scan of the pterygo-maxillary index; direction of cross-sections and measurements.*

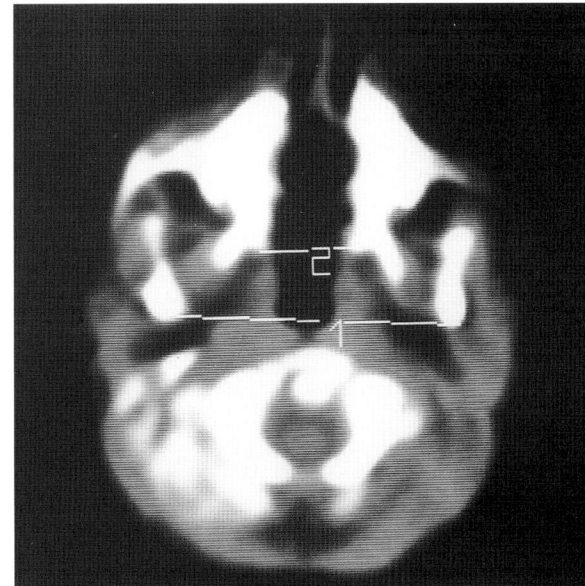

a

b

Fig. 17.20 *(a and b) Normal versus pathological pterygo-maxillary index: (0.33 in a compared with 40+ in b).*

early primary veloplasty. However, we do not have comparable data on infants operated on at a later date (12–18 months), and therefore cannot confirm until what age this condition is still reversible.

Nasal structures

In addition to the septum, which has already been discussed, the other nasal structures are also deformed by muscle imbalance and the displacement of underlying bone. However, it is customary to consider (perhaps wrongly) that they are not in fact malformed, the contention being that there is no hypoplastic malformation in this case.

The bony pyramid (nasal bones) is deflected towards the non-cleft side, following the deviation of the cartilaginous septum (Fig. 17.21a).

The nasal septum follows this displacement, but also presents deformities of its own. It balloons into the cleft like a sail inflated by the wind.

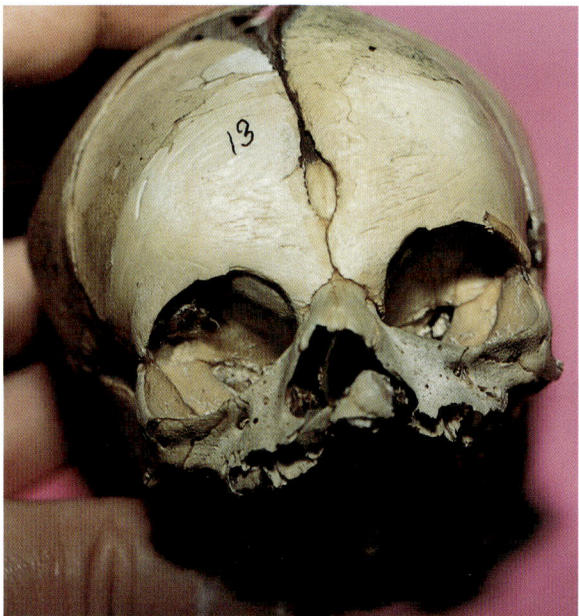

Fig. 17.21a *Bone deformities.*

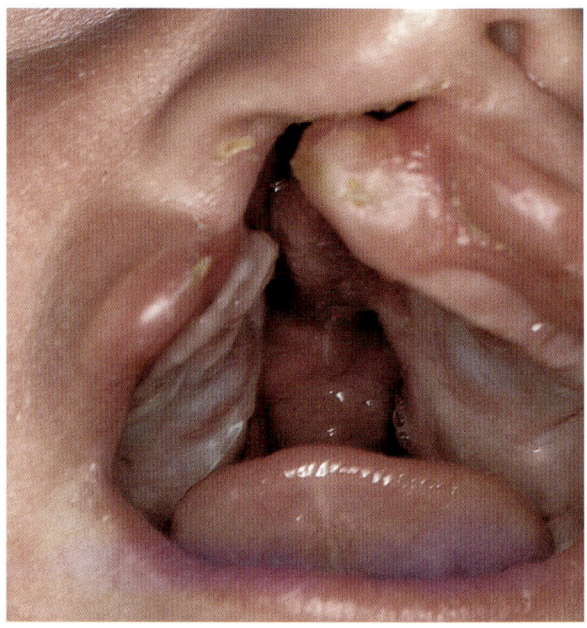

Fig. 17.21b *Nasal tip distortion.*

The outer wall of the nasal fossa on the cleft side nears the creased zone of the septum (Poutriquet's ridge). Thus, the nasal obstruction frequently observed on the cleft side is not caused by protrusion of the septum into the cleft, but rather by the inward movement of the outer wall of the nasal fossa as it follows the displacement of the minor segment (Fig. 17.21b).

It is clear that if correction of the nasal deviation as a whole includes 'straightening' the septum in the same direction, this may aggravate the obstruction of the nasal fossa, which will later require treatment by resection of the nasal concha.

The triangular cartilages are also deflected so that the inferior border of the cartilage on the cleft side appears to be lower than its counterpart.

The most characteristic deformities are those that affect the alar cartilages. As we have seen, interruption of the muscle layer produces diverging forces at the cleft nostril sill. The maxillary nasal spine and the base of the columella are pulled towards the non-cleft side, while the outer base of the alar wing and, consequently, the nasal tip are drawn towards the cleft side: the domes of the alar cartilages are no longer on the same level. Thus, the columella slants towards the cleft. The lower margin of the septal cartilage which is dislocated from the nasal spine is visible in the normal nostril opening.

At its junction with the triangular cartilage, the alar cartilage tends to slip downward. The outer alar base is everted for the reasons discussed in the section on the periosteal junction (Fig. 17.22a) (see Chapter 18).

Facial structures

Taken as a whole, the facial structures present two types of deformity. These were codified by Jean Psaume (1950, 1975) as follows:

1. Distortion of the maxilla into an oblique oval on a horizontal plane, which includes the alveolar ridges. The arch is deformed into an ellipse. Its main axis is slanted from back to front and towards the non-cleft side (Fig. 17.22b).
2. Arciform distortion of the face represents the second large-scale deformity. It is observed in the frontal or coronal plane.

   This phenomenon may be confirmed objectively by marking three reference points on the theoretical midline (Fig. 17.22c):

   • A medial point in the inter-ocular region.
   • The point corresponding to the anterior nasal spine of the upper maxilla, which can be palpated in the normal nostril sill.

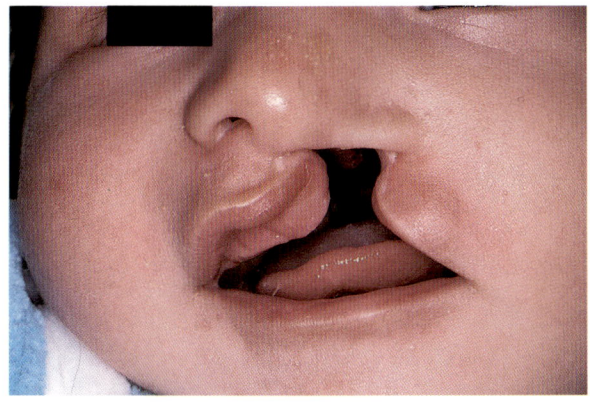

Fig. 17.22a *Typical deformities of nose cartilages.*

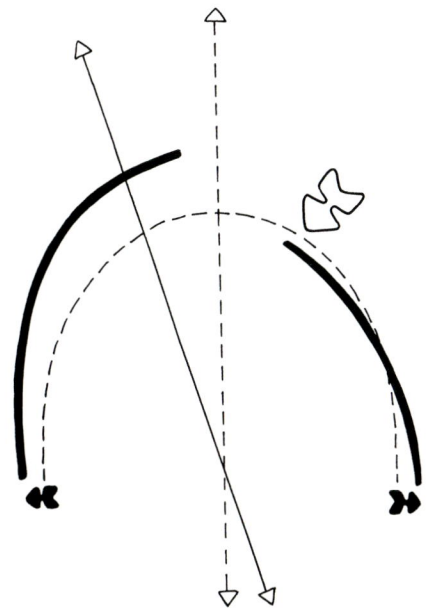

Fig. 17.22b *The oblique oval deformation of the maxilla.*

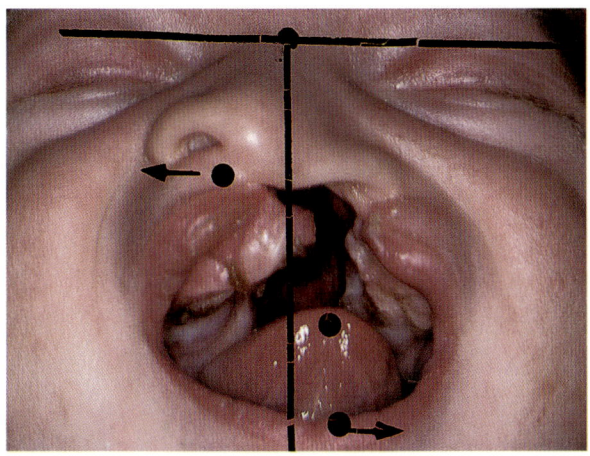

Fig. 17.22c *Arciform distortion of the face.*

- Lastly, the point that marks the center of the chin. The chin itself is deviated towards the cleft side because it follows the lateral displacement of the lingual mass which, as we have stressed, penetrates into the cleft.

The distortion of the theoretical midline is therefore obvious.

These two types of distortion do not take into account possible deformities of the face as a whole due to local hypoplastic malformation and therefore microsomia related to defective malar and maxillary development. Nor do they cover the effects of downward displacement of the bone structures on the cleft side, or of associated anomalies of the jaw.

To conclude the discussion of osteo-cartilaginous deformities in unilateral clefts, we must again stress the importance of mucosal and periosteal anomalies linked to the existence of the gap itself. It is absolutely essential to correct these disorders.

BILATERAL CLEFTS

In the most characteristic symmetrical forms, the bone deformities are radically different.

The premaxilla and the septum together are isolated from the upper maxilla. In the absence of pressure from the lip, the vomer and the premaxilla grow forward. This leads to what can often be very striking antero-posterior misalignment with the front ends of the small lateral alveolar segments on either side (Fig. 17.23).

The lower border of the vomer is located in a high position, no doubt due to direct pressure from the tongue, which intrudes into the cleft. At times it is even perched above the free borders of the palatal shelves, although they themselves are on a steep slant (Fig. 17.24).

This portion of the skeleton (premaxilla and vomer) shows considerable lateral mobility because the bones and cartilages that attach it to the base of the skull are particularly frail. The septum itself is not always set in the center of the cleft even if the form is symmetrical or if no bridges of soft tissue are present. The premaxilla is sometimes deflected to one side, in which case the septum may seem scoliotic (Fig. 17.23). The explanation for this deformity may

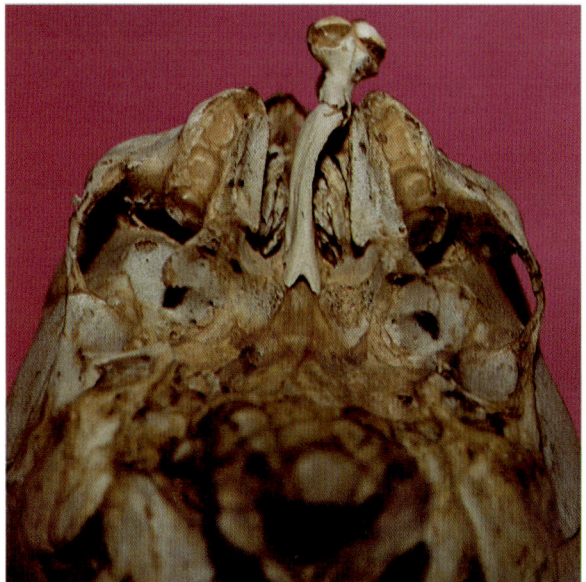

Fig. 17.23 *Antero-posterior misalignment of the fragments in bilateral case. Scoliotic aspect of the vomer and premaxilla.*

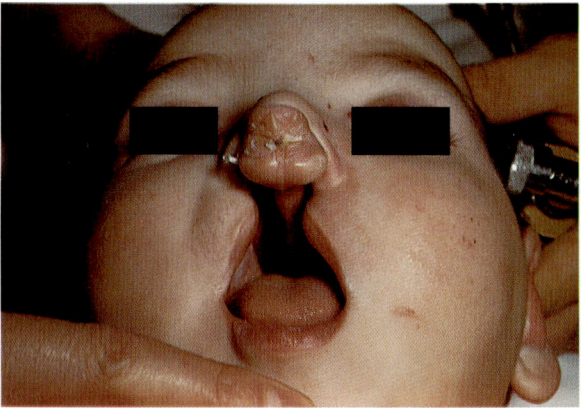

Fig. 17.24 *High location of the inferior border of the vomer.*

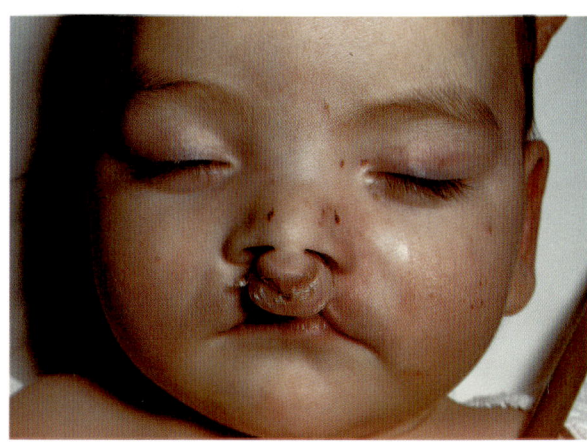

Fig. 17.25 *The short columella and the flattening of the nose.*

lie either in tongue intrusion, which tends to favour one side over the other, or, more probably, in the particular position of the face of the fetus in its mother's womb. Naturally, the existence of bridges may also create asymmetrical muscle forces which modify the position of the premaxilla.

The lesser segments of the maxilla are separated from one another and from the midline to a variable degree. Their morphology is similar to that of the small segment in unilateral forms. They too are subjected to pressure from the superficial muscle mass, and tend to present anterior collapse as compared with an ideal articulation with the inferior arch.

Bone misalignment and medial hypoplasia, which is often significant in these cases, are responsible for the abnormally short columella. The domes of the alar cartilages are 'unrolled', so to speak, by diverging muscle traction. The nasal tip appears to be foreshortened as well as flattened and broadened (Fig. 17.25).

The slanted palatal shelves and the enlarged pharynx are also factors in bilateral clefts. The vomer, as stated, is in a high position. The lower border of the bone shows no angulation with the posterior border.

18. Lesions of the nose

It is customary to consider that there is no malformation of the nose in labio-palatal clefts. Obviously this is not the case, since there is a gap in the nasal floor.

As a rule, the normal ring formed by the nostril is no longer intact, and the muscles that surround its opening have lost their midline insertions. It is true, however, that the deformities observed predominate over hypoplasia of the osteo-cartilaginous structures, and that the nasal pyramid merely seems deviated. Nonetheless, the nasal septum numbers among these structures and rectifying its deformities represents an essential aspect of surgical repair.

A present trend advocates early repair of nasal deformities during primary surgery. In our opinion, the nature of the bone deformities involved precludes this policy. They are such that the nose cannot be straightened without osteotomies. On the other hand, if the bone anomalies are not corrected and the cartilages alone are repaired, this is bound to result in an abnormal anatomical structure. It is impossible to predict the effects of growth on its future development.

Prior to any discussion of corrective techniques, it is essential to understand the precise nature of the anatomical lesions that affect the nasal structures. These are significantly different in unilateral and bilateral clefts.

UNILATERAL CLEFTS

Deformities of the bones and cartilages are basically standard from one case to another, although they may vary in degree. These deformities are the result of muscular action exerted during the early formation of the facial structures – to be more precise, of the traction or pressure generated by the superficial facial muscles on one hand, and by the muscle mass of the tongue on the other.

Bony structures

In these children, the tongue is retropositioned. It also undergoes lateral displacement compared with the sagittal midline of the face, since it intrudes into the maxillo-palatal cleft. This causes lateral deviation of the mandible, which is intimately associated with the tongue. The tongue is responsible for increasing the gap between the bony segments of the cleft maxilla (Fig. 18.1). Tongue pressure also causes the

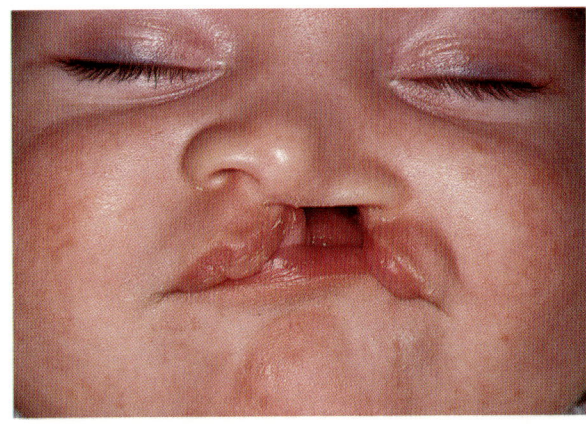

Fig. 18.1 The tongue intrudes into the cleft and increases the gap between the segments.

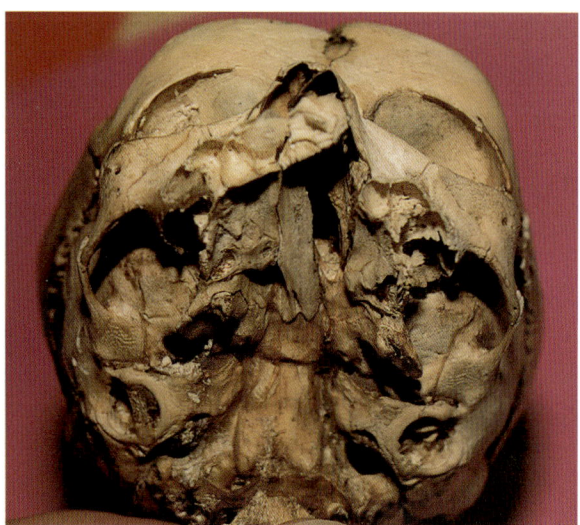

Fig. 18.2 Deformities of the vomer.

1.   *Poutriquet's ridge*
2.   *Un-named furrow at the base of the septum.*

palatal shelf of the lesser segment to slant at a latero-medial and inferior-superior angle.

The side of the vomer facing the cleft is also subject to the same abnormal tongue pressure. The vomer turns on its longitudinal axis and is rotated so that its lateral aspect faces downward (Fig. 18.2). As a result a fold is formed on the vomer, and bulges along about two-thirds of its posterior portion. This rounded prominence is known as the vomerian or

Poutriquet's ridge. The nature of this ridge (or crest) is complex because it corresponds to a crease in the vomerine bone, which is inserted into the sphenoid, near the posterior border while further forward it is found at the junction between the upper border of the vomer and the perpendicular plate of the ethmoid bone. Here, Poutriquet's crest can form a ridge of bone corresponding to the upper border of the vomer.

This ridge marks the virtual summit of the roof of the cleft oral cavity. It is therefore located on a level facing the free border of the palatal shelf of the small segment, which is set on a steep upward slant (Fig. 18.3).

The separation in the facial muscle layer also leads to bone displacement on the superficial level of the facial skeleton. Normally, the contractions of the orbicularis oris function as a sphincter. Here, however, the gap in the muscle fibers at the level of the nostril sill creates new diverging forces which are diametrically opposed to normal physiology (Fig. 18.4).

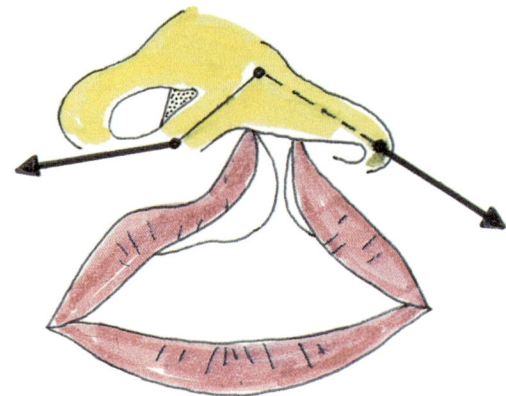

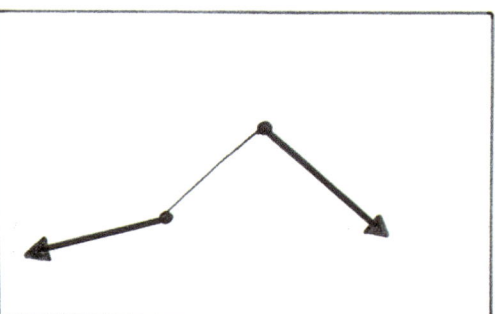

Fig. 18.3 Slant of the palatal shelves. The border of the palatal shelf of the small segment is on a level with Poutriquet's ridge.

Fig. 18.4 Diverging forces created by gap in the muscle layer, and their coupled effect on the orifice of the nostril.

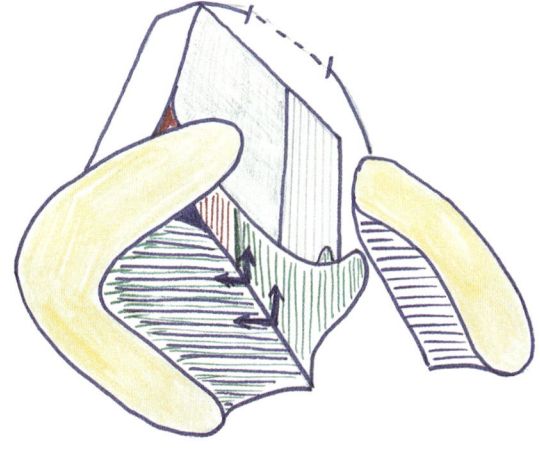

a

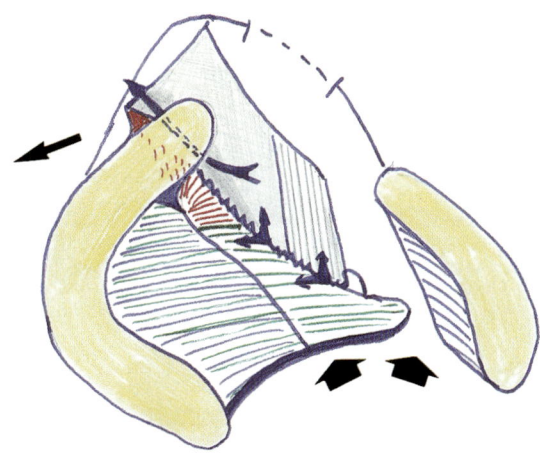

b

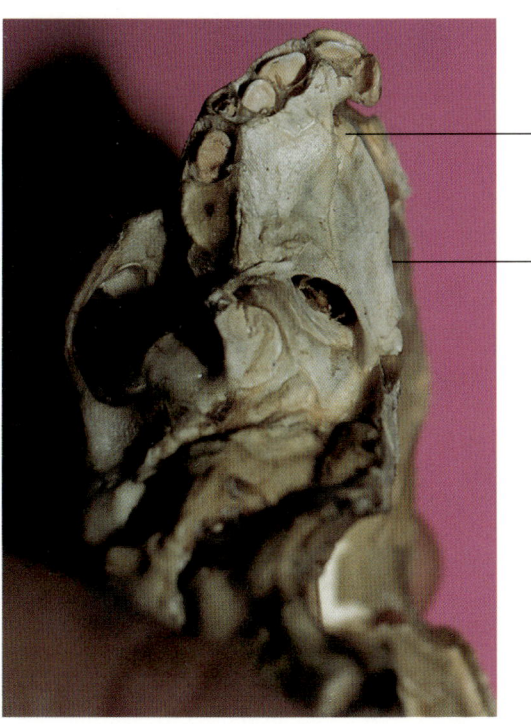

c

Due to the continuity between surface and deep structures at the cleft, the outer fibers which insert into the periosteum of the small segment ('periosteal junction') have a two-fold effect. They produce an eversion of the outer alar base and, to a lesser degree, displace the anterior portion of the small segment to the side. Vertical continuity of the muscle layer, which subsists despite the cleft, brings antero-posterior pressure to bear on the anterior extremity of the bone. This pressure prevails over the outward displacement, and tends to deform the anterior alveolar arch into the shape of a *J*. The impression created is that the cleft has discreetly narrowed (cf. Chapter 17).

The inner fibers have an effect on the greater or major segment. They pull the anterior nasal spine from the midline towards the normal side, and this deflection causes the premaxilla to rotate so that its lateral aspect on the cleft side faces upward.

Thus, the premaxillary bone undergoes considerable torque. Its posterior portion follows the deformation of the vomer to which it remains attached, so that it faces downward. Its anterior portion containing the incisive structures twists in the opposite direction until its lateral aspect on the cleft side faces upward. This torque effect dislocates the junction between the premaxilla and the septal cartilage. The septum is automatically deviated towards the normal side, since it follows the displacement of the anterior nasal spine and the premaxillary bone. The torque effect on the premaxilla itself also creates a deep, narrow furrow, which is clearly visible on the side towards the cleft at the juncture between bone and cartilage (Fig. 18.5). The cartilage tends to slip out of

Fig. 18.5 *Deformities of the septum and premaxillary bone:*
a. Diagram of a normal septum (the cleft shows the normal angle between shelf and vomer).
b. Under lingual pressure, the vomer is found in the extension of the palatal shelf of the major segment. The nasal spine twists in the opposite direction, which produces the torque effect on the premaxilla.
c. On the portion of the skeleton that contains the large segment, Poutriquet's ridge and the un-named furrow are visible.

1. *Poutriquet's ridge*
2. *Inominate sulcus*

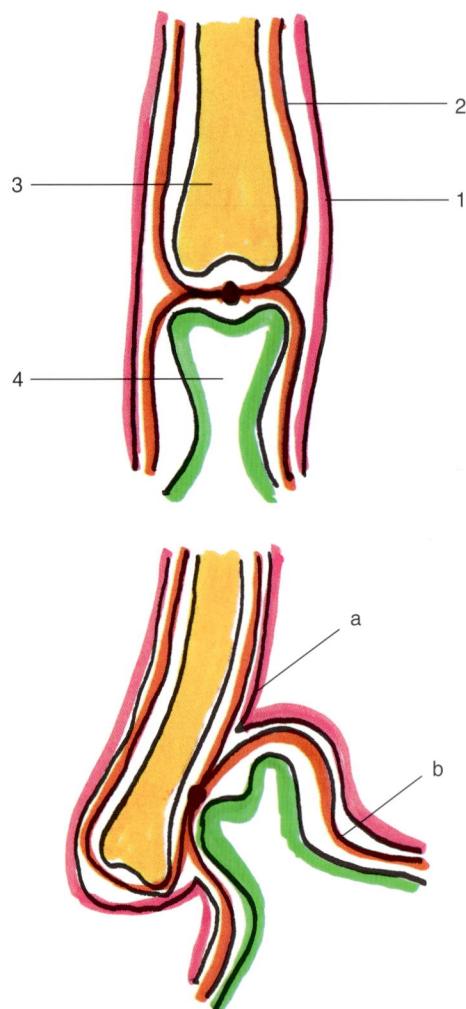

Fig. 18.6 *Dislocation of the septal cartilage. A second furrow (a) appears up to the un-named furrow (b).*

1. *Mucosa*
2. *Periosteum*
3. *Septal cartilage*
4. *Anterior nasal spine*

the upper groove presented by the two premaxillary bones like a tire coming off its rim (Fig. 18.6).

This furrow, different from the un-named furrow just described, runs in a continuous line with Poutriquet's ridge, is sharp and deep. As a result, the septum takes on a highly characteristic shape. Its posterior portion seems to balloon like the sail of a ship, while the anterior portion is deflected towards the non-cleft side where its lower end is visible in the normal nostril opening (Fig. 18.7).

The gap in the superficial muscle layer has additional anatomical repercussions. Its main consequence concerns the misalignment of the bone structures on the borders.

When the antero-posterior pressure normally exerted on the peripheral surface of the bone structures

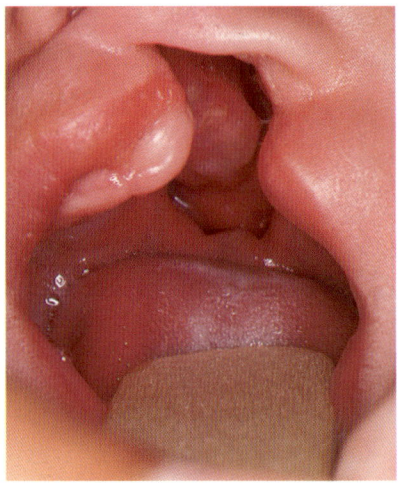

Fig. 18.7 *Septum bulging into the nasal fossa on the cleft side.*

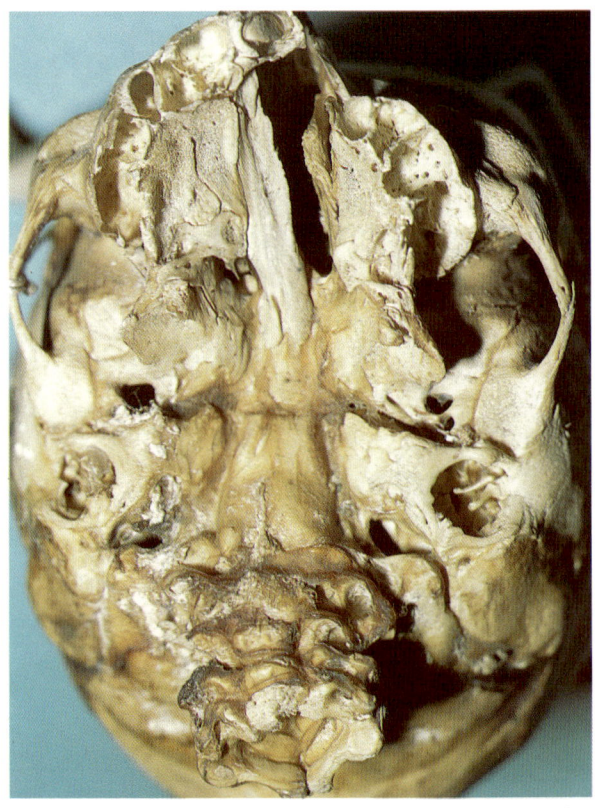

Fig. 18.8 *Misalignment of the alveolar borders.*

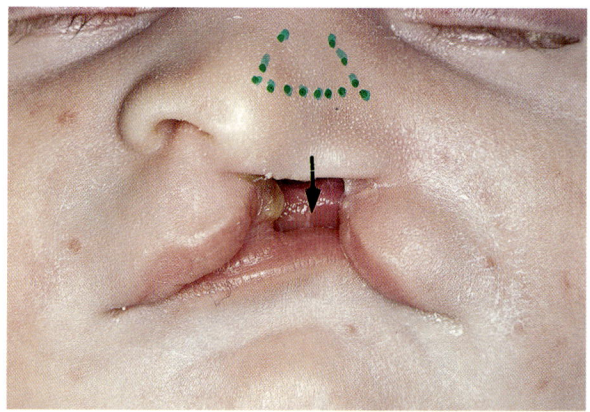

Fig. 18.9 *Lowering of the soft tissues contributes to nasal deformity.*

by the facial muscle fibers is absent or significantly reduced, there is no longer a limit to forward growth of the vomer. Thus, the premaxilla shifts forward compared with the normal frontal plane of the face. The antero-posterior misalignment of the bony segments is linked to this advance of the premaxilla and to the retraction of the lesser segment described earlier (Fig. 18.8).

The loss of midline muscle insertions on the anterior nasal spine results in a general lowering of the lateral soft tissues, which are subjected to the downward muscle pull most frequently produced by such movements as the opening of the mouth or contractions of the neck muscles. Therefore, the corner of the lip is found below its normal level on the cleft side, as is the outer alar base (Fig. 18.9). (See Chapter 6.)

Cartilaginous structures

Abnormal insertions, modified muscle action and subsequent lowering of the soft tissues combine with the misalignment of the bony borders to depress or flatten the cartilaginous structures.

The tip of the nose and the axis of the columella are deflected towards the cleft side. The dome of the alar cartilage is 'unrolled' or flattened on the cleft side. Its prominence corresponds solely to the existence of the normal alar cartilage.

A general lowering of the soft tissues on the cleft side causes the alar cartilage to slip down the ipsilateral triangular cartilage on which its upper portion

normally rests. The medial crus is hypoplastic, and its lower end is flattened towards the nostril opening at the base of the columella.

The lower end of the septum no longer fits into the space between the medial crura of the alar cartilages, and the cartilaginous structures can truly be described as dislocated. We have already drawn attention to the fact that the lower edge of the septum is visible in the non-cleft nostril.

The lateral crus is virtually collapsed in the nostril vestibule, and contributes to the formation of naso-vestibular infolding. The alar rotation and eversion of the alar wing produce a visible fold in the free border, which is continued within the nostril by the bulge of the outer portion of the alar cartilage. This creates a naso-vestibular fold totally distinct from the normal plica nasii, which corresponds to the edge of the maxilla (Fig. 18.10).

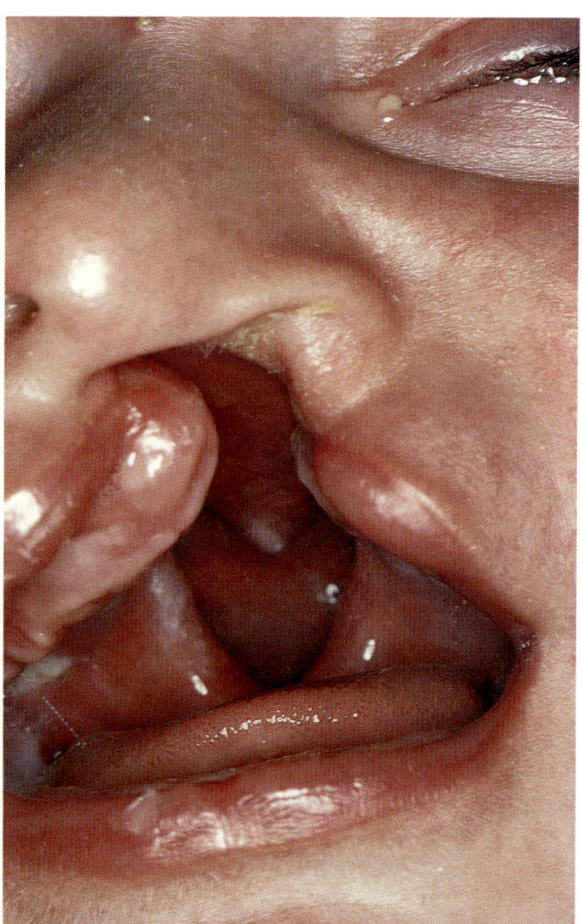

Fig. 18.10 *Deformities of the cartilages in the tip of the nose and formation of a naso-vestibular fold.*

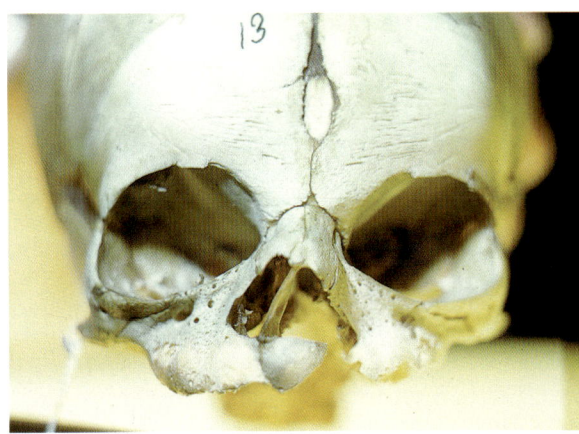

Fig. 18.11 *Deflection of the bony pyramid towards the non-cleft side.*

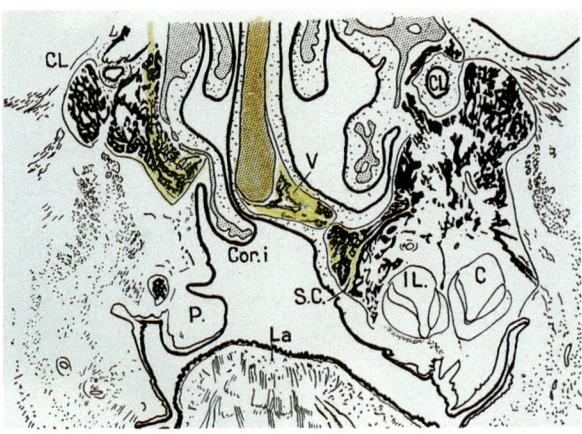

Fig. 18.12 *Coronal section shows decrease in height of nasal fossa and hypertrophy of inferior nasal concha (Veau).*

The pyramid made up of the nasal bones and the triangular cartilages is also deformed by the many displacements described above. It follows the deflection of the anterior portion of the septum towards the normal side (Fig. 18.11). Due to this displacement, the triangular cartilage seems unusually broad. Its lower border droops below its normal level.

Other effects

Unilateral clefts can also cause other defects of the anatomy of the nose and nasal fossae.

Contrary to what might be expected, the volume of the nasal fossa is not diminished, nor is its permeability affected by deviation of the septum towards the non-cleft side. This will no longer be the case, however, after cleft repair. Closure of the cleft does not automatically reverse the process of displacement which took place during the embryological development of the facial structures. The inferior nasal concha is generally hypertrophic, and its free border is way below its normal level. This can be easily detected on CT scan coronal views. The slant of the palatal shelves and the displacement of the lateral surface of the vomer facing the cleft side into the oral cavity reduce the vertical height of the nasal fossa (Fig. 18.12).

Tongue pressure exerted towards the back of the oral cavity reduces the size of the choanal opening on both sides. The velar stumps are now close to the upper wall of the nasopharynx. This partially obstructs the airway, and this factor must be taken

into account once the oral vault is reconstructed. During the swallowing process the velar stumps develop a very peculiar pathological physiology, which is clearly visible on videofluoroscopic studies. The stumps rotate on a slanted line starting anteriorly at the inner summit of the palatal shelf (normal

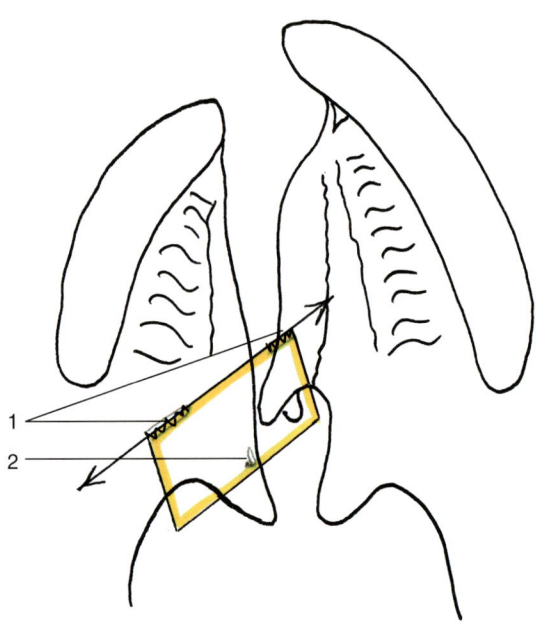

Fig. 18.13 *'Swinging door' movement of the velar stumps obstructs the choanae due to pressure from the tongue during swallowing.*

1. *Hinge-pins*
2. *Handle*

location of the posterior nasal spine, which is cleft in this case) and extending as far back as the levator palatini. Under pressure from the tongue the velar stumps partially or completely obturate the choanae, which do or do not open downward depending on the nature of the cleft. This prevents or at least limits nasal reflux of the alimentary bolus (Fig. 18.13; see also Chapter 10). This constant constriction of the airway, combined with the width of the gap, helps to explain why children with cleft palate are usually oral breathers. In a later section, further discussion will be devoted to the need for early repair in order to eliminate this undesirable respiratory habit. Once the reflex becomes integrated into neuromotor patterns, it is extremely difficult to suppress.

The lowering and eversion of the outer alar base on the cleft side and the lowering of the inferior border of the triangular cartilages affect the nostril vestibule. We have already pointed out the development of a naso-vestibular fold. Furthermore, a portion of the pilous endonasal skin pertaining to the ala comes into view and seems to belong to the upper part of the cutaneous lip. This can be a source of error when the reference points are plotted for cutaneous plasty, and may lead to placing the reference point for the nostril sill of the outer border too high.

BILATERAL CLEFTS

Nasal lesions in bilateral clefts are radically different. In symmetrical forms, which are the most typical, the nose is straight and is not deflected from the midline. The nasal tip is characteristically flattened and broadened (Fig. 18.14).

As a rule, there is no deviation of the septum. The absence of normal lip pressure on the underlying bone structure explains the projection of the premaxilla, which flares forward due to unchecked growth of the vomer.

The two lesser segments are set far back from the premaxilla. This misalignment of the bone structures is accentuated by the pressure exerted on their anterior portion by the superficial muscle layer (Fig. 18.15). On either side, there is a tendency towards ptosis of the soft tissues previously described in the section on unilateral clefts.

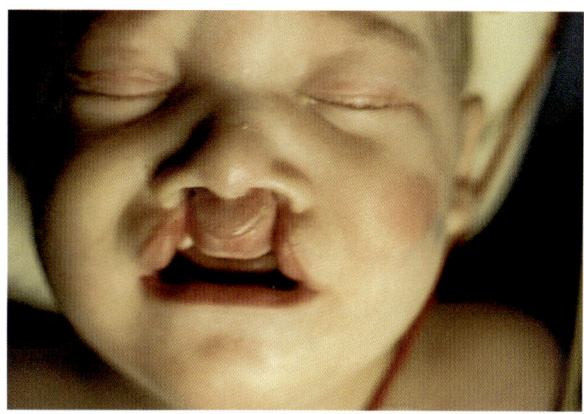

Fig. 18.14 *In symmetrical bilateral clefts, the nose is broadened but remains straight.*

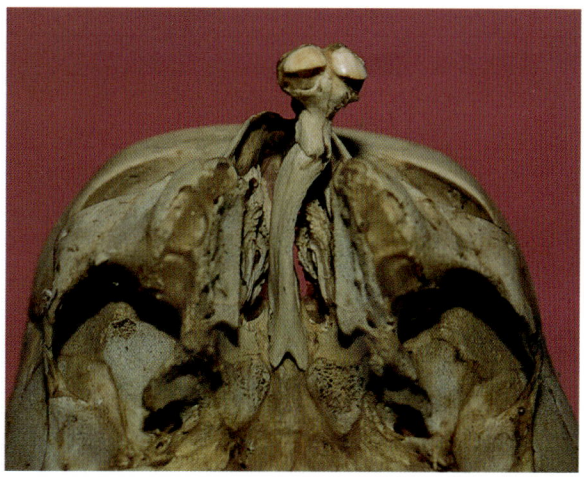

Fig. 18.15 *Misalignment of bony borders is considerable.*

Diverging lateral pull exerted on either side by the facial muscles, which have lost their midline insertions on the nasal spine, 'unrolls' the domes of the alar cartilages. The nasal tip is flattened and at the same time broadened.

In addition, the medial crura and soft tissues are hypoplastic (it is thought that the mesenchyme which progresses from the sides towards the midline must have failed to penetrate this zone during embryological development). The resulting lack of columellar development is a hallmark of bilateral clefts (Fig. 18.16). This hypoplasia extends to the antero-inferior portion of the septal cartilage, which no longer supports the alar domes. It is associated with hypoplasia of the prolabium, which is often reduced to a small, biconvex mass, and with the absence of a medial labial vestibule.

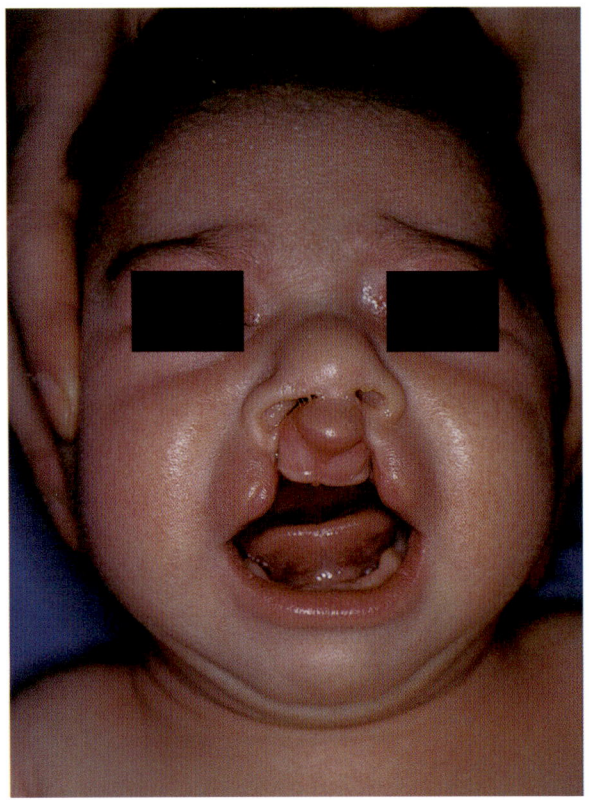

Fig. 18.16 *Hypoplasia of the columella and prolabium.*

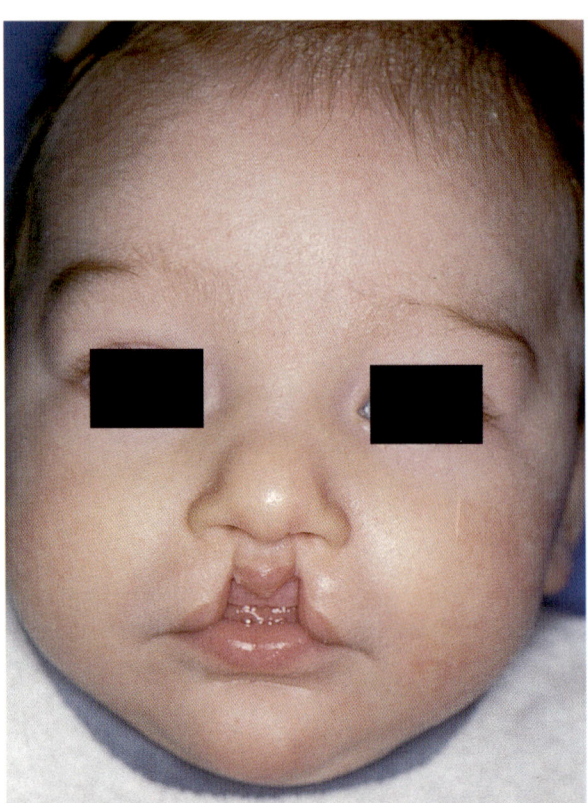

Fig. 18.17 *In simple bilateral forms, nasal deformity is minor despite pronounced hypoplasia of the prolabium.*

The bone structures of the nasal pyramid may show deficient development as well. As a rule, they are only moderately broadened except in the case of orbital hypertelorism or median cleft face syndrome, which is not uncommon.

There is no particular effect on the triangular cartilages.

Lastly, the height of the choanae is also reduced.

In bilateral clefts with a bridge of soft tissue, nasal deformities are less pronounced but they are comparable in nature (Fig. 18.17).

In asymmetrical forms, the deformities are similar to those found in unilateral clefts (deviated septum and nasal spine, distorted alar cartilages) but they are compounded by the signs of more or less pronounced medial hypoplasia.

19. Guidelines for primary treatment

This chapter is essential since it focuses on the tremendous differences in the various therapeutic methods applied nowadays. There is no consensus of opinion, either on the right age for surgery or on the surgical techniques themselves.

The age at which repair is first undertaken varies widely from one surgeon to the next. A number of criteria must be taken into account when determining the best age for surgery – the anatomical form, the extent of anesthetic and surgical risk, the inevitable iatrogenic effects inherent to surgery and their repercussions on the growth process, and the degree of technical difficulty involved (which depends on the patient's anatomical development). One of the most important factors is that of functional development, which is disrupted by the existence of the gap – above all in the case of palatal clefts.

The sequence of the stages of surgery, which often involves multiple operations, also represents a highly controversial point.

The choice of therapy must be made immediately after birth. This is a very difficult decision for the parents, who are not always in a position to grasp the surgeon's reasoning. The ordeal of having to consult a series of different practitioners, as is usually the case in large cities, tends to overwhelm the parents who are already deeply distressed. The obstetrician and pediatrician therefore have a key role to play in helping the parents to come to a decision. Needless to say, they themselves must be familiar with cleft pathology.

Only the long-term results of the methods of treatment proposed can serve as a valid basis for judging their respective merits, and a thorough knowledge of the lesions and of their repercussions on physiology is also required to justify any changes in the treatment prescribed. Lastly, in our profession we cannot expect positive results from a therapeutic method that is not true to a certain logic.

It is wise to be extremely wary of new trends based on presentations which are inevitably rushed and incomplete due to the rising numbers of conventions and symposiums organized in the past few years. Before launching into what is bound to be a long and arduous program of treatment, the best attitude to adopt is one of serious reflection on the basic notions: normal versus pathological anatomy, physio-pathology.

No one can presume to have a monopoly on truth, however, the outlook is always brighter if a therapeutic consensus can be reached (there is room for evolution, of course, in the treatment agreed upon). For the time being, unfortunately, the lack of consensus puts an extra burden on the parents who, after consulting several specialists, are faced with the dilemma of conflicting opinions.

20. Early primary palate repair

ARGUMENTS IN FAVOR

Now the anatomical lesions of complete clefts have been described, we can turn to the physiological disorders they generate. These troubles stem from palatal division, which is the major factor of the malformation, as Veau clearly stressed. Their consequences have already been outlined in Chapter 10 devoted to isolated cleft palate. However, since the cleft affects the bone structures, we must also include the consequences of muscular imbalance on the alignment of the segments. Their growth pattern is also seriously altered.

Before presenting our technique and its results, let us first examine the anatomical and physiological arguments that motivated the new therapeutic approach established jointly with Jean Psaume, our former team orthodontist, and applied from 1975.

Until 1975, the guidelines set up by Veau had been followed – in other words, the 'classical' method – with slight modifications to the calendar as suggested by Petit. These included closure of the lip, the alveolar site and the adjoining anterior vault at 6 months (Fig. 20.1a), and repair of the palate (velum and remaining vault) using the palatal mucoperiosteum at 18 months (Fig. 20.1b).

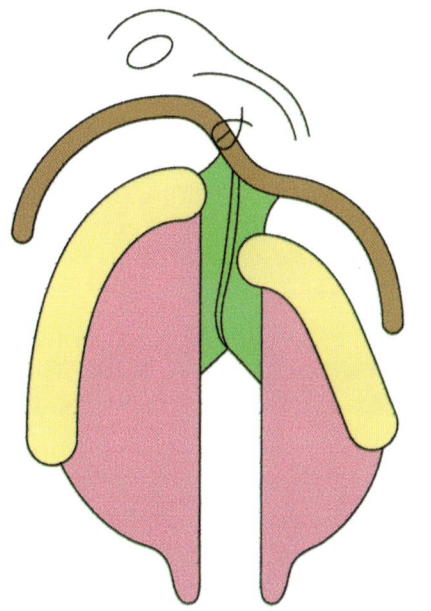 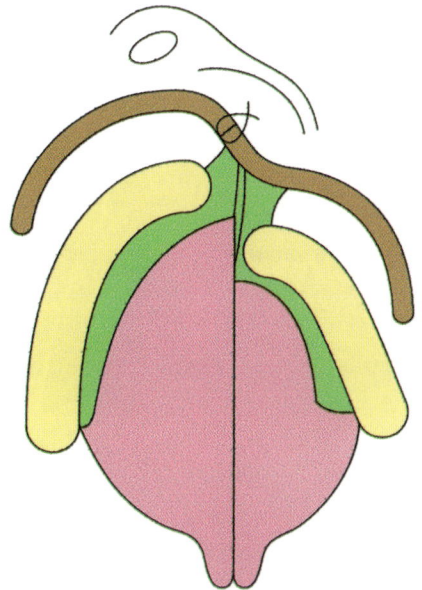

Fig. 20.1 The 'classic' method: Veau and Petit.

a 6 months

b 18 months

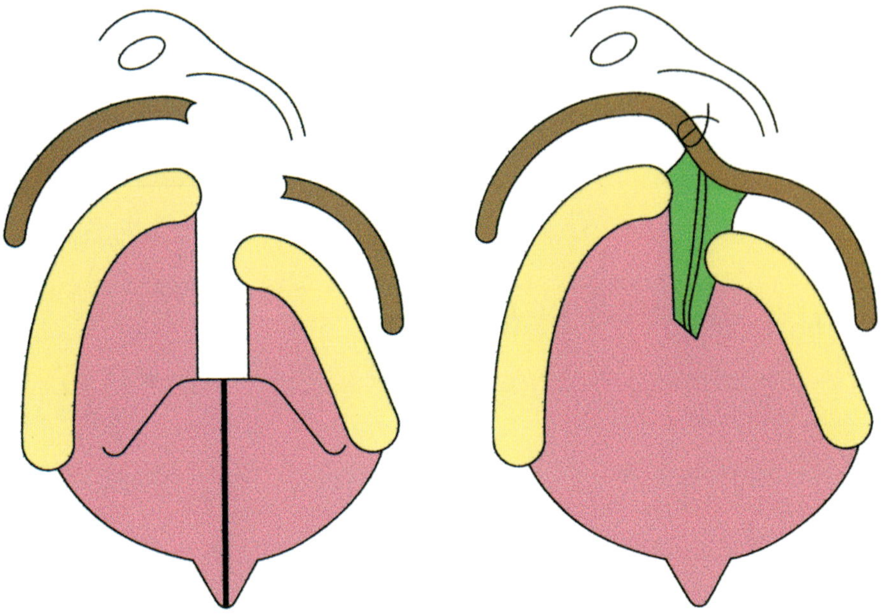

a 3 months   *b 6 months*

Fig. 20.2 *The early primary palate method.*

According to the new approach, the early primary palate method, we now proceed in the following order: first, the soft palate is corrected at 3 months (Fig. 20.2a) and second, the lip and the anterior hard palate are repaired at 6 months (in unilateral forms). It is important to note that we no longer resort to elevation of the palatal mucoperiosteum for closure of the vault due to the iatrogenic risk (Fig. 20.2b).

The term 'early primary palate' was initially chosen to highlight the fact that palatal repair is performed at a much earlier age than the 'classical' methods. The abbreviation PP1 (for the French 'palais précoce') is the reference customarily used to designate the first stage of our method (i.e. veloplasty), as opposed to PP2, which refers to early palatal closure in cases of isolated cleft palate.

As will be demonstrated, a valid case can now be made for this method based on the supporting evidence of a large number of patients with favorable long-term results. We feel fully confident in recommend it as the ideal procedure for complete cleft surgery.

The arguments in favor of our modified therapeutic approach can be grouped under three headings:

1. Skeletal or maxillo-dental reasons
2. Reasons for performing surgery early
3. Reasons for inverting the surgical sequence.

Skeletal or maxillo-dental reasons

Initially, our main goal was to improve maxillo-dental results. Even under ideal technical conditions, the 'classical' procedure produced results that left much to be desired. True, since statistics were not the fashion at the time, little data on this period is available; however, to judge by the feedback from our own patients in Petit's Department, over half the cases presented mediocre or poor results despite long-term orthopedic and orthodontal treatment (Fig. 20.3a and b). A considerable number of patients eventually required corrective osteotomies of the maxilla (Lefort 1).

During the 1960s, surgeons throughout the world were confronted with the same lack of success.

The major problem was apparently linked to transverse approximation of the maxillary segments (essentially due to collapse of the small segment) and retrusion of the upper jaw compared with the lower because of deficient maxillary growth (pseudo-mandibulary prognathia). Various solutions were suggested:

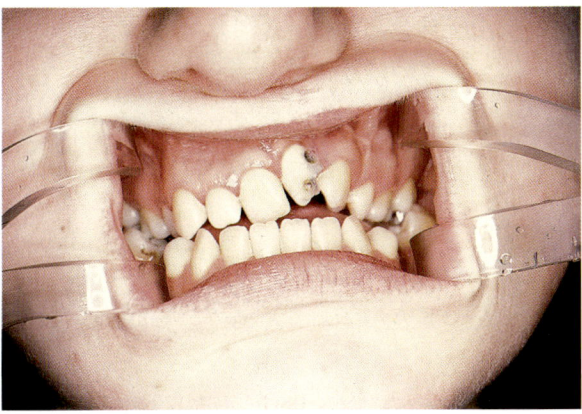

a

Fig. 20.3 *Mediocre results of the classical schedule despite long-term orthodontic treatment:*

a. Poor occlusion

b. Poor profile related to retrognathism of the maxilla. **b**

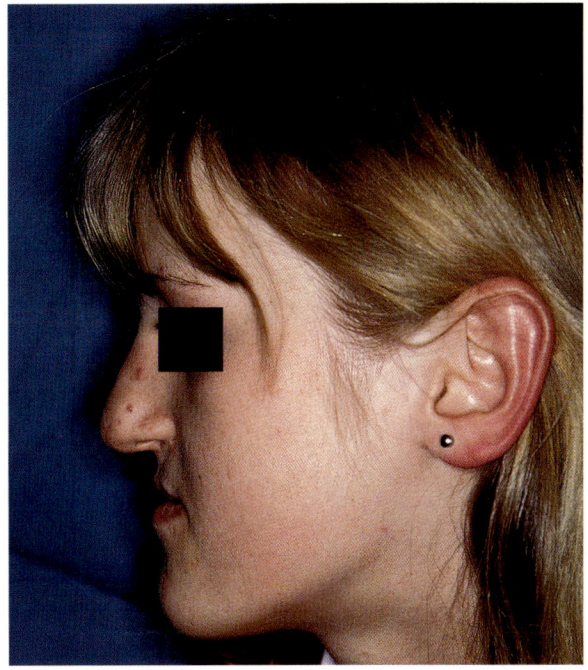

1. There was a certain hasty tendency to automatically incriminate an inevitable hypoplastic malformation. At one time a bone graft was recommended to block this process of transverse narrowing, which tended to become even more accentuated after treatment. The technique was widely applied, but soon feel into disfavor, even among its original advocates, since it clearly jeopardized normal growth (Fig. 20.4) (Friede and Johanson, 1982).

2. Other surgeons, including Gillies and, above all, Schweckendieck, cautioned against the iatrogenic risk of raising the mucoperiosteum during closure

Fig. 20.4 *Primary intermaxillary bone graft.*

a. Configuration of the rib grafts.

b. Vomerian mucosa used as lining (Stellmach, 1959, Scrubble and Stellmach, 1959).

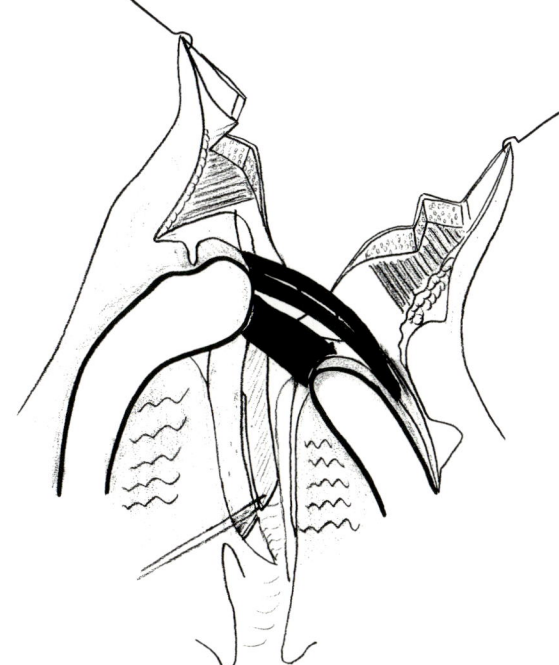

a **b**

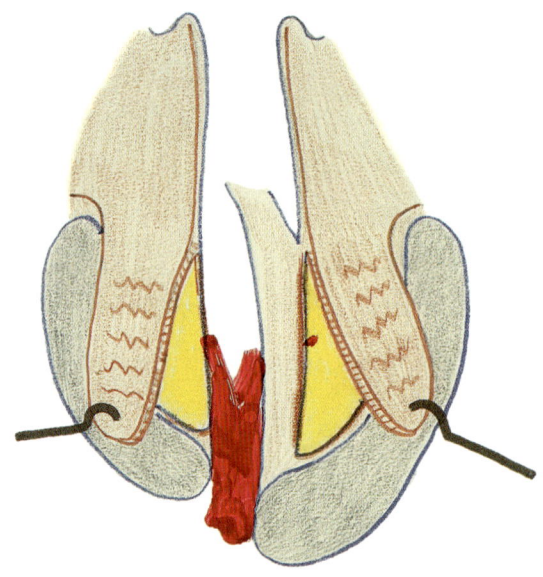

Fig. 20.5 *Iatrogenic effects of elevating the palatine mucoperiosteum are largely responsible for the poor results.*

of the palate (Fig. 20.5). They advocated postponing this step until maxillary growth was well advanced. No precise age or date was set for this stage of surgery, and it varied widely from one surgeon to another – from 5–13 years of age! (Fig. 20.6a,b,c). Many experimental studies were carried out using this method (Herfert, 1958; Kremenak *et al.*, 1967, 1970a, 1970b), and the convincing results led to its adoption world-wide. It is still in use today.

At the time, our medical team, in complete agreement with Petit, were concerned that the development of proper speech patterns might suffer if the palatal vault were left open over such a long period. Hence, while retaining the principle of leaving the periosteum intact, we determined to close the entire cleft. Once the appropriate technique had been perfected, we were in a position to modify the surgical schedule as well.

Reasons for performing surgery early

The second reason for modifying the operating agenda resulted from our determination to effect early repair of the palatal cleft (essentially of the cleft soft palate). This is because of the functional disorders it generates, which we were anxious to eliminate as quickly as possible, and because of the role played by the palatal cleft in the onset and unfavorable evolution of anatomical lesions which, after only a short length of time, can no longer be reversed.

Surgery during the first weeks of life presented itself as the obvious solution and, despite the slightly greater technical difficulties involved, the progress made in pediatric anesthesia justified the decision to operate on very young infants.

Nevertheless, it was considered advisable to delay closure of the soft palate until the velar stumps (which are tiny and frail during the early weeks of life due to congenital hypoplasia and, no doubt, to lack of use as

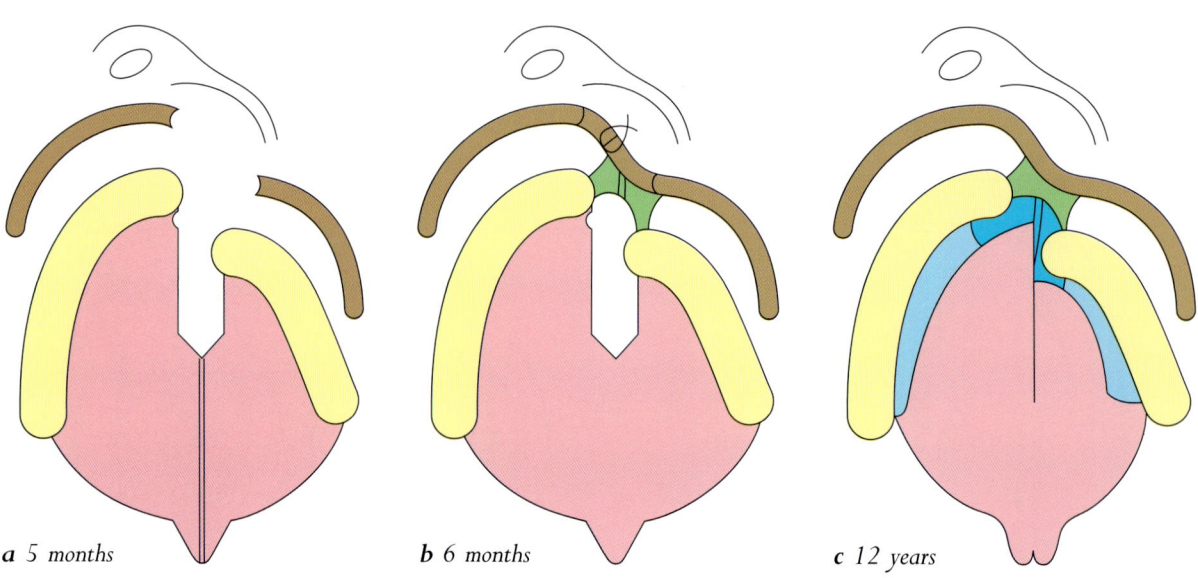

a 5 months   *b 6 months*   *c 12 years*

Fig. 20.6 *Schweckendieck method. Secondary closure of the interalveolar region is difficult without re-opening the lip.*

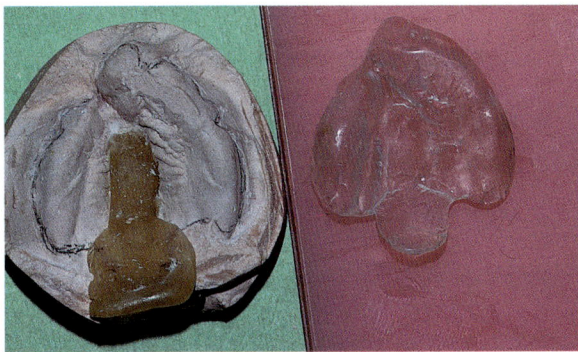

a

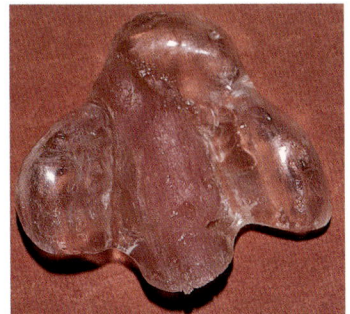

b

Fig. 20.7 First palatal appliance with velar extension.
a. Unilateral cleft.
b. Bilateral cleft.

well) had taken on a certain volume. It is undeniable that the velar stumps do develop to some extent over the first few weeks of life. Although they do not actively participate in the actual swallowing process, the muscles do still contract and grow more sturdy. There was clearly a need to leave an initial interval before veloplasty, and we arbitrarily set it at 3 months.

In the meanwhile, it was judged wise to fit the infants with a palatal appliance which would partially close the cleft (Fig. 20.7a and b).

Advantages of an appliance (plate)

Along with Jean Psaume, we initially believed that the plate would serve a two-fold purpose: first, it would prevent the tongue from penetrating into the back of the cleft; secondly, since the infant willingly sucks the appliance, this would contribute to moving the tongue forward. Thus, the plate should limit the risk involved in spontaneous narrowing of the anterior portions of the alveolar rims.

Other advantages include easier bottle-feeding, since the nipple can be compressed against the plate, and parental relief, since the appliance gives the impression that treatment of their infant has now begun.

Despite the benefits that may be involved, these points remain open to discussion.

Reasons for inverting the surgical sequence

As explained, the surgical sequence begins with veloplasty, followed several weeks later by lip repair. This inversion of the conventional steps calls for an additional explanation, and this is where the problem of muscular imbalance enters into play.

Several reminders are called for in this context:

1. The maxillary cleft means potential *mobility of the bone segments*. Only thin, malleable lamellae of bone now attach these segments to the rest of the facial skeleton.

2. The position and normal action of *the tongue* are modified by the existence of the cleft. Because the palate is no longer intact, swallowing disorders develop. At the back of the oral cavity, the tongue penetrates into the nasopharynx in the process of moving the alimentary bolus towards the esophagus (Fig. 20.8). Posterior lingual pressure enlarges the nasopharynx (a phenomenon attested by the increased distance between the pterygoid processes) as was explained in the section on anatomy. Videofluoroscopic studies have shown the role of the tongue. The Thornwall bursa is clearly seen and the elevation of the tongue is proven. The two halves of the velum are pushed

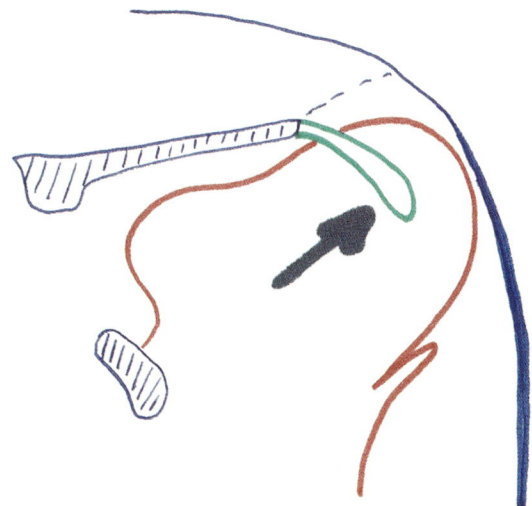

Fig. 20.8 When the tongue penetrates into the nasopharynx, the velar stumps are pushed outward.

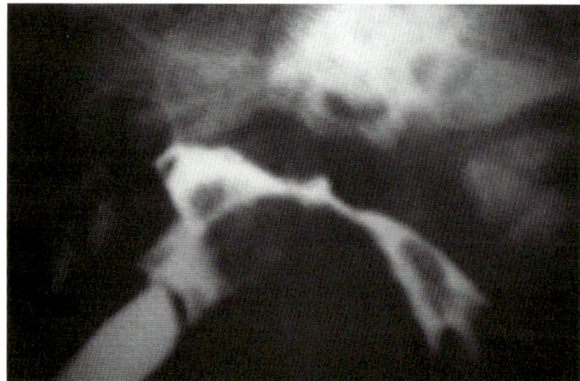

Fig. 20.9 *Videofluoroscopic view of deglutition.*

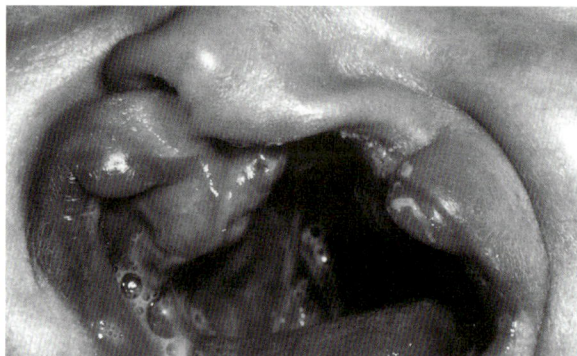

Fig. 20.10 *Diverging mechanical forces generated by the gap in the muscles.*

laterally (Fig. 20.9). It is widely acknowledged that the tongue plays a significant role in moulding the maxilla, and it therefore seems logical to assume that if its action shifts towards the back of the mouth, there is bound to be a decrease in the pressure that the tongue normally brings to bear on the anterior portion of the inner surface of the bone segments.

3. The insertions of the *superficial facial muscles* are modified by the cleft. Normally, the orbicularis oris acts as a sphincter with converging pull, but the gap created by the cleft obviously leads to altogether new mechanical forces which pull apart rather than together. These diverging forces are exerted primarily on the greater segment, which includes the nasal spine where the muscles on the non-cleft side have retained their midline insertions (Fig. 20.10). However, despite the cleft, the

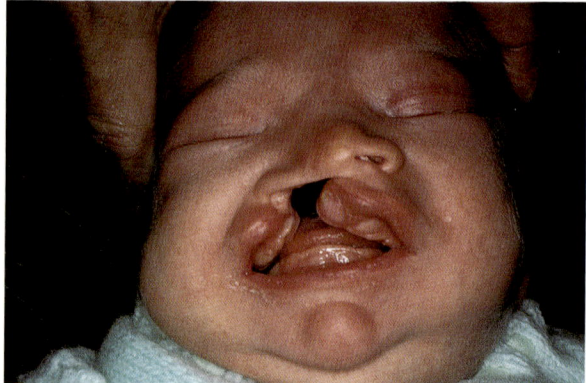

a

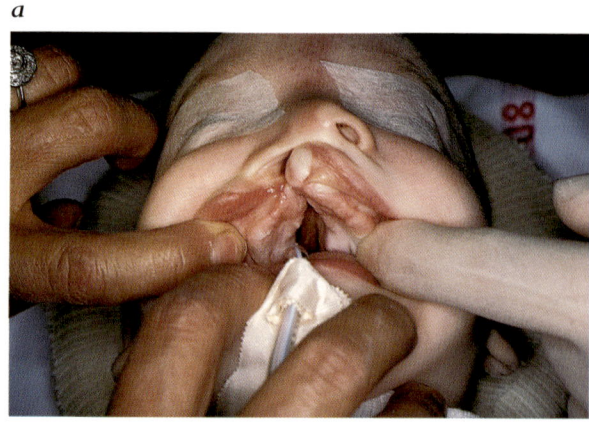

b

Fig. 20.12 *Spontaneous narrowing of the borders of the cleft:*
a. At birth.
b. At 4 months of age.

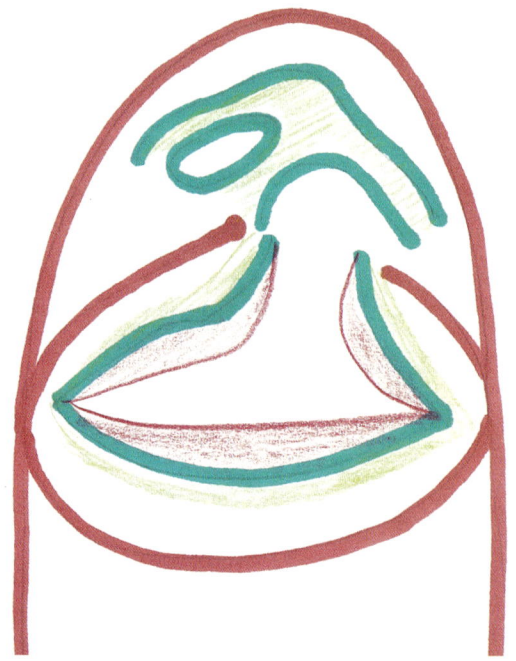

Fig. 20.11 *Muscular continuity subsists above and below the mouth; hence the forces exerted on the surface of the bone structures.*

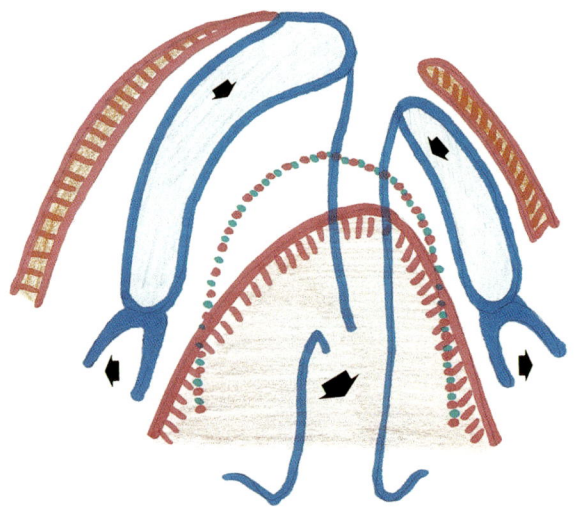

Fig. 20.13 *Orientation of diverse forces exerted on the maxillary segments.*

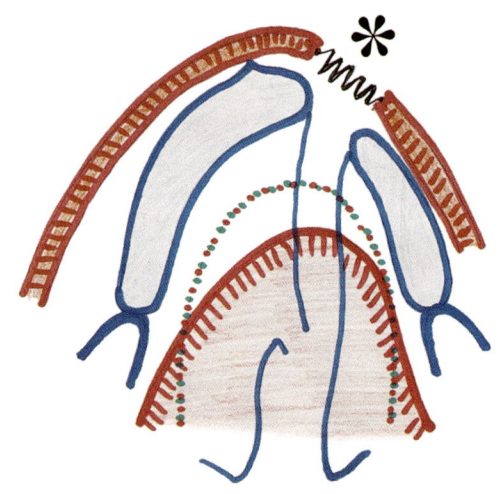

Fig. 20.14 *If the lip is closed first, the concentric forces are increased.*

superficial muscles continue to generate converging forces on the surface of the segments due, in this instance, to the intact muscle layer that subsists above and below the mouth and on the level of the nose and chin (Delaire) (Fig. 20.11). These forces are not wholly offset by the tongue, and the lesser segment, which is the most mobile, may shift inward. It may also be submitted to outside influences with a convergent effect (mothers tend to rest the infant's head on the cleft side to hide the deformity).

Therefore, even before steps are taken to treat the cleft there is a likelihood of small segment collapse and of spontaneous approximation of the borders of the cleft. The risk increases as facial muscle activity develops (feeding, expressions, etc.) (Figs 20.12a and b, 20.13).

OUR THERAPEUTIC HYPOTHESIS

If the lip is repaired first (in other words before the palate), this produces an immediate increase in the anterior concentric forces. This is bound to aggravate displacement of the small segment. The tongue cannot oppose sufficient resistance to offset these forces, since the pressure it exerts is primarily centered towards the back of the mouth during swallowing (Fig. 20.14).

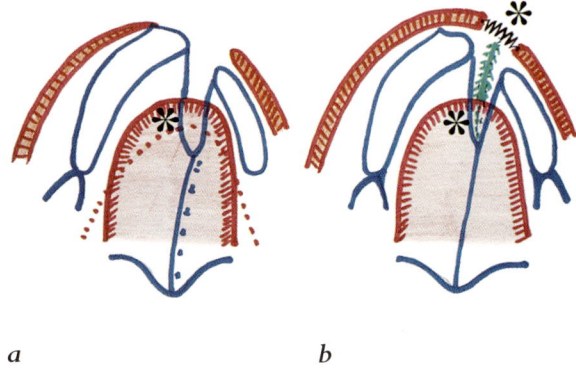

a   *b*

Fig. 20.15 *If the soft palate is repaired first, the tongue is more likely to find a better position (a) and a more satisfactory balance of forces can be anticipated for the stage of cheiloplasty (b).*

If, on the contrary, the palate is repaired first, the tongue is better able to exert anterior pressure on the inner surface of the segments (Fig. 20.15a). When lip repair is performed several months later, a virtually normal balance of antagonistic forces can be expected (Fig. 20.15b). Thus, it is possible to obtain a harmonious development of the upper jaw despite the continued existence of the bony cleft.

The interval between veloplasty and lip repair (second interval) is established as arbitrarily as the first. It can be justified for two reasons.

First, the recovery of normal tongue function cannot happen overnight. It takes a certain length of time (this is a perfectly plausible theory although it cannot as yet be proven). Indeed, the return to normal coincides with narrowing of the pharynx. We have observed the phenomenon with CT scans performed 3 months after veloplasty, which clearly show a normalization of the pterygomaxillary index (Fig. 20.16a and b).

Second, as stated earlier, we were determined to close the entire cleft for functional reasons, but without running the risks involved in using the mucoperiosteum. We needed a means to guarantee safe and reliable closure.

Reconstruction of a nasal mucoperiosteal layer offered one technical possibility, but this is often difficult to suture and may prove unreliable in the long run. This would predispose to residual fistulae.

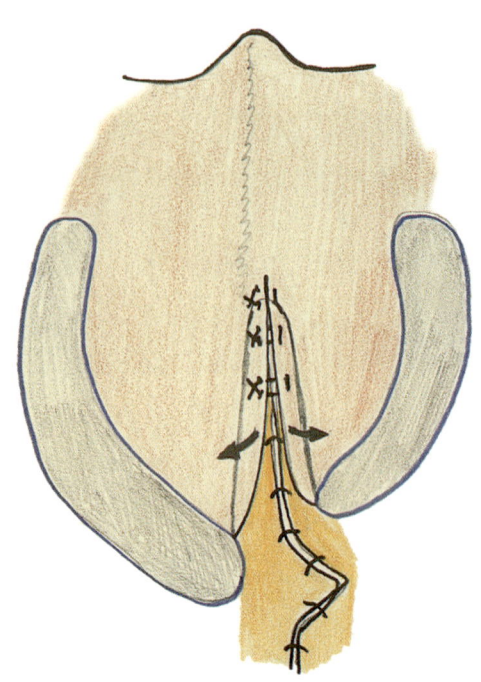

Fig. 20.17 *Two-layer closure represents the most effective way of preventing residual fistulae of the vault.*

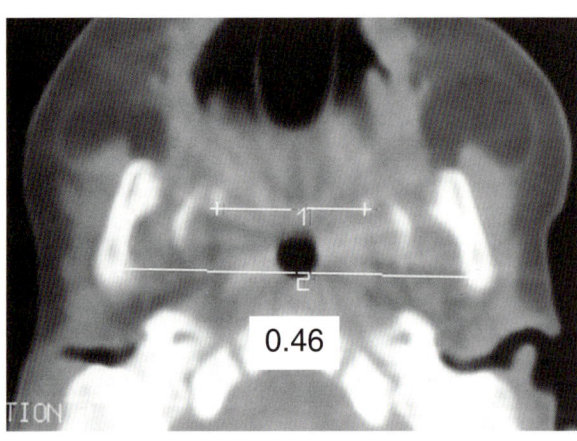

a

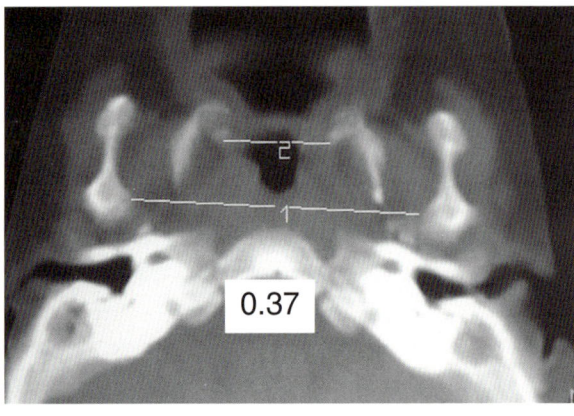

b

Fig. 20.16 *Enlargement of the pharynx can be reversed as demonstrated by successive CT scans at 3 months (a) and, before lip repair, at 6 months (b).*

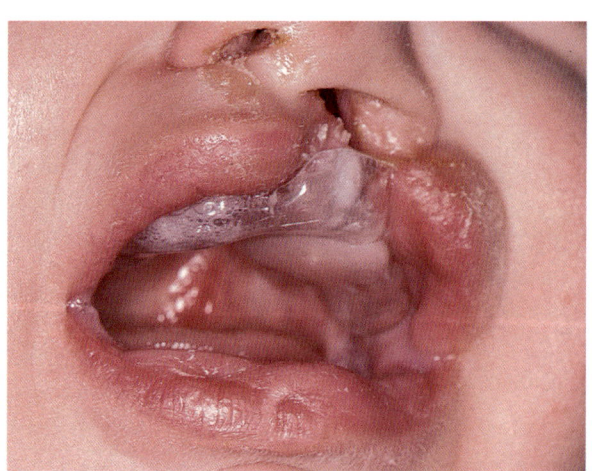

Fig. 20.18 *The second palatal appliance protects the sutures and limits narrowing of the borders after lip repair.*

In our experience the best way to avoid this problem is to use a second oral layer comprised of buccal mucosa, which is thicker and better vascularized. However, unless undermining is extensive, this procedure cannot be applied as long as the edges of the cleft remain too far apart.

We have observed that the width of the cleft diminishes considerably after veloplasty. It is quite often possible to create a second oral layer simply by stitching the borders to one another after only minimal undermining (Fig. 20.17). As an added precaution, a palatal plate is used to protect this layer (second plate) (Fig. 20.18).

We have had many discussions with our orthodontists in an attempt to determine precisely why the cleft narrows after veloplasty. There is no doubt that it can be attributed to the fact that the bone structures themselves draw closer together. This may be linked either to growth of the free margins of the palatal shelves, or to the fact that the shelves themselves straighten out horizontally and are no longer as steeply angled. Then again, the mucosa along the margins may simply thicken. There does not seem to be any one clear conclusion.

Whatever the case, narrowing of the cleft definitely serves our purpose by permitting complete closure of the palatal vault based on two secure layers. Above all, to judge by our cases, there are no harmful repercussions on maxillo-dental development. This alone amply justifies the second interval we have chosen to respect.

It also clinches the argument for our new surgical schedule, which can be applied to all complete forms, whether uni- or bilateral.

OTHER THERAPEUTIC APPROACHES

Our choice of procedure is based on the arguments just discussed.

The approach we have settled on seems all the more justified in the absence of long-term statistics on the results of alternate methods, none of which meet with our unconditional approval. However, a brief review of the other therapeutic methods will permit a useful comparison of their respective principles.

The 'classic' method

The 'classic' method (Veau–Petit) of cheiloplasty at 6 months followed by staphylorraphy at 18 months involves elevation of the mucoperiosteum with its repercussions on maxillary growth, and palatal closure. The procedure is risk-free, but intervenes at too late a stage in the development of speech.

Advancing the age at which staphylorraphy is performed does not provide the solution to the problems of bone growth. On the contrary, the younger the patient, the more serious the consequences of elevating the mucoperiosteum.

This is equally true of the earlier date set for cheiloplasty according to the current policy of postnatal surgery.

The Schweckendieck method

The Schweckendieck method in three stages does not impair bone growth, but since the bony vault must be left open, the consequences for speech development are just as serious as those of a large residual fistula.

Single-stage closure

Closure of the entire cleft in a single stage spares the mucoperiosteum, but does not permit the tongue to adjust gradually to the narrowed pharynx.

This presents technical difficulties in very young infants, since it precludes the use of two-layer closure on the bony vault. All too frequently it leaves a residual fistula, whatever the technical ingenuity deployed.

If the mucoperiosteum is, in fact, elevated, the drawbacks are compounded.

If surgery is performed too soon, the disadvantages of early labial repair tend to show up. These have already been pointed out (Chapter 8).

21. First stage: early primary veloplasty

Early veloplasty is performed as of the age of 3 months. As established in our PP1 timetable, which schedules veloplasty before lip repair, this is the appropriate age for the first step of surgery on most labio-palatal clefts.

In complete labio-palatal clefts, a small flap of vomerian mucosa is used. It is cut according to a different pattern depending on whether the form is uni- or bilateral.

PREPARATION

The infant is installed in the customary position. The surgeon stands at the end of the operating table with the assistant on his or her right.

The infant's head is placed in a hyperextended position, and must rest firmly on a stable, ring-shaped support. This hyperextension allows convenient access to the palate, prevents the passage of fluids into the trachea and, in most cases, dispenses with the use of gauze.

A handy new mouth-gag (manufactured by the Leibinger Establishments, Oswald Leibinger Gmbh, Muhlein-Stetten, Germany, according to our design and specifications) has greatly simplified the operation (Fig. 21.1). The dimensions of the blades are adapted to the small-sized mouths of very young infants, and the slot in the middle of the blade prevents it from compressing the preflexed endotracheal tube against the lower jaw.

The oral cavity is cleansed with a solution of quaternary ammonium and an anesthetic adrenaline solution is infiltrated along the lines of the incisions.

UNILATERAL FORMS

Incisions

Two incision lines are drawn (Fig. 21.2).

On the outer border, an initial curved lateral incision is made. This starts immediately behind the posterior maxillary tuberosity and curves inward directly below the posterior edge of the palatal shelf (usually clearly perceptible by touch or located, if need be, by palpating the divided posterior nasal spine beneath the mucosa). It then curves forward, thus marking off (as it follows the free margin of the cleft) a small triangular flap with its apex towards the front. A second incision slits the half-velum lengthwise. The curved blade (No. 12) should follow the easily recognized dividing line between the nasal and oral mucosae, which are not of the same color.

On the inner or large segment, the two incisions are basically similar to those just described. However, due to the junction between the palatal shelf and the vomer, the longitudinal incision which splits the half-velum must be continued further forward over the flat surface presented by the vomer at this point. On this surface, a small quadrangular flap with a posterior pedicle a few millimetres wide by a few long is elevated from the vomerian mucosa. The pedicle of this rectangular flap must be situated on a level with the posterior edge of the palatal shelf. First, it will serve to fasten the vomer to the palate securely. Secondly, thanks to its width, its sturdiness and its inclusion in adjacent nasal mucosa on the posterior rim of the shelves, it offers the significant advantage of reducing transverse tension on the suture

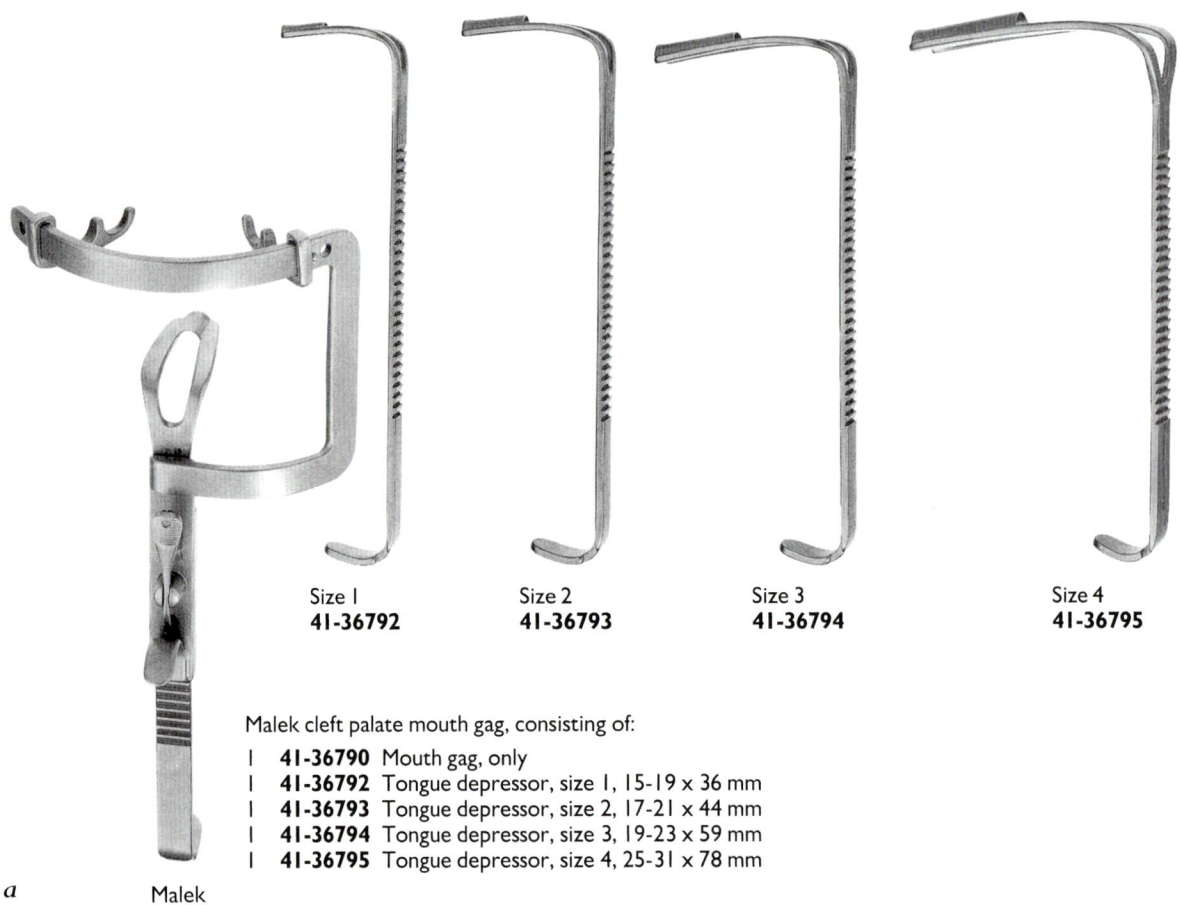

Size 1
41-36792

Size 2
41-36793

Size 3
41-36794

Size 4
41-36795

Malek cleft palate mouth gag, consisting of:
I   **41-36790** Mouth gag, only
I   **41-36792** Tongue depressor, size 1, 15-19 x 36 mm
I   **41-36793** Tongue depressor, size 2, 17-21 x 44 mm
I   **41-36794** Tongue depressor, size 3, 19-23 x 59 mm
I   **41-36795** Tongue depressor, size 4, 25-31 x 78 mm

a   Malek

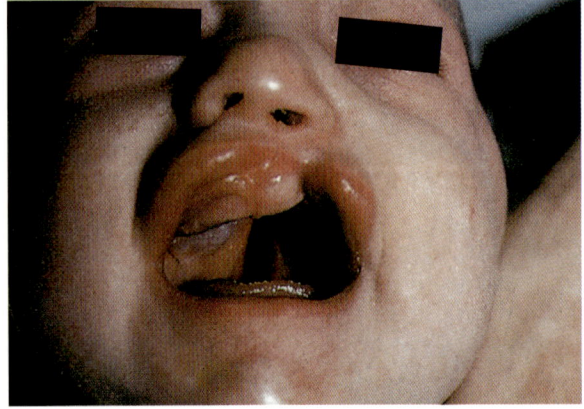

b   Three-months-old CLP patient, preoperatively.

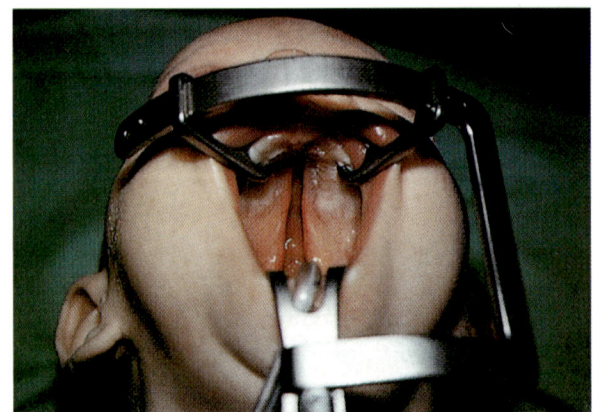

c   The same patient with mouth gag in position.

Fig. 21.1 *Mouth-gag manufactured to our specifications. It is adapted for the size of very young infants, and does not compress the endotracheal tube.*

between the two separate halves of the palate, where stress is at its highest.

Undermining

Both sides are undermined with a Veau elevator (Fig. 21.3).

Small or minor segment

Initial undermining involves the small triangular flap described above. This is where contact must be established with the underlying bone structure. Towards the rear, it is important to locate the posterior margin of the palatal shelf.

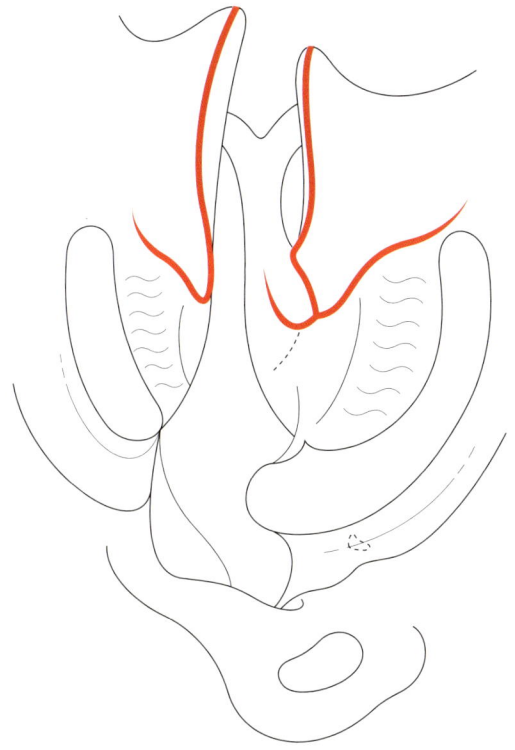

Fig. 21.2 *Pattern of incisions for complete unilateral cleft involving dissection of a vomerian flap with a counter-incision to permit its rotation. Note displacement of inner edge towards the rear. Dotted line corresponds to a little counter-incision.*

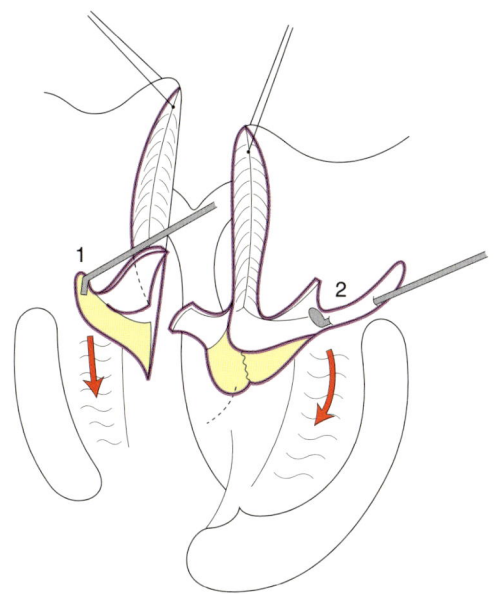

Fig. 21.3 *Undermining of mucoperiosteal flaps. Using the Trelat skin-hook, the pterygoid hamulus is fractured (1), and muscle attachments on the palatal shelf are sectioned behind the neurovascular bundle (2).*

Below and beyond the edge of the shelf, the elevator meets the lateral wall of the medial ala of the pterygoid process. This is where undermining begins.

Next, on the very outside of the incision, two slender, blunt hooks are used to expose the tensor veli palatini tendon. The hamulus is located and fractured. The neurovascular bundle is left intact. The muscle fibers to its rear (in mid-incision) are lifted using a Trelat elevator, and are carefully sectioned behind the vessels with a scalpel. The half-velum is thus completely detached from the bone and can be drawn inward for later suturing.

Lastly, the muscle fibers that seem to be oriented anteriorly near the edge of the cleft (Veau's fissural muscle) are detached from the nasal periosteum with the tip of the scalpel. No further muscle dissection is undertaken. Despite the continuity of the nasal mucosal layer, which must not be disrupted, there appears to be a certain withdrawal of the half-velum. This may or may not subsist after healing.

Large or major segment
Undermining on the major segment methodically follows the same pattern.

When the cleft in the palatal vault is strictly unilateral, the small triangular zone of the incision is adjacent to the quadrangular flap drawn on the flat surface of the vomer. The latter flap is lifted and folded towards the back of the mouth. It is rather difficult to draw the velum inward due to the existence of the fixed point at the junction between the vomer and the palatal shelf on the non-cleft side; nonetheless, since this point does represent the normal midline it must be respected, however off-center it may appear at the time of suturing.

A short counter-incision is made in the anterior portion of the flap area so that the vomerian mucosa can be folded towards the palatal shelves and sutured to the nasal mucosa of the small segment.

When the cleft in the bony palate is bilateral and extends forward to some degree (this is reasonably common in unilateral labio-palatal clefts), lateral undermining of the flaps is identical, step by step, to the small segment procedure. The vomerian flap, however, must be undermined separately. The base of its pedicle should be situated at the posterior margin of the palatal shelves. The nasal and vomerian mucosae must be carefully sutured together on both

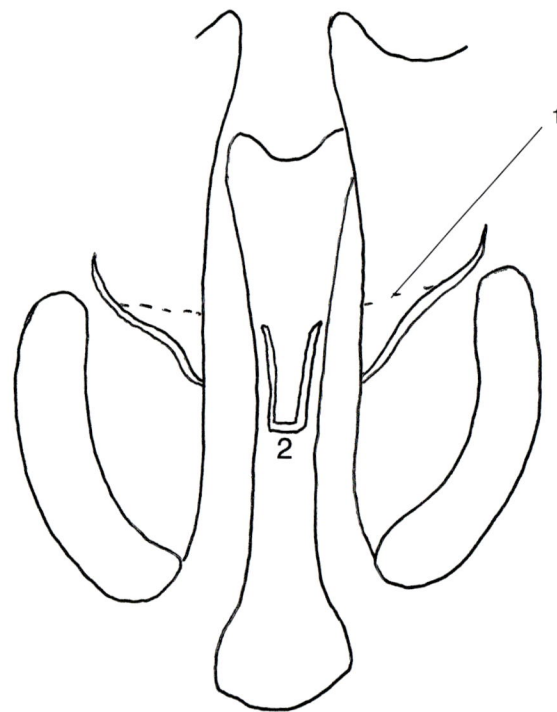

Fig. 21.4 *Pattern of incisions and vomerian flap for bilateral complete cleft.*

1. *Level with the posterior border of the palatal shelf*
2. *Vomerian flap*

sides to prevent a residual fistula on the large segment, which would be difficult to correct at the time of lip repair.

BILATERAL FORMS

Incisions and undermining of the two segments follow the procedure described above (Fig. 21.4). Of necessity, the vomerian flap is isolated. On either side, an elevator is used to lift the vomerian mucosa. The lower rim of the vomer is often unusually high because septal development may be deficient due to antero-posterior growth of the vomer or to lingual pressure towards the back of the oral cavity. Care must be taken not to dissect a vomerian flap with a pedicle that is placed too high; this would attach the velum in an unsatisfactory position. At times, as a precaution (particularly in the case of a wide cleft) a

longer flap should be cut so that once it is sutured to the two halves of the palatal shelf, it will not pull them upward towards the roof of the nasal cavity.

SUTURING

Suturing begins with the nasal layer using atraumatic needles and absorbable thread (4/0) (Fig. 21.5).

The hard palate is closed about half-way; in other words, as far as the base of the flap. Next, each edge of the flap is sutured to the nasal mucosa all the way to its summit. This is the point where the first stitch is taken to unite the mucoperiosteal nasal layer of the velum. This initial stitch should be anchored in the periosteum at the extremity of the flap to avoid tearing in an area of maximal stress.

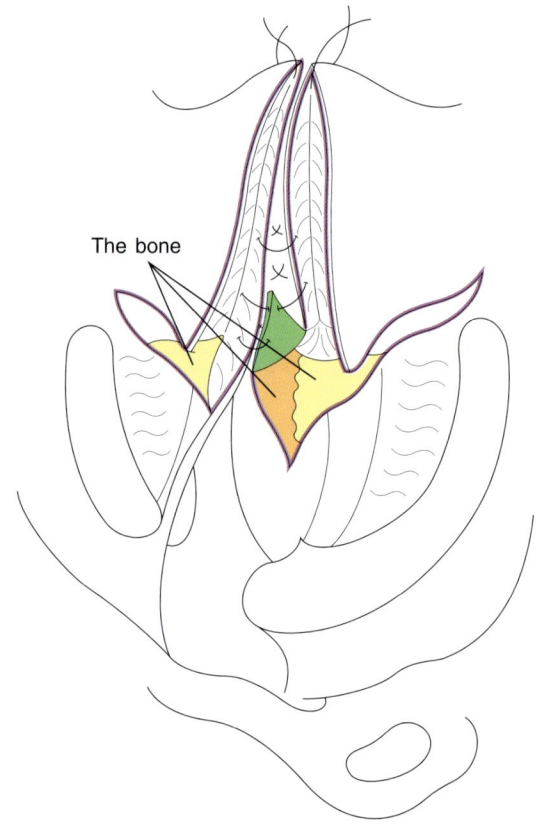

Fig. 21.5 *Suturing of the nasal layer and positioning of the vomerine flap.*

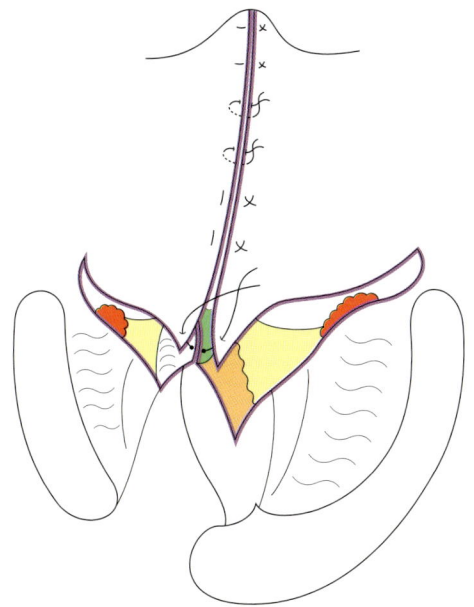

Fig. 21.6 *End of veloplasty.*

The nasal layer is closed as far as the uvula. Each stitch should gather a small amount of mucosa and a greater thickness of muscle fiber to ensure a strong hold.

From the base of the uvula, Donati stitches must be used to obtain proper apposition. At the tip of the uvula, a length of thread is left as a drawstring to permit symmetrical joining. The oral layer is then sutured exclusively with Donati stitches (Fig. 21.6).

Suturing is completed by three stitches which apply the flaps to the roof of the palate. The first is taken at the apex of the triangular flaps, and the other two are placed on either side to reduce the amount of raw area left between the edges of the incised mucosa and encourage quick healing.

22. Second stage: cheiloplasty

STEPS OF CHEILOPLASTY

A detailed discussion of these steps appears in Chapter 7, which focuses on complete clefts. However, to help the reader we will repeat some of the technical points already exposed above.

The procedure is always carried out in the same order.

1. Plotting and placing the reference points.
2. Calculation of plasty and tracing the plasty onto the lip.
3. Infiltration.
4. Cutaneo-muscular and mucosal incisions. Undermining of outer mucosa.
5. Periosteal undermining of nasal spine and submaxillary fossa.
6. Preparation of upper portion of the muscle on the outer border. Undermining of nostril and septal cartilages, if necessary.
7. Suturing of nostril sill and reinsertion of muscle on the nasal spine.
8. Suture of cutaneous stitch at nostril sill.
9. Muscular suturing, especially key points at angles of plasty.
10. Cutaneous suturing starting at skin–vermilion line.
11. Mucosal suturing at vestibular furrow.
12. Adjustments of mucosa and suturing.
13. Adhesive strips on lip. Insertion of endo-nasal tube.

UNILATERAL CLEFTS

Operating procedure

According to the procedure known as the early primary palate method, the stage that involves lip repair also includes closure of the bony palatal vault. The soft palate and part of the hard palate have already been corrected during the stage of veloplasty, which is performed at 3 months.

The lip is repaired at **6 months**, since there must be an interval between veloplasty and cheiloplasty for the reasons previously listed in Chapter 20. In the meantime, the borders of the cleft in the hard palate have generally drawn closer together.

This approximation originally sparked a difference of opinion between the orthodontist and the surgeon on our team. The orthodontist contended that the palatal shelves come closer together due to their growth (particularly along the border which was free of any attachments, i.e. the small segment), and because the shelves themselves become more horizontal (i.e. less steeply angled). These two phenomena are linked to the fact that, after veloplasty, the tongue can no longer penetrate as far into the cleft.

This evolution seems to be even more striking if the child has worn a palatal plate over a certain length of time (provided the plate does not rest on the margins of the gap) (Fig. 22.1).

In actual fact, the horizontality of the shelves is purely hypothetical. It is not confirmed on CT scans, which are routinely taken at 6 months and therefore 3 months after veloplasty (coronal or frontal views). Rotation of the vomer, which has already been discussed at length, remains unchanged. The impression that the shelves have swung downward is generally created by an increase in the thickness of the mucoperiosteum, which is no longer subject to pressure from the tongue.

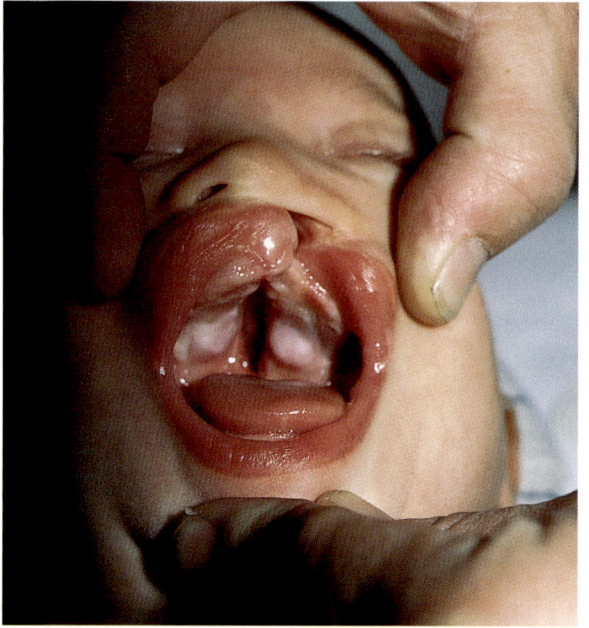

a

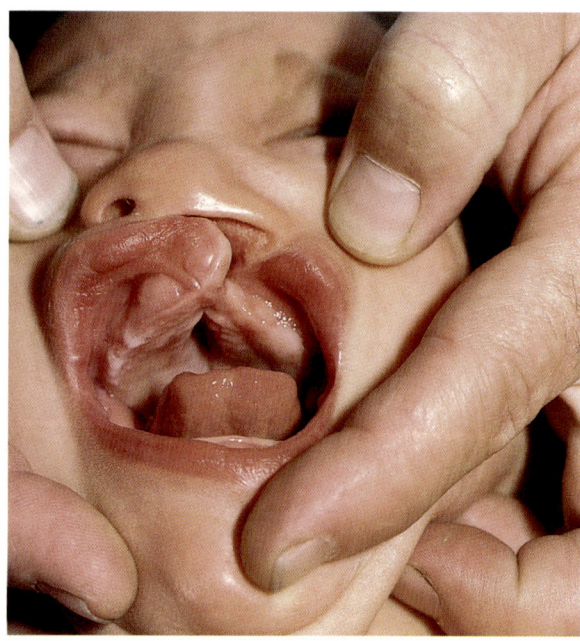

b

Fig. 22.1 *Approximation of borders after veloplasty.*
a. Configuration of segments at time of veloplasty.
b. Three months later during cheiloplasty.

As far as lateral growth along the borders of the shelves is concerned, there is no solid evidence to substantiate this theory.

Consequently, we must accept the fact that the maxillary segments themselves have come together despite the presence of the plate, which is intended precisely to prevent any such displacement. It seems clear that when a plate is fitted, as is customary to keep it from working its way into the cleft, it can do little to combat lateral displacement. At best, it may help to keep such displacement at a minimum. Plates continue to be used because their true benefits lie elsewhere, as has already been explained.

In most cases, therefore, there is an undeniable approximation of the borders of the cleft after veloplasty. However, this does not necessarily compromise the prognosis as far as bone development is concerned. Even in those instances that aroused concern for future dental development because approximation was such that it verged on collapse, we were consistently reassured by the spontaneous evolution.

If approximation does exist, it seems to be a reversible condition, at least over a period of a few months following primary veloplasty.

Incisions and undermining

We will not enlarge here on the nature of the labial incision, which varies from case to case according to the repair required (cf. Chapter 7).

Lip incisions

A pointed knife (No. 11 blade) is used to make the lip incision. If the surgeon is right-handed, the entire thickness of the border should be held firmly between the thumb and forefinger of the left hand for the tissues to the left of the cleft. Then, to the right of the cleft, a finger is used to steady the tissues by pressing them against the bone structures (left-handed surgeons reverse the maneuvre).

To avoid any mistakes in the position of the reference points, particularly if the ink is blurred or erased when the time comes for suturing (a frequent occurrence in the final stages of the operation), tiny punctures can be made with the tip of the knife at the two points that correspond to the nostril sill.

It is also advisable to place the mark for the lower reference point of the lip slightly above its exact location, so that the incision will always be perfectly perpendicular where it crosses the skin–vermilion line. Veau always used a double needle which straddled the skin–vermilion line, but the practice has been discontinued despite the handiness of this device.

Care must be taken to section both skin and muscle without cutting into the mucosa. This becomes easier with practice, since the inside finger can easily follow the tip of the knife from underneath.

The knife should be held perfectly perpendicular to the skin, particularly while incising the triangle(s) for the repair on the outer border. The thickness of these flaps is what determines whether they are sturdy enough to keep the shape that corresponds to the original calculations.

If the surgeon is experienced, the vertical segment of the incisions can be slightly bevelled towards the deep surface so that suturing of the muscle layer will create a strip of tissue that imitates a philtral ridge.

Vestibular incision

The next step involves the vestibular incision, which meets the lateral cutaneous incision in the upper portion of the lip. The very bottom of the vestibular sulcus is left intact; the incision is made 2 mm above it and must cut cleanly through the underlying periosteum.

On the inner border the incision automatically sections the frenum of the upper lip, which is always abnormally short and thick, before reaching the vestibular sulcus on the non-cleft side. A number of authors object to the practice of sectioning the frenum on the grounds that this cuts through essential fibers (Latham and Deaton, 1976), but experience shows that this step is necessary to obtain satisfactory fullness of the vermilion.

Undermining the vestibular mucosa

Once the incisions are made, the vestibular mucosa is undermined and separated from the deep muscle layer. A hemostat is placed at the tip of the mucosa, where the vestibular and cutaneous incisions form an angle, and a Gillies skin-hook is positioned in the incision of the skin–vermilion line. Moderate diverging traction can be exerted on these two instruments so that, between them, it is possible to penetrate the submucosal layer, which is easy to recognize thanks to the rounded acini of the labial salivary glands which remain embedded in the mucosa.

This is the level on which the blood vessels that course upward along the cleft are located. They 'lock' the cleft borders at a certain height, so to speak. They must therefore be identified and sectioned, after electrocoagulation, so that additional height can be gained thanks to the Z-plasty incisions.

For the same reasons, the inner surface of the triangular musculocutaneous flap(s) must be thoroughly undermined so that nothing will hinder their subsequent rotation.

The mucosal plasty that is needed to complete the superficial musculocutaneous repair involves the transfer of outer mucosa to the inner surface. The mucosal flap is fitted between the edges of the inner vestibular incision. To facilitate this transposition, particularly in cases that present a broad cleft with significant misalignment of the bone structures, a small vertical counter-incision should be made at the outer end of the vestibular incision. This can prove extremely useful.

Undermining the periosteum

The periosteum is then undermined with a Veau elevator, which is perfectly adapted to this procedure because its rounded end does not tear the tissues.

Undermining involves the entire sub-orbital fossa. The sub-orbital vascular bundle is clearly visible, and should be left intact. The processus frontalis of the upper maxilla is also denuded. It presents a sharp edge on the level of the piriform sinus (Fig. 22.2).

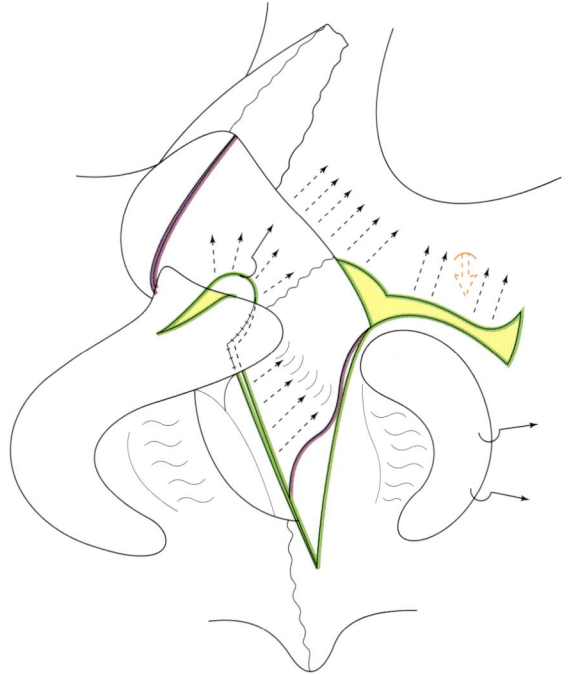

Fig. 22.2 *Periosteal undermining. The minor segment is artificially shifted outward to permit display of the mucoperiosteal incisions, which must often be performed blind.*

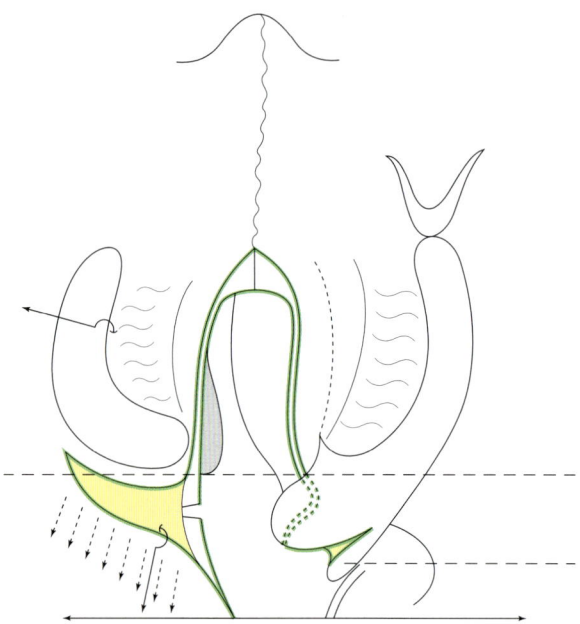

Fig. 22.3 *Incisions in operating position. Enough vomerian mucosa is retained to permit closure of the oral layer. The periosteal incision of the frontal process is not on a line with the vertical counter-incision made in the nasal mucosa in front of the inferior concha.*

A reasonably long vertical incision should be made here in the periosteum so that the soft tissues can be moved forward without being distorted, and so that the two tissue borders can be brought into line to compensate for the antero-posterior misalignment of the bony segments. This periosteal incision is therefore always a necessary step. To make it easier, a counter-incision is made in the nasal mucosa on the lower portion of the frontal process. This is also intended to correct the difference in length between the borders of the nasal floor caused by misalignment of the bone structures.

Situated in front of the inferior nasal concha, the vertical counter-incision is equivalent to the intercartilaginous incision used in rhinoplasty. It follows the outermost contour of the triangular cartilage, which is left intact. Details of the procedure will be discussed below.

The premaxilla on the inner border is also partially denuded. The vestibular incision which cuts through the frenum is extended backward along the border of the cleft in a semi-circle until it meets the incision in the mucosa on the intermaxillary bone to

form a triangular flap with a superior pedicle. This triangle of mucoperiosteal tissue is elevated and rotated so that it can be fitted between the edges of the counter-incision in the outer nasal mucosa (remember that this is destined to correct the uneven borders) (Fig. 22.3).

At the base of the columella and the immediately adjacent part of the cleft nostril sill there is a small portion of septal perichondrium extending from the periosteum. The tip of a Trelat skin-hook is inserted into the undermined zone to permit a vertical incision.

The bony vault and interalveolar zone

This step is followed by dissection of the borders of the cleft in the bony vault and interalveolar zone.

The Veau toothed-rack mouth-gag is installed, and the mouth is opened to its maximum width.

On the outer border the elevator, which is maintained in contact with the bone where the processus frontalis was undermined, is inserted horizontally and from front to back below the inferior concha. The anterior end of the inferior concha is clearly visible in the cleft. Thus, the elevator is actually on the upper surface of the palatal shelf of the small segment, where it is in a position to undermine the mucosa near its free border on the nasal side.

No incision is needed because the tip of the elevator is used to separate the nasal mucosa from the mucoperiosteum on the oral side. Thus, the entire mucosa and the periosteal junction on the outer border of the cleft in the hard palate are now incised (Fig. 22.4).

Using a Gillies skin-hook inserted on the oral side, moderate downward traction is exerted on the edge of the mucoperiosteum, which is easily detached provided the sub-periosteal space has been properly infiltrated. This undermining (over a very limited width) is necessary so that the two borders (which have usually drawn considerably closer together, as observed earlier) can be sutured. It does not jeopardize growth because the mucoperiosteal blood supply is left intact and neither incisions nor undermining have been performed near the alveolar rim.

Lastly, a short lengthwise incision is made at the back of the cleft in the zone that was originally reconstructed during veloplasty. This incision allows the outer border to be split for a few additional millimetres, which completes its division.

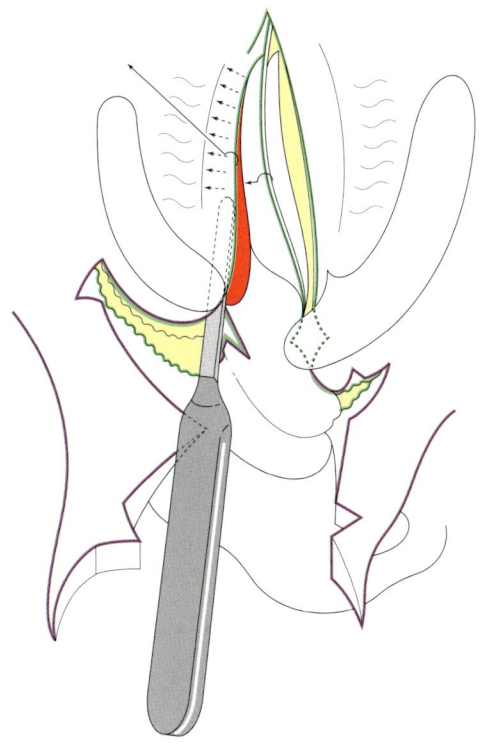

Fig. 22.4 The Veau elevator is inserted from front to back above the free border of the palatal shelf to permit the division of the mucoperiosteum, which is discreetly detached on the oral side. The short incision in the soft palate, which has already undergone repair, helps to isolate the nasal and oral layers properly.

This outer mucosal border is too short compared with the inner border due to the antero-posterior misalignment of the bone surfaces, and it must be vertically incised to lodge the triangular flap elevated on the inner border. Its location has already been discussed, but a few details on technique are in order.

First of all, the muscle layer must be separated from the mucocutaneous lining of the nostril vestibule. If a No. 15 blade is passed gently under this lining, the muscle layer is easily identified. Short pointed scissors are then introduced (the separation of their handles isolates the muscle from the superficial plane). The vertical incision begins in the mucosal layer and continues along the naso-vestibular fold.

The elevator is used to free the edge of the processus frontalis of the upper maxilla. A second vertical incision is made a short distance from the first, at the piriform aperture. These two vertical incisions permit realignment of the borders.

The separation of the musculo-periosteal from the mucocutaneous plane at the nasal vestibule permits the upper portion of the muscle layer from the outer border to be transposed inward and inserted into the periosteum of the nasal spine without affecting the size of the nasal orifice. This step is the key to correcting any forward roll of the deformed alar wing. It is also essential to the reinsertion of the facial muscle layer on the nasal spine, as stressed by Jean Delaire.

On the inner border, undermining starts with a horizontal incision in the vomerine mucosa. It is important to leave enough mucosa on the oral side for it to be sutured to the mucoperiosteum of the outer border without requiring undue traction. This horizontal incision starts towards the rear in the thickness of the scar tissue formed after primary veloplasty, which is incised lengthwise for several millimetres. Towards the front of the mouth (in the retro-alveolar region) it meets the semi-circular premaxillary incision mentioned earlier. As already seen, this is where a furrow has been formed by the torque effect on the intermaxillary bone. Undermining may pose a problem here. It is essential to verify that the junction between the two incisions has been properly cut, and this can be checked with a laryngeal mirror and completed if necessary with the tip of a No. 11 blade. Undermining is less difficult in this zone if it has been carefully and thoroughly infiltrated (Fig. 22.5).

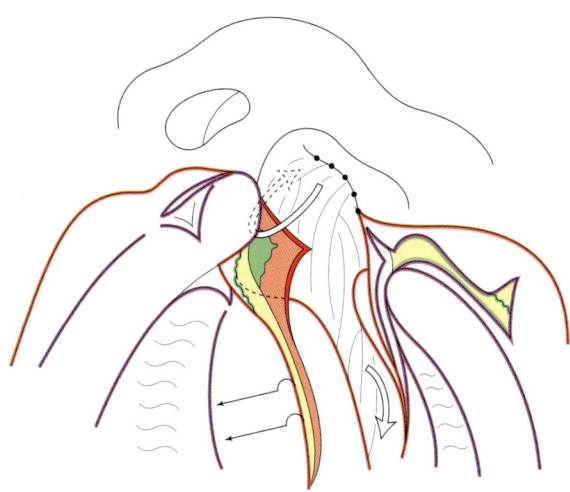

Fig. 22.5 In the anterior portion of the incision on the inner border, the junction between the perichondrium and periosteum is detached from the furrow and incised vertically to facilitate displacement of the columellar base.

Towards the mouth, the mucosa comes off easily. Detaching the septal perichondrium presents more of a problem. It is cautiously incised with the scalpel from front to back, guided by sight, and from the mouth towards the nose. The perichondrium, which is continuous with the periosteum, is then sectioned. As Veau used to stress, if the elevator is used proceeding from top to bottom, there is a danger of perforating the mucosa or of fracturing the edge of the bone because the instrument tends to catch on the bony groove of the premaxillary bone. One element worthy of note is the presence of Jacobson's small cartilage, which comes off with the perichondrium, but this does not create any particular problem.

Closure

After this extensive undermining there is no longer any abnormal continuity between the superficial and deep tissues – a pathological condition initially created by the cleft itself.

As of this point, provided the tissues can be properly approximated, suturing is carried out on two layers.

Suturing of the lip is generally problem-free. The same holds true for the hard palate, since the borders have drawn closer together spontaneously as pointed out earlier.

This is not the case, however, for the inter-alveolar region within the oral cavity, where suturing is not feasible. A number of authors have described the alternative of resorting to a flap of labial mucosa. However, these vestibular flaps have the drawback of anchoring the deeper portion of the lip, which may deprive it of satisfactory mobility. Orthodontists do not encourage this procedure and nor does it produce favorable cosmetic results, so we tend to avoid it.

It is easy to understand why *residual fistulae* can occur in this zone, and they probably result from the high intra-buccal air pressure that the child is capable of producing once the oral cavity can be closed completely. It is worth mentioning that there were virtually no anterior fistulae when operations were scheduled according to the 'classic' agenda, which started with lip and hard palate repair but left the soft palate open until the age of 18 months. Under these circumstances, it was impossible for the child to create high positive or negative air pressure.

This emphasizes the care that must be taken in suturing the nasal layer, including closure of the inter-alveolar region.

We have experimented with various means of improving the airtightness of this zone, at least during the period necessary for proper healing. Use of a film of absorbable material (vicryl/collagen) seemed to offer a good solution, but the occurrence of bovine spongiform encephalopathy has put an end to our supply of this product, which is based on bovine gelatine. Freeze-dried dura mater is also no longer commercially available.

We are reluctant to go to the lengths of using a graft of free skin or of tibial periosteum, as Stricker

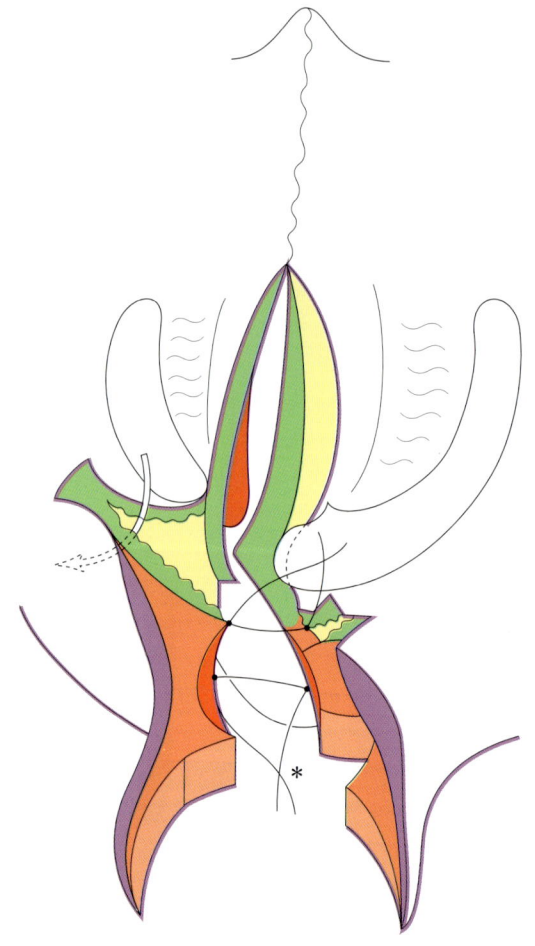

Fig. 22.6 *Closure is carried out from back to front. The stitch that anchors the muscular layer to the periosteum of the anterior nasal spine is of utmost importance. Traction stitch* at the reference points for the nostril sills permits satisfactory placement of the sutures needed to correct misalignment of the borders.*

and Raphael (1983) advocate, let alone of epicranial tissue. Excising this type of graft adds pointless complications to the surgical procedure, for a result that is not guaranteed to hold up within the oral environment.

Suturing of the nasal layer of the hard palate is greatly simplified by the use of needles with mobile eyes which we call Petit needles (equivalent to a very small sized Reverdin needle). Introduced through the nasal fossa, this type of needle permits suturing of the outer nasal to the vomerian mucosa with the knots tied inside the nose. The stitches hold fast provided a good bite is taken of both mucosa *and* periosteum, which, as we have seen, is the only tissue sturdy enough to offer reliable resistance. Simple or U-shaped stitches can be used. Suturing of the nasal layer of the hard palate is continued anteriorly with that of the nostril floor and of the cutaneous portion of the lip. Since the uneven borders must be adjusted using the triangular flap of mucosa described above, in order to avoid distortion of the tissues a length of suture material for traction is set in place but left untied at the site of each of the punctures that correspond to the superior reference points for the nostril sills. Traction exerted on this suture with a forceps brings the two borders face to face (Fig. 22.6).

Suturing of the oral layer is performed using absorbable thread. As many U-shaped stitches as possible should be used to guarantee an airtight seal. This suture necessarily stops at the inter-alveolar region.

Reconstruction of the lip

The next step concerns reconstruction of the lip, which begins with suturing of the muscle layer starting at the traction stitches placed at the superior reference points. Above these lie muscle fibers that do not correspond to the lip itself but to the muscles of the alar wing. These muscles must be reinserted on the nasal spine. It has been seen that proper reinsertion is the key to satisfactory repositioning of the entire facial muscle layer. Anchorage is ensured by a single non-absorbable suture. On the inner side, a good bite is taken of the periosteum corresponding to the nasal spine, which was elevated when the premaxilla was denuded. The muscle fibers must be isolated and dissected from the mucocutaneous layer so that anchorage will not modify that portion of the lip below it, and so that there is no risk of reducing

the size of the nostril orifice. Pointed scissors are inserted between the muscle and the lining of the nostril vestibule in order to detach the muscular layer, which can then be transferred inward without affecting the nostril floor and the alar base. This procedure does not interfere with the plasty intended to lengthen the lip. Lastly, it gives a nice symmetrical roll to the ala, which is a very important step.

The next phase involves reconstruction of the orbicularis oris. The distance between the reference point for the nostril muscles and the first point of the orbicularis oris must be sufficient to permit the reproduction of the right-angle that normally exists between the lip and the nasal floor. Several nylon sutures which gather a good amount of tissue are placed at strategic points of the incision and at the skin–vermilion line. As a rule, no muscular sutures are used here to avoid hindering the adjustment of flaps on the vermilion.

Cutaneous suturing is performed next, starting with a suture at the skin–vermilion line. This is essential to a satisfactory end result. The stitches are tied loosely to prevent the formation of scalariform scar tissue. This also explains why the skin–vermilion suture is never used for traction, since asymmetrical tension might produce misalignment. The stitch immediately below it is the one that serves this purpose. The angles of the incision are sutured, and closure is completed by a few stitches along the intermediate segments.

The final step is suturing of the vestibular mucosa and the vermilion. To give the lip a certain amount of body, the vestibular mucosa is repaired first. On the level of the bone structures, the divided frenum is corrected with a suture and resection of the mucosa below it. Hemostasis is generally called for at this point. The tip of the outer mucosal flap is anchored to the summit of the inner incision at the bottom of the vestibule. The first one or two vestibular stitches take a bite of the muscle to create a clearly defined vestibule and avoid ptosis of the mucosa detached from the deep muscle surface (Fig. 22.7). For the same reason, once the mucosal sutures are completed, a U-shaped stitch that transfixes the lip can be used to apply the mucosa to the deep surface of the lip in the inter-segmental region. This stitch is loosely tied over a roll of gauze, and is removed within 48 hours of surgery to avoid leaving a scar.

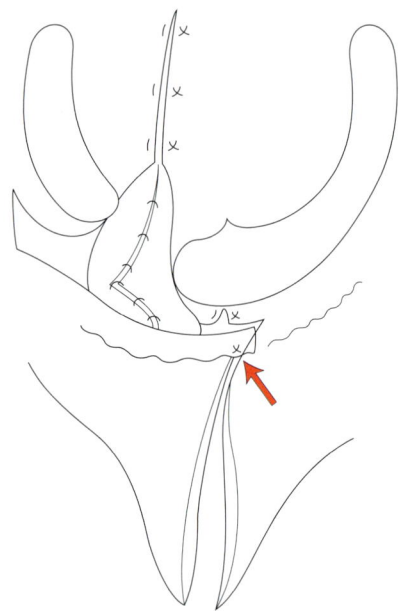

Fig. 22.7 *Suturing of the lip on the mucosal side. The outer mucosa is advanced beyond the frenum as far as the bottom of the vestibule. A stitch or two (arrow) takes a good bite of the deep muscle layer.*

The scar tissue in the vestibular mucosa is what gives the vermilion its fullness. It takes a good deal of experience to obtain a satisfactory degree of symmetry. It is important to retain the notion that the further inward the mucosa is transposed, the fuller the resulting lip will be. Conversely, the closer the suture is to the outside, the thinner the lip will be.

The final touches concern adjustments to the vermilion (Fig. 22.8). Here again a type of Z-plasty is used. An oblique incision that slants outward is made below the skin–vermilion line. This opens the stub of the lip, which is generally rounded due to the increasingly severe degree of hypoplasia that affects the tissues nearer to the cleft.

A flap of excess inner mucosa is fitted into this incision. Veau used to contend that this 'sterile' inner mucosa should be resected. On the contrary, not only is resection uncalled for, it would actually prevent the flap procedure we are now describing (Fig. 22.9).

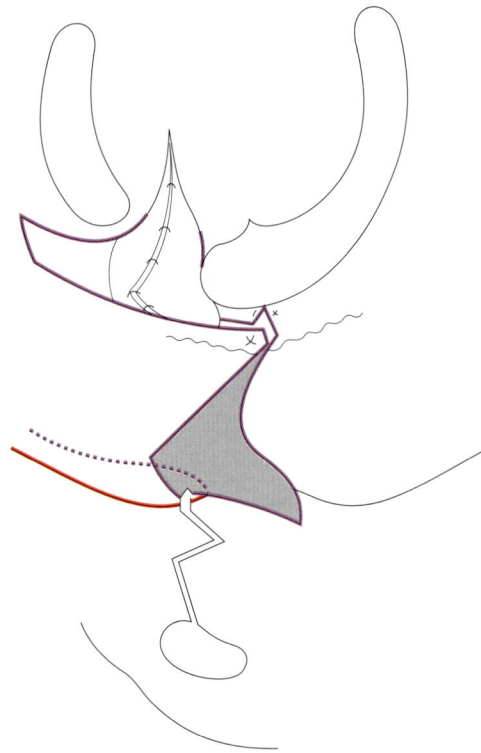

Fig. 22.8 *Adjustments of the vermilion and mucosa. An oblique incision is made below the skin–vermilion line which ends at the junction between dry and moist portions of the vermilion. The shaded zone indicates the area that should be resected.*

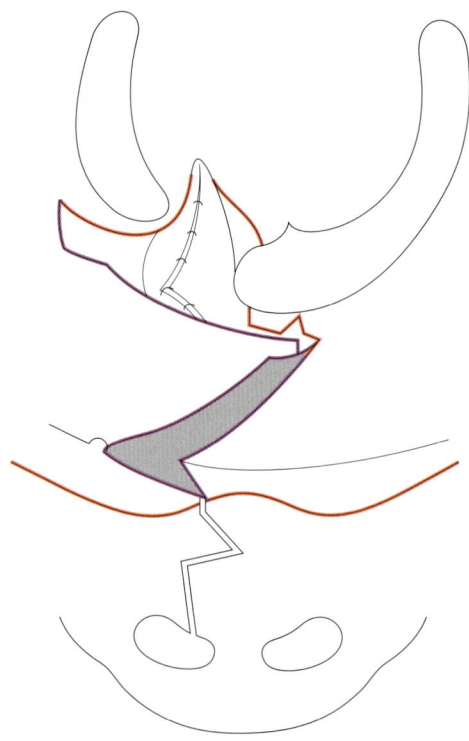

Fig. 22.9 *Resection on the inner border spares a triangular portion destined to be inserted between the edges of the incision on the outer border. The shaded zone indicates the area that should be resected.*

Between the outermost point of the vermilion incision and the innermost point of the vestibular suture, it is always necessary to trim some excess tissue. However, it is essential to remember that a little extra tissue can always be resected, whereas a lack of tissue may produce an irreparable defect.

End of surgery

At the end of surgery, the pharyngeal gauze is removed. Adhesive strips come in handy to limit post-operative edema and protect the skin from nasal secretions.

Summary

The steps discussed above show that no specific procedure is performed to correct **nasal deformities**. This is because nasal deformities consistently persist or recur if the bone structures are misaligned, or if the septum is severely deviated and presents the skeletal deformities discussed elsewhere.

Any attempts to correct deformities during primary repair necessarily remain incomplete or, worse still, create abnormal anatomical relationships (for instance, by separating the cartilaginous septum from the septal bone structures).

There seems to be a general consensus of opinion against osteotomy in very young infants to avoid compromising the growth process. In actual fact, this attitude may be debatable. Paul Tessier in particular contests it (personal communication), and has performed a large number of osteotomies on small infants to correct cranio-facial malformations. However, we must admit that the fear of creating irreparable damage has always made us reluctant to operate on the bone structures.

Thus, these deformities persist or soon recur, making later repair inevitable. This is bound to be complicated by the presence of any fibrotic scar tissue left by earlier surgery on the nasal structures.

Over a short period of time it is a good idea to insert a rubber endonasal tube, which takes advantage of the undermining automatically performed on the bone and cartilage and prevents stenosis of the nostril opening. Although its volume temporarily improves the appearance of the nostril, it will not produce a durable curve in the contour of the ala, which generally appears webbed after cheiloplasty.

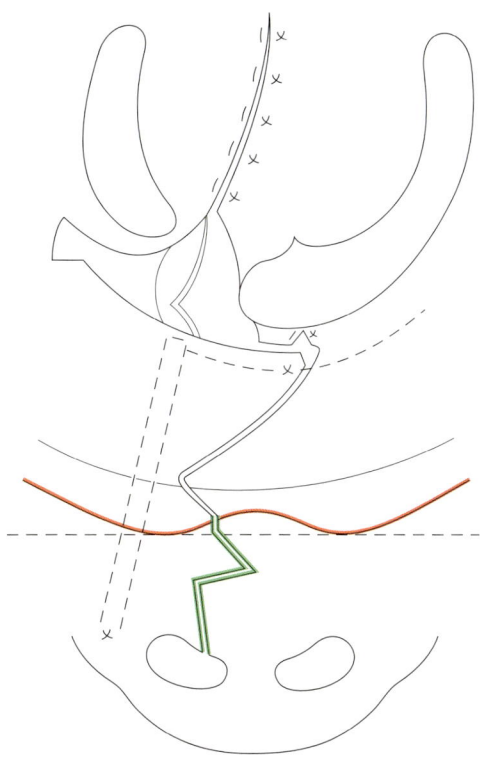

Fig. 22.10 *Pattern of sutures at the end of surgery.*

The protective appliance or plate (moulded a few days prior to surgery) is fitted as soon as the operation is over.

Post-operative care

Feeding is resumed that same evening. As is the case after veloplasty, bottle-feeding is proscribed to avoid lip contact with a nipple and to discourage sucking efforts, which produce negative pressure in the oral cavity. This strict diktat has been challenged, perhaps rightly so, but we would rather avoid taking any chances. Those surgeons who advocate bottle-feeding are generally those who leave the hard palate open (the Schweckendieck procedure), and we do not necessarily share the same concerns.

Elbow restraints are used to prevent infants from sucking their thumb or fingers.

In the winter, when infants are most susceptible to upper airway infections, short-term antibiotic therapy is prescribed. Petit advocated this practice to prevent any post-operative infection, which would be catastrophic for the sutures. Aside from such cases of superinfection, which are now a rarity, there is virtually no danger of labial rupturing. This only occurs when there is direct trauma, and we customarily caution mothers not to hold their infant's head too close to their own, particularly in a vehicle which may have to stop suddenly.

The patient is released after the fourth post-operative day. The stitches are removed on the seventh day, without the need for anesthesia; the child is merely rolled up in a sheet and held firmly while one assistant restrains the head and another prevents movement of the lower limbs.

The elbow restraints, protective plate and veto on bottle-feeding are maintained for about a month, at which time the patient is recalled for a check-up.

BILATERAL CLEFTS

Protocols

We have establish a set of rules, presented here as a preamble. Some of them have already been exposed.

1. During cheiloplasty of complete clefts, we consistently close the alveolar cleft as well as the cleft in the palatal vault. A 'curtain' closure, which leaves all the structures open behind it, is never performed.

2. We always use the technique of the inferior equilateral triangle flap to repair the lip. This is the best means of obtaining satisfactory lip height, even in those forms where the prolabium seems severely hypoplastic. There is always an astounding improvement in this medial portion once the bilateral clefts are repaired. The calculation of those references that determine the desired height is necessarily arbitrary since there is no normal side to furnish a basis of comparison; the height is calculated on a vertical line with the outer alar base of the nose. In asymmetrical forms, the measurements are made on the less affected side.

3. As a consequence of these two first rules, we never correct both sides in the course of the same operation. This would endanger the blood supply to the premaxilla in complete forms, and to the central portion of the prolabium whatever the form. The prolabium and the portion of skin–vermilion line it contains must be preserved at all costs, even if there is no visible trace of the Cupid's bow. Under no circumstances should it be

resected or used for correction other than of the lip. Otherwise, the result is bound to involve excessive transverse tightness of the upper lip, as well as repercussions on the bone structures which will be discussed in a later section.

4. We do not attempt any of the procedures destined to correct the short columella during the cheiloplasty stage, and are careful to avoid any scar formation at the labio-columellar junction so that secondary repair of this height deficiency will not be compromised. The Millard techniques (types 1 or 2) or the inverted equilateral triangle are therefore not proposed.

5. Despite the absence or sparsity of muscle fibers in the prolabium, we never undertake to suture the two portions of orbicularis oris on the outer borders together directly. This would in any case only be feasible during the second phase of cheiloplasty, since the operation is not performed in a single stage. The fibers are anchored to the subcutaneous elements of the prolabium.

6. We find it necessary to respect a waiting period between the two stages of cheiloplasty. An interval of 2 months suffices.

7. Contrary to the practice advocated by Petit, we start with the widest side when the cleft is asymmetrical or when the premaxilla shows obvious lateral displacement. This is to reduce the transverse tension, which must be overcome when the second side is repaired.

8. Retrodisplacement of the premaxilla is always obtained within a few months thanks to reinsertion of the muscle fibers on the nasal spine and reconstruction of a satisfactory vestibule, which determines proper mobility of the lip. This is the case even when misalignment of the bone structures is extremely pronounced at the start. This result is achieved without ever resorting to preoperative orthopedic treatment, let alone osteotomy of the premaxillary bone.

First stage of cheiloplasty

The operating procedure is identical to that described for unilateral clefts.

The height measured on a vertical line with the outer alar base serves as a reference for calculating the dimensions of the plasty (always an inferior

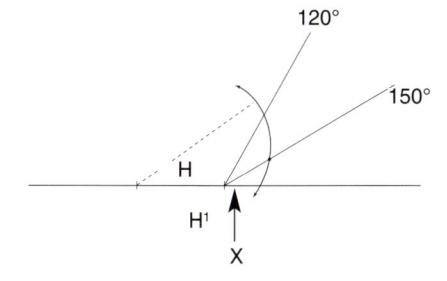

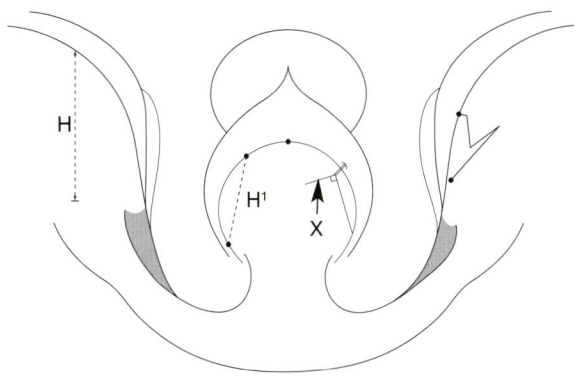

Fig. 22.11 *Measurements for equilateral triangle plasty (150°) used for first side of lip.*

reinforced by an oral layer. There is often a band of whitish mucosa on the lower border of the vomer which resembles oral mucosa and contrasts with the red of nasal mucosal tissue.

Even when clefts have remained wide open after primary veloplasty, closure of the vault does not present a problem thanks to the vomer's extreme transverse mobility (Fig. 22.12).

The muscular suture follows the same principles outlined for unilateral clefts. After the outer border has been incised anterior to the lower concha, the muscular portion corresponding to the facial layer is dissected on both surfaces. It will be sutured to the periosteum of the premaxilla at a point corresponding to the anterior nasal spine, which may not be well developed. The stitches for the orbicularis take a good bite of subcutaneous tissue from the prolabium, which does not present readily recognizable muscular characteristics.

When cutaneous suturing is performed, special care must be taken to re-establish the skin–vermilion line. This is often hard to detect on the side towards the prolabium.

equilateral triangle). Potential adjustments must be allowed for; the incision of the prolabium should not cross over the midline. This is to prevent it from meeting the incision that will be required during the second stage. Even if there is no longer a vascular risk to the portion of the lip thus delimited, the cosmetic result would be anything but perfect (Fig. 22.11).

For the labial incision, the blade is held perpendicular to the skin. The flap of mucosa which borders the prolabium must be of a certain thickness, since it will serve for vermilion repair.

The incision of the medial mucosa cuts through the frenum, which is almost always present, and continues upward for a bit on the opposite side.

It is easier to denude the premaxilla and undermine the septal cartilage than it usually is in unilateral forms, since there is no furrow to mark their junction. However, the sheet of periosteum that is interposed between the bone and cartilage must be broken down with the elevator or, better still, slit with the knife blade. When the vomerian mucosa is incised, a few millimetres of tissue are left on the free border of the vomer so that the nasal layer will be

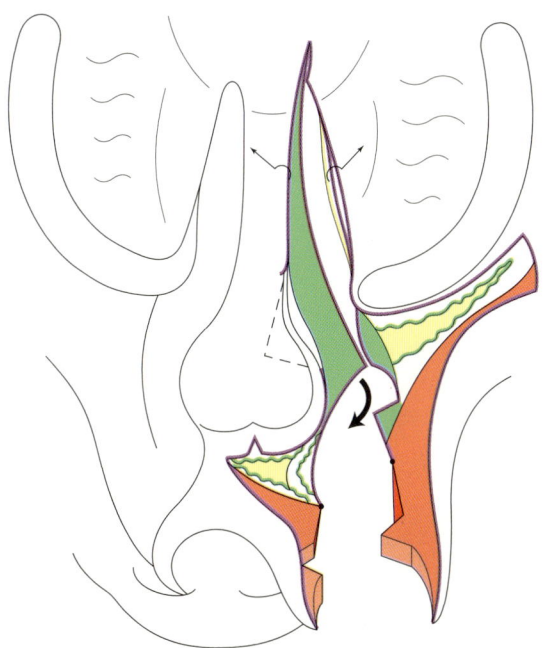

Fig. 22.12 *Closure of palatal vault: nasal layer including the flap of retroalveolar mucosa to be fitted into the outer counter-incision. The aim is to correct the misalignment of borders, which is often very pronounced.*

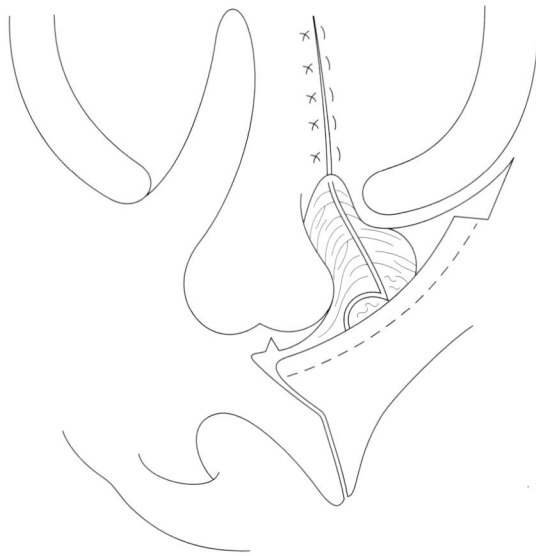

Fig. 22.13 *The oral layer is feasible thanks to the mobility of the vomer. The beginnings of a vestibule have been prepared (dotted line).*

Reconstruction of the vermilion is completed by the two plasties described earlier. During resection of the excess mucosa on the outer side it is advisable to conserve as large an amount as possible of subcutaneous tissue, which is composed of the glands and muscle fibers that originally ran up the length of the outer border. This tissue will serve to bolster the inner mucosa, which is far less substantial, and thus contributes to the prevention of the whistling deformity often found in bilateral forms.

The opposite side remains open after this first stage of cheiloplasty on bilateral labio-palatal clefts. The impression left should be that of a unilateral cleft, however hypoplastic the original prolabium. The beginnings of a medial vestibule are already in place (Fig. 22.13).

Second stage of cheiloplasty

The next stage shows a closer resemblance to unilateral cleft repair. However, a considerable amount of tension may exist if the cleft is reasonably broad and if the first stage of surgery has pulled the highly mobile lip components and the premaxilla towards the side initially corrected. Undermining of the suborbital fossa, periosteal incisions and counter-incision of the mucosa must therefore be extensive enough to allow for this tension.

It is essential to spare the vomerian mucosa, even more so than during the first stage, so that the two-layered suturing necessary to guarantee secure closure of the bony vault can be carried out.

As a rule, it is necessary to go beyond the zone of scar tissue left by primary surgery on the premaxilla in order to eliminate any deep-lying adhesions.

The mucosal incision must also be extended for a considerable distance in the vestibular furrow created in the course of the first operation (Fig. 22.14).

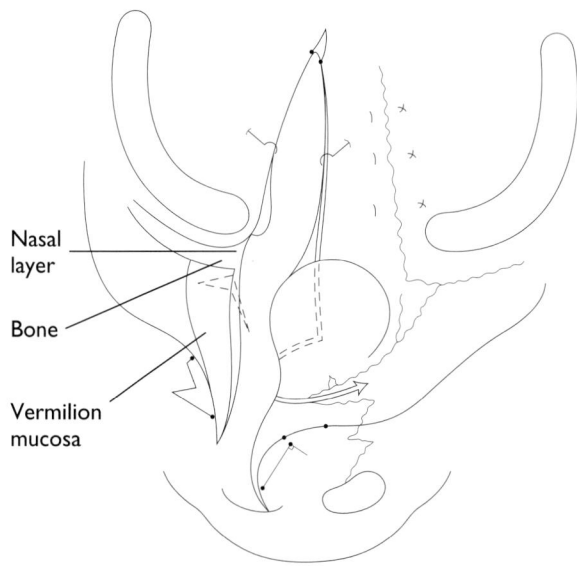

Fig. 22.14 *Pattern of incisions during second stage of labial surgery. The vestibular incision on the premaxilla is extended significantly towards the side previously repaired.*

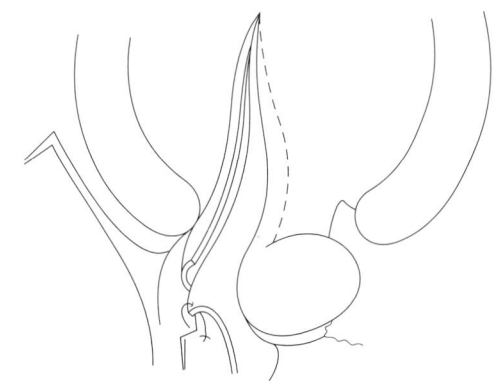

Fig. 22.15 *Plasty needed to correct misaligned borders. The oral layer is only possible if a considerable amount of mucosa has been retained on the lower edge of the vomer.*

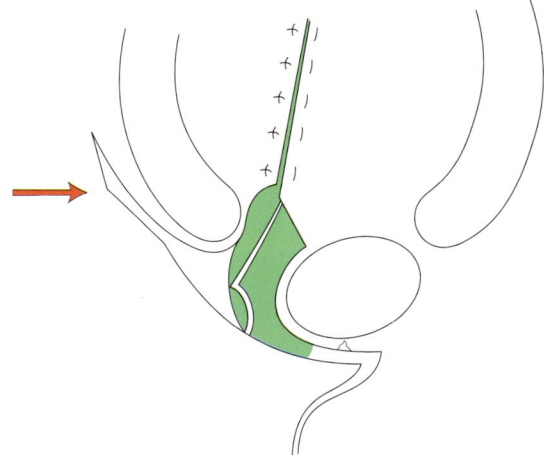

Fig. 22.16 Large outer counter-incision of vestibular mucosa (arrow), so that it can be advanced towards the premaxilla. Since there is no lining to cover the interalveolar region, it is susceptible to residual fistulae.

Despite the added difficulty caused by tissular tension, we know of no case where the second side of a bilateral cleft could not be closed under satisfactory conditions even when an important misalignment exists (Figs 22.15 and 22.16).

We must repeat that even a very tiny prolabium can gain considerable length after repair. Although medial hypoplasia undeniably exists, this is no excuse for a poor result and, in particular, for leaving a whistling deformity due to a lack of medial vermilion. This can perfectly well be avoided.

Age for surgery in bilateral complete cleft lip and palate

Whether the form is symmetrical or not, veloplasty is performed at 3 months. The first cheiloplasty is performed at 6 months and the second side is closed at 8 months.

FISTULAE AND THE EARLY PRIMARY PALATE METHOD

As we said, the residual fistula of the palate represents the major complication in the early primary palate technique. It is difficult to estimate its frequency, since the fistula may not be detected until long after surgery if the symptoms are particularly discreet. In some cases, it is only discovered during an operation undertaken to correct an altogether different problem (cf. rhinoplasty). However, the occurence of fistulae in our own experience is only 10–15%.

Statistics concerning the classic technique employed by Veau and Petit contain little data on this subject, but it would seem that fistulae used to be far less common. Needless to say, Schweckendieck's delayed palatal closure or related procedures always leave a residual communication. A certain number of authors believe that this has adverse consequences, and emphasize the fact that the surgeon's logical objective should be complete closure of the palate. However, even an attempt at complete closure carries a significant risk of leaving a fistula of some kind, if only a mere slit.

These fistulae do not appear to be linked exclusively to a defective surgical technique. A weakness in the sutures may obviously represent a contributing factor. Single layered closure of the nasal mucosa on the bony vault often made fistulae more likely. Nevertheless, when we used to apply Veau's method, there was never a breakdown providing the nasal mucosa was sutured far enough to the rear during cheiloplasty because the soft palate was left open.

A second layer of closure on the oral side significantly reduces the incidence of fistulae, but does not eliminate them altogether. Yet, at least in the retroalveolar region of the vault, suturing of the oral mucosa should be satisfactory since it is better vascularized and richer in conjunctive tissue than the nasal mucosa, which is reduced to a thin layer of mucoperiosteum.

The use of a protective plate does not totally cancel the risk either. Since it does not hermetically seal the mucosa, fluids and air can leak into the nose above it.

In actual fact, all of these factors contribute to a variable degree. The major cause seems to lie in the positive and negative pressure which the child is capable of producing in the oral cavity once it can be completely closed. In the classic procedure, even a mediocre suture of the nasal mucosa did not result in a breakdown since the presence of the palatal gap precluded a build-up of intra-oral pressure.

Conversely, in the early primary palate technique (which repairs the soft palate first), high pressure can be built up once the second stage of the operation has closed the lip and bony vault. The aspiration created by the tongue, particularly behind the alveolar ridge, causes air, saliva and nasal secretions to pass through the sutured zone, which is not hermetically sealed.

In an attempt to guard against fistulae we experimented with a wide range of procedures in addition to the plate, which is routinely used after surgery. However, they either added undue complications to the surgical procedure (a graft of tibial periosteum, for instance, which tended to leave an unsightly scar on the leg) or were not risk-free (the use of sheets of collagen, which have now been withdrawn as have all products of collagenic origin, or sheets of absorbable artificial tissue, which are prematurely eliminated).

The best preventive measure is a painstaking suture technique based on double-layered closure, which is feasible thanks to narrowing of the cleft after veloplasty. However, in the customary technique there is always a zone in the interalveolar region that is not covered by the oral layer. Although the potential risk is not great, it does subsist to some extent in this area.

A flap of labial mucosa with either an inner or an outer pedicle (Burian, 1954) can be used to provide an oral lining. Petit was not in favour of this type of flap because he found that it inevitably hampered the mobility of the lip to some degree. His orthodontist, J. Psaume, was even more adamant. In his opinion, these flaps resulted in a shallow vestibular sulcus and compromised the stability of prostheses.

Be that as it may, these flaps can prove highly useful in the treatment of sequelae during secondary surgery. It is better not to use them during primary surgery.

A number of therapeutic theories have been elaborated to help prevent these fistulae, which are caused primarily by problems of pressure. One simple solution might lie in prosthetic obturation based on a graduated plate, which is thick enough at a given point to prevent complete closure of the mouth. This could be left in place for the short period of time necessary for satisfactory healing. It is up to the younger generation of surgeons to trial this method.

When a fistula does exist, it is reasonably small as a rule, and subsists with no major changes unless surgery is performed on the maxillary segments. There is no such thing as spontaneous closure, since two mucosae back-to-back will not heal together. The fistula may be so insignificant in size that it does not produce any of the following disorders.

Disorders due to fistulae

There may be leakage of fluids or soft food matter such as milk, soup, puréed fruit and so on. In older children, we speak of the 'tell-tale chocolate sign' as food oozes from the nostril on the cleft side. This leakage must be distinguished from reflux, where food matter goes up the nose the wrong way – a common occurence in all children. Passage of food the wrong way is particularly frequent in cases of a short soft palate. The food generally exudes through the healthy nostril in unilateral clefts, because the other nostril is partially obstructed by the bulging septum and by the distortion of the opening itself into an oblique oval shape.

There are grounds for uncertainty as to whether the matter passes through the nasopharynx or through a fistula when the palatal cleft involves the bony vault on the normal side to any degree. Often, the mere volume of matter regurgitated tips the balance in favor of reflux.

Visual inspection of the palate does not always provide conclusive evidence, since the orifice of the fistula may be hidden or may open horizontally. In the retro-alveolar region, a mirror may be needed to detect it.

In older children, speech defects represent a second consequence of residual fistulae. There is nasal escape of air; here too, in less severe forms, it is difficult to tell the difference between velar incompetence and air escaping through a fistula. Nonetheless, speech therapists are well equipped to detect defective closure of the nasopharynx. As will be seen, this plays a major role in determining whether fistular closure or pharyngoplasty is called for. To further complicate matters, it is thought that the presence of a fistula diminishes the functional potential of a velum that would otherwise be considered adequate.

Permanent irritation of the nasal mucosa, chronic rhinorrhea and serous otitis can also all be linked to the existence of a communication between the oral and nasal cavities.

The indication for fistular closure depends on the severity of the disorders just listed. To avoid one operation too many (in case pharyngoplasty might prove necessary later on) we tend to postpone fistular closure until 3–5 years of age. The speech therapists are confident that the phonetic results will be satisfactory at this point. This operation can either be isolated or combined with a lip touch-up or with early rhinoplasty.

As a matter of principle, this technique of closure of a fistula should exclude elevation of the mucoperiosteum. It is thus within the framework of the early primary palate method, which proscribes this during the phase of growth. However, in those rare cases where the defect is large in size and particularly in width (above all in the case of children who live far from the hospital and for whom a successful operation is all the more important), we resign ourselves to using the mucoperiosteum. The term 'cross forms' serves to designate these cases in evaluating the results of the early primary palate procedure, as is also the case when pharyngoplasty has been performed.

It is preferable to close the fistula with small local flaps. Here too, double-layered suturing offers the best guarantee.

23. Long-term results

APPRAISAL

What is the best way to collect and present the results so that the finished product is both objective and applicable to other experiences, a *sine qua non* of progress in the field?

This is no easy task, involving assessment of cosmetic and functional results over a long period.

Cosmetic result

The cosmetic result is a matter of appraisal by both the surgeon and the parents of the infant.

For the surgeon in particular, this assessment is obviously subjective in nature; it is neither easy to quantify nor to communicate to others. There is no way to make valid comparisons. By definition, photographs are static: the picture can vary according to its dimensions, lighting, contrast, etc. Even multiple views are not enough to judge the dynamics of the lip, which is a particularly mobile region of the anatomy both in speech and expression.

It is possible, however, to show greater objectivity in evaluating the symmetry and suppleness of a lip or straightness of a nose.

The parents are always very demanding. They place great faith in the results of cosmetic surgery 'later on'. What they do not always recognize is that the cleft surgeon, who is extremely deft and painstaking, is in a position to obtain excellent cosmetic results from the start.

The notion of rating both parental and surgeon's satisfaction on some hypothetical scale amounts to pseudo-scientific fraud.

Once patients are old enough to be aware of the situation, their psychological reaction enters into their own assessment of the cosmetic result. These results, in turn, have an impact on the psychological consequences of the deformity, which can be vastly different from one case to another.

The reasons just developed help to explain how difficult it is to compare the cosmetic results of two different techniques unless, of course, they show consistent and flagrant defects.

Functional results

The situation is altogether different regarding the functional results, which can be assessed far more easily within a framework of statistical studies of dental results, which include the analysis of occlusion and cephalometrics, speech results and hearing results.

Nowadays, statistical data based on a large sample size have become compulsory. However, only a certain number of specialized centres can boast the staff necessary to provide valid figures for comparison. In this regard, the current tendency for purely financial reasons to increase the number of local centers providing treatment is regrettable. It is true that if the baby is operated on at a hospital near to the parents' home, costly travel expenses can be avoided; however, the number of cases operated on by each center per year is necessarily smaller, and this has an impact on the surgeon's experience, and makes the development of a multidisciplinary team devoted to this pathology an unlikely option.

The assessments must be made by each of the various specialists involved in the program of treatment. Here again we must stress the essential role of the multidisciplinary team, which continually monitors patients throughout the entire period of growth.

Time frame

The results cannot be validly assessed without respecting the necessary timeframe.

To assess results on the skeleton and the teeth, the growth phase of the patient must have come to an end. This takes 15–20 years for each case. Thus, when a new method is to be tested, it must be possible to follow-up patients throughout this entire period. If the experiment under study is spread over a number of years, then the total follow-up time must be multiplied by as much as two. This represents an additional obstacle that few teams can overcome.

Lastly, the statistics of other teams must be available for comparison in order to furnish justifiable grounds for a change in technique or method. However, publications on long-term results are few and far between. Furthermore, the technical prowess of individual surgeons may vary considerably and thus the scientific caliber of the assessments is not always guaranteed.

Still, a cross-comparison of results bolstered by a thorough knowledge of the lesions and the disorders they generate is essential if we are to justify certain changes which help to advance along the path of progress.

Key periods of observation
1. Immediate results: 0–2 years
   * Cosmetic appearance and dynamics of lip
   * Appearance of nose
   * Complete closure of the cleft, alveolar region and palate
   * Emergent speech.
2. Intermediate results: 2–9 years
   * Same as above, plus effects of growth
   * Dental and orthopedic results
   * Phonetic evolution
   * Evolution of hearing
   * Psychological impact.

3. Late results: 9–18 years
   * Same as above
   * Results of secondary treatment: surgery, therapy, orthodontics
   * Evaluation of sequelae
   * Psychological make-up and personality development.

Statistics on the early primary palate experiment

It is instructive to study our statistics presented at the most recent International Convention on facial clefts and cranio-facial deformities in Broadbeach, Queensland, Australia (November 1993). The figures were based on 700 cases of complete clefts, uni- or bilateral, and, of these, 642 case studies were retained where the follow-up was thorough over a number of years. The patients operated on since this date have not been included, to guarantee a minimum timeframe of at least 6 years.

These statistics cover 433 cases of unilateral clefts (67 per cent) and 209 bilateral clefts (33 per cent).

This research is based on a total number of 1493 operations which can be broken down into:

* 642 primary early veloplasties
* 851 cheiloplasties
* 808 closures of the bony palatal vault performed at the same time as labial closure.

Virtually all these operations were performed by the author, thus conferring a certain unity to the experiment.

MORPHOLOGICAL RESULTS

Morphological results of the lip and nose in complete labio-maxillo-palatal clefts depend on the maxillo-dental results, which will be discussed in a later section.

Labial results are not modified by growth. This includes lip height, successful alignment of the skin–vermilion line, and the appearance of the vermilion and vestibule.

The only modifications that may develop over the course of time are those linked to correction or aggravation of the skeletal lesions (antero-posterior misalignment of the segments, collapse of the small segment, defective growth of the upper jaw) and to deformities of the nose and septum which, as has already been pointed out, cannot be wholly corrected during primary surgery.

Nasal surgery

Needless to say, many of the techniques performed during primary cleft lip surgery concern the nose:

- Reconstruction of the nasal floor with closure of the interalveolar region
- Reconstruction of the nostril.

Whatever the case, routine procedure involves:

- Undermining of the perichondrium on the septal cartilage
- A vertical incision of the periosteum of the small maxillary segment after reasonably extensive dissection to free the outer alar base
- An incision at the junction between the alar and triangular cartilages in the vestibule of the nares.

These steps permit symmetrical repositioning of the structures found on either border of the cleft. Reinsertion of the outer muscle layer in the periosteum of the nasal spine contributes to the correction of alar eversion and helps to re-orient the outer alar base.

It is true that these basic surgical acts do not qualify as rhinoplasty in the strictest sense, although perhaps wrongly so. The surgeon's attention is focused on correcting the deflection of the nose, the distortion of the nasal tip (misalignment of the domes) and the deviation of the septum.

In the chapter on lesions of the nasal bone structures and cartilages, particularly of the septum (Chapter 18), we explained why total rhinoplasty should not be performed at an early age, and under no circumstances during primary cleft repair. If rhinoplasty were undertaken, it would require either various stages of bone surgery, to correct the nasal pyramid (osteotomy of the nasal bones) or to treat the deviated septum (resection of the vomer which has undergone the rotation described earlier), or the creation of an abnormal anatomical structure (for instance, if the septal cartilage is straightened without first correcting the malpositioned vomer and anterior nasal spine).

The objections are less categorical where the cartilaginous structures, especially the alar cartilages, are concerned. These can be dissected and adjusted. Deformities of the tip of the nose can be attenuated, if not totally corrected, without unduly compromising the growth process.

The psychological impact of this corrective measure answers an insistent demand on the part of both parents and child. Early rhinoplasty is therefore generally proposed around the time for starting grade school, at about 6–8 years of age.

In this context, one might wonder why we do not agree with those surgeons who advocate the self-same acts during primary cleft surgery. There are several reasons for our attitude:

1. These acts may not prove necessary in the long run. If the prime cause of the lesions (abnormal insertion of the facial muscles) is properly treated and satisfactory bone development is obtained, then the normal growth process will take over and the defects will partially correct themselves (Fig. 23.1).
2. The psychological need varies according to the individual and to the environment. The child does not usually become acutely aware of residual defects until he or she reaches school age, and the operation we propose will therefore be most beneficial to the child at this stage.
3. Technically speaking, sub-perichondrial dissection of the cartilages grows simpler as the child matures.

In all events, there is nothing final about early rhinoplasty. Few patients escape definitive nasal repair once the growth phase is over, and there is no doubt that final surgery can be seriously complicated by the sequelae of an earlier operation. This argument should be made clear to the parents when the surgical agenda is under discussion.

Early rhinoplasty in unilateral clefts

Correction of cartilage deformities of the nasal tip always calls for a midline columellar incision. The incision is made along the entire height of the columella, and then curves over the dome of the lateral cartilage on the cleft side (Fig. 23.2). This opening exposes the cutaneous surface of the alar cartilages, as well as the zone where the medial crura meet, for dissection. Hemostasis is necessary on the larger blood vessels.

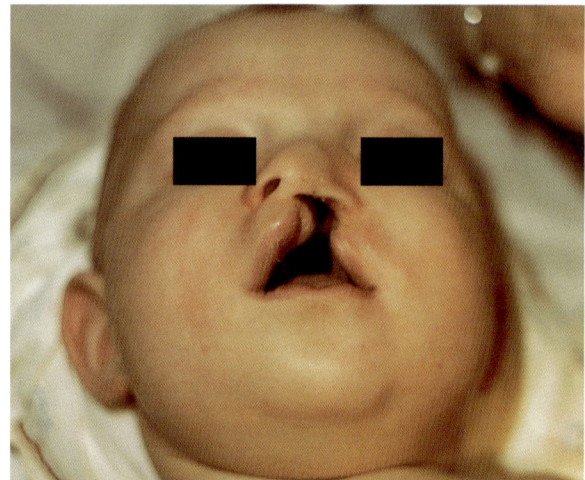

a

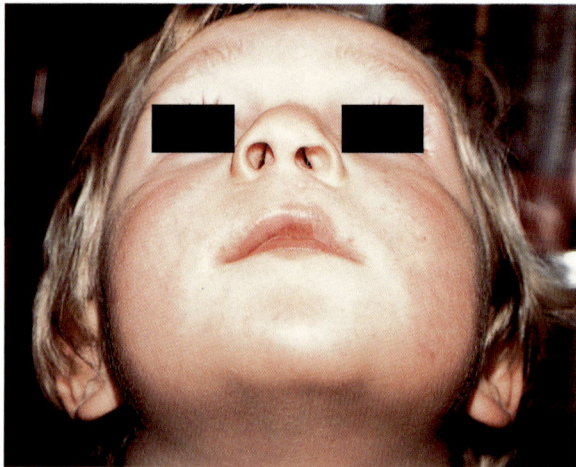

b

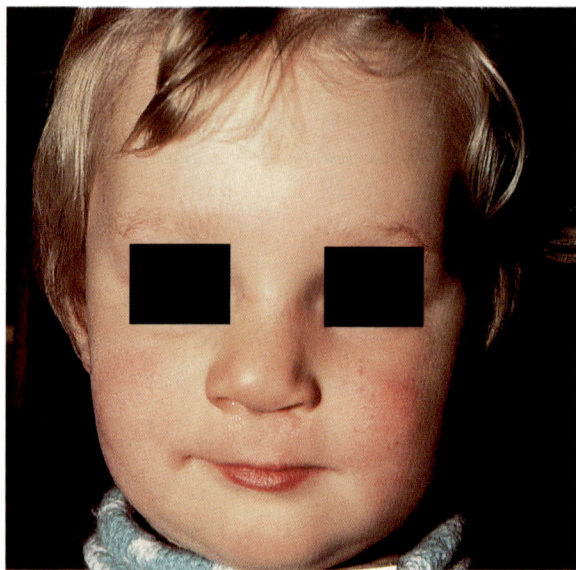

c

Fig. 23.1 *Nasal results obtained without intervention on tip of nose in complete cleft without bridge.*

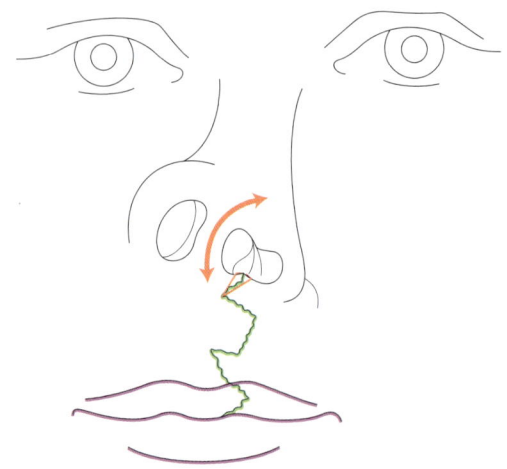

Fig. 23.2 *The cutaneous medio-columellar incision permits rhinoplasty of the nasal tip. This is often combined with a high labial incision to perfect reinsertion of the muscles.*

The lower margin of the septal cartilage, visible in the nostril on the non-cleft side, is then freed. On either side of this margin, a No. 11 blade is used to incise the perichondrium so that the septal cartilage and the maxillary spine can be dissected beneath it (this step is known as sub-perichondrial dissection of the septum).

The septum rests against the nasal spine, which should be undermined to isolate the premaxillary bone and the vomer. Bearing in mind the rotation the vomer has undergone, it is important to proceed with caution at the bottom of the un-named furrow and in the area of Poutriquet's ridge.

Undermining is continued upward, using a Veau elevator or a blunt spatula, as far as the angle between the septum and the triangular cartilages. This junction is incised lengthwise along the nasal crest (Fig. 23.3).

The septum is generally dislocated compared with the anterior nasal spine, and rests against it facing the non-cleft side. The septal cartilage is therefore too long, and the excess tissue at its lower margin must be trimmed carefully without overdoing it. Since it is not possible to resect the nasal spine at this early age, the septal cartilage is relocated towards the cleft side.

If a cosmetic touch-up is being performed on scar tissue in the upper portion of the lip at the same time, the lower edge of the septum can be anchored

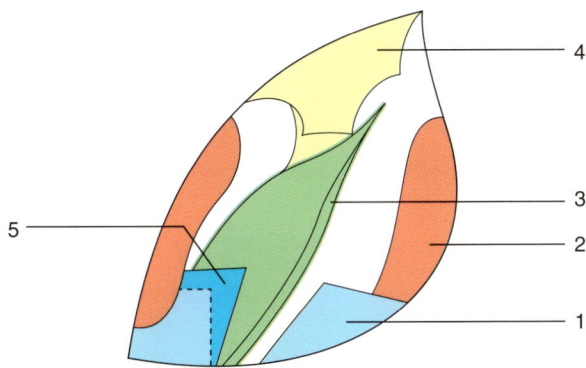

Fig. 23.3 *View of anatomical elements through the medio-columellar incision. The septum is freed from the triangular cartilage on either side.*

1. *Triangular cartilage*
2. *Alar dome*
3. *Septal cartilage*
4. *Premaxilla and anterior nasal spine*
5. *Resection of a portion of triangular cartilage on cleft side*

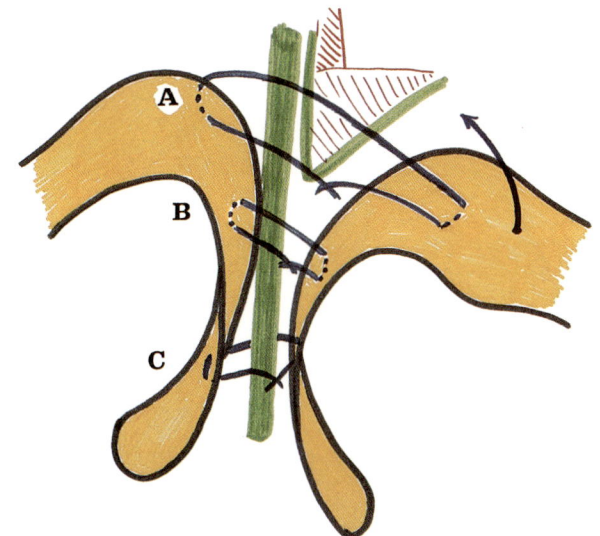

Fig. 23.5 *Correction of misaligned domes of alar cartilages. Stitch A, simple or double, is the most crucial. Stitches B and C can serve to anchor the mesial crura and permit forward projection of the nasal tip.*

to the outer muscle layer with a nylon suture which passes under the mucous membrane (Fig. 23.4).

If no additional work on the lip is scheduled, then the septum may receive sufficiently stable support from the nasal spine itself.

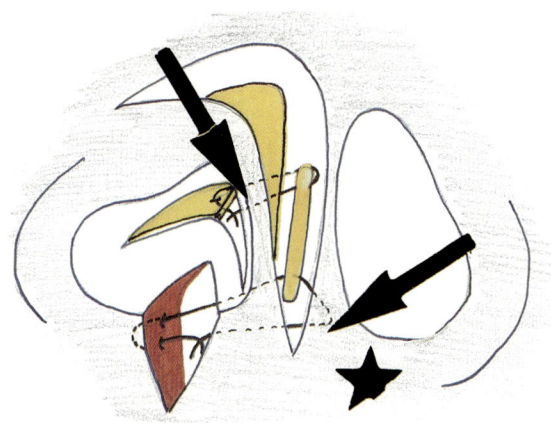

Fig. 23.4 *Correction of deviated septal cartilage. The arrow shows anchorage of the lower margin (after resection of the part dislocated from the anterior nasal spine) to labial muscle, thanks to a counter-incision in the upper portion of the scar as well as that of the upper edge of the triangular cartilage, a portion of which has been resected.*

To permit straightening of the septum, a thin strip of triangular cartilage should be removed along the entire height of the incision on the cleft side. Once corrected, the exposed edge can be held in place with a fine nylon suture (Fig. 23.4).

After the septum has been dealt with, the deformity of the alar cartilage is corrected. The individual structures are clearly exposed thanks to the outer incision. Through this incision, it is possible to cut the connective tissue between the alar and triangular cartilages to correct the downward slippage of the former. An additional short intercartilaginous incision may be necessary to allow satisfactory dissection of this zone.

The next step concerns correction of the misaligned domes or cupulae. A fine nylon suture (10/1000) is placed in both domes. A second is then positioned to form a U directly below the apex of the dome on the non-cleft side and, on the cleft side, angled quite a bit further out on the cutaneous surface of the cartilage. This stitch serves to elevate the ala and attempts to correct the customary infolding that generally subsists after cheiloplasty (Fig. 23.5).

The lower edge of the septum should be situated between the medial crura of the alar cartilages. The

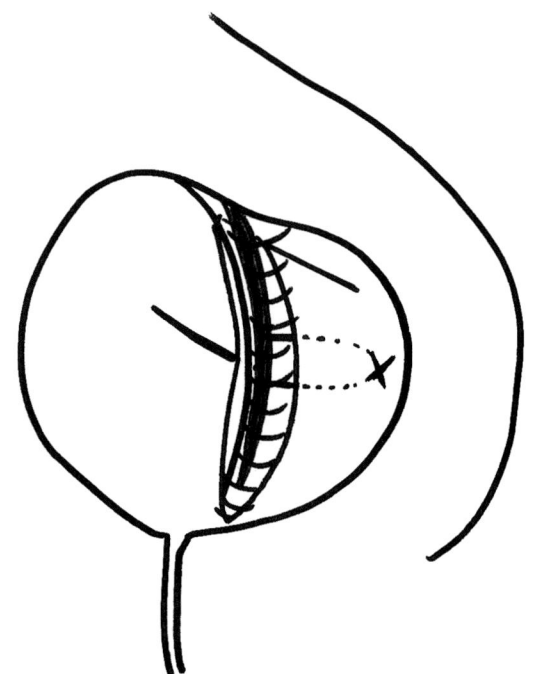

Fig. 23.6 *Naso-vestibular fold corrected by elliptical resection of the mucosa, often combined with a Z-plasty.*

septum normally supports the tip of the nose and when its development is deficient, the forward projection of the nasal tip can be enhanced by stitching the medial crura and the septum together. At times, a cartilaginous graft is indicated (using the resected septal tissue).

The skin edges are carefully approximated and sutured on a single plane with 6/0 nylon. Discreet resection of the skin on the border of the normal side can help to elevate the free border of the ala on the cleft side.

It may prove necessary to correct a naso-vestibular fold, which indicates continued eversion of the outer alar base with ptosis of the alar cartilage. In most cases, simple elliptical resection of the mucosa will suffice (Fig. 23.6).

To complete this section on early rhinoplasty, we feel bound to stress once again that there is nothing final about this method although it may ease the wait for definitive surgery (Figs 23.7, 23.8). We will also let Veau emphasize our point about the risks involved in performing rhinoplasty during primary cleft surgery:

I beseech all those who read these pages never to dream of resecting the septum of an infant: otherwise they are bound to incur the worst catastrophes; until their patient's dying day, there will always be someone to curse their memory.

Early rhinoplasty in bilateral clefts

Principles

Unlike in unilateral clefts, the nose is not deviated in bilateral forms. The major lesion corresponds to a flattened nasal tip associated with a short columella (Fig. 23.9).

Very early on, the link was established between this deformity and congenital hypoplasia. 'Classic' authors used to say that this medial hypoplasia involved both the prolabium and the columella. In the course of their reflection on methods of treatment, they demonstrated that if an attempt was made to lengthen the lip by pulling its central portion downward, flattening of the nasal tip was thereby accentuated. Conversely, if the tip of the nose was lifted, the columella was lengthened at the expense of the lip, which seemed to be absorbed into the columellar base (Fig. 23.10). Thus, they produced conclusive evidence that a flap was needed to lengthen the medial portion of the nose. Either the prolabium can provide the tissue, which is replaced by an Abbe–Estlander flap taken from the lower lip, or, as proposed by Morel-Fatio and Lalardrie (1966), a portion of skin can be slid from the nose to lengthen the columella.

As another resort, local flaps can be used to lengthen both lip and columella at their junction, but the results are not always satisfactory from an esthetic point of view.

On both a pathogenic and a therapeutic level, the concept itself deserves additional discussion.

Without presuming to deny that medial hypoplasia does indeed exist, although it varies in degree, we believe that the basic causes of nasal tip deformity need to be re-examined. Due to the gap created by the cleft, the two lateral portions of the orbicularis oris develop divergent action. This divergent muscle action pulls the alar bases outward, and the rounded domes of the alar cartilage are, in a sense, 'unrolled'. This tends to flatten the tip of the nose, which is

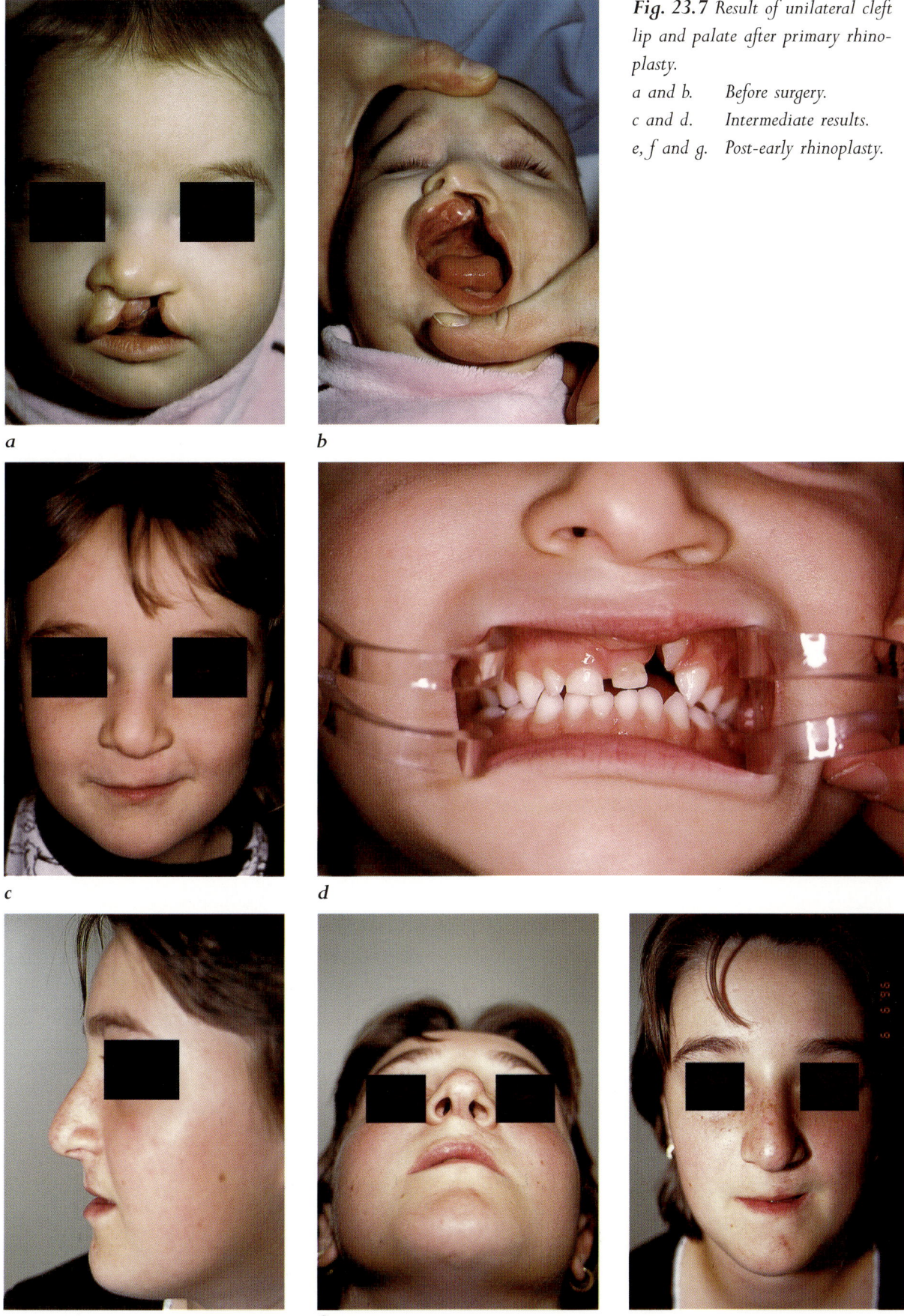

a

b

c

d

e

f

g

Fig. 23.7 *Result of unilateral cleft lip and palate after primary rhinoplasty.*

a and *b*.	*Before surgery.*
c and *d*.	*Intermediate results.*
e, f and *g*.	*Post-early rhinoplasty.*

Fig. 23.8 *Results of unilateral cleft lip and palate after primary rhinoplasty.*
a and b.   At birth.
c and d.   At 5 years.
e and f.   At 9 years.

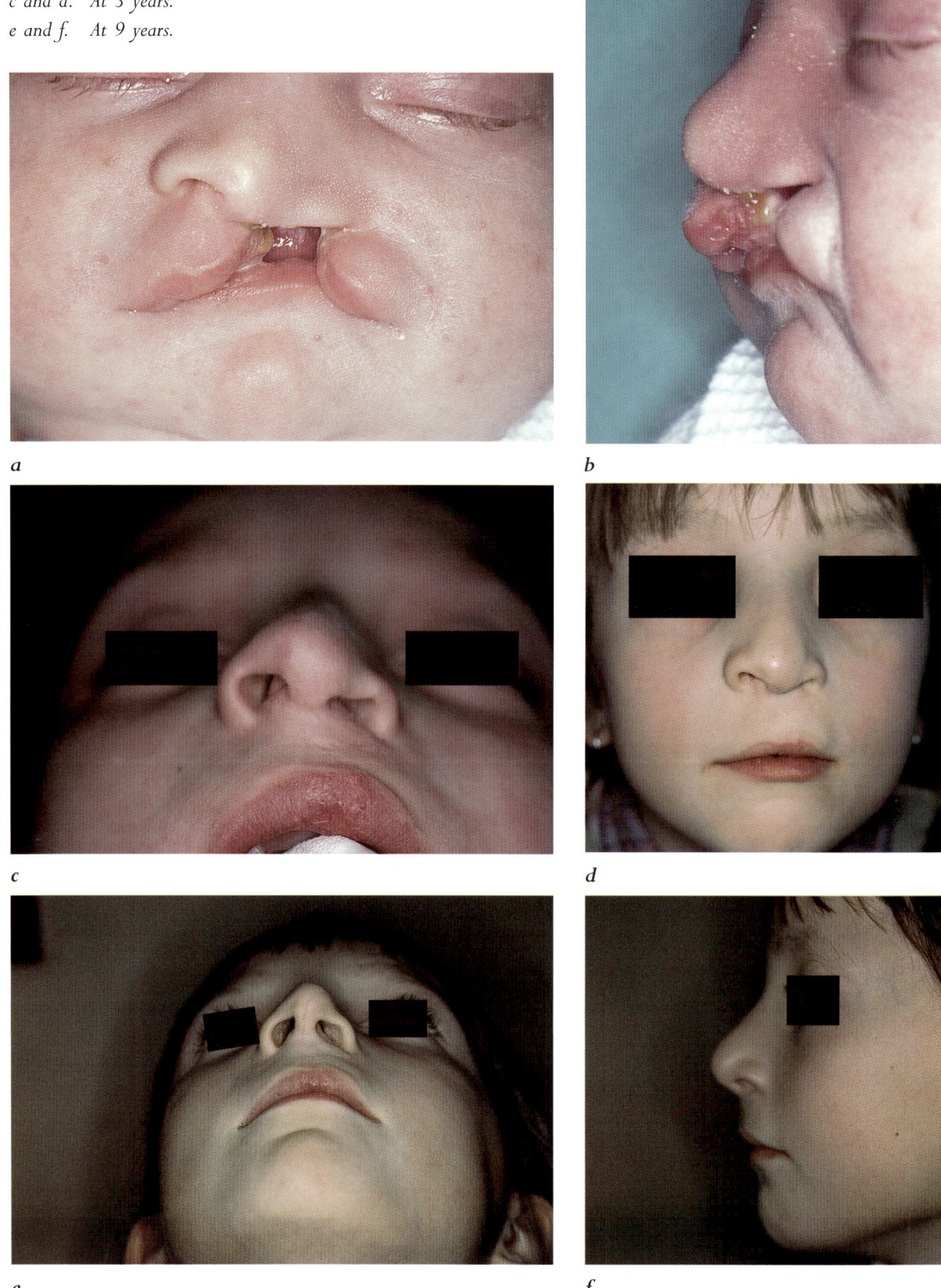

a

b

c

d

e

f

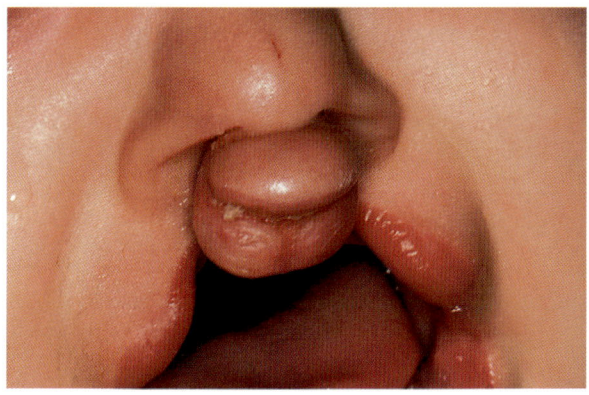

Fig. 23.9 *Usual shortness of the columella in bilateral cases.*

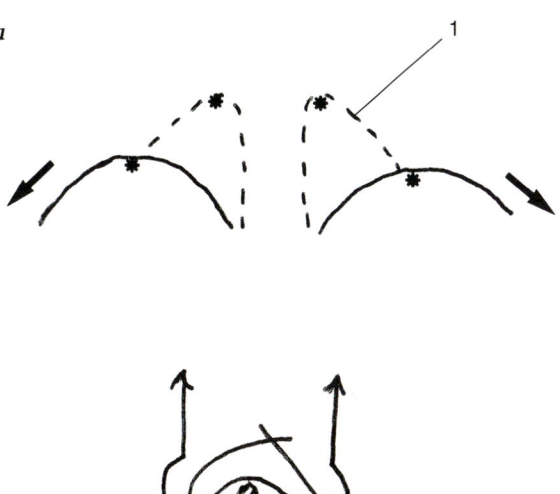

Fig. 23.11

a. *Flattening of the tips of the nose is due to lateral displacement of the domes of the alae.*

1. *Normal situation of alar cartilage.*

b. *Correct suture of the domes after lateral undermining with supporting graft.*

2. *Graft from septal cartilage.*

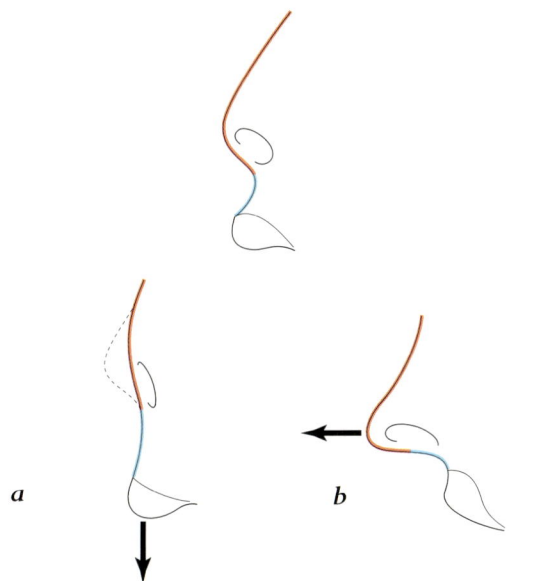

Fig. 23.10 *Classical maneuvers to show the balance between lip and columella:*

a. *If the lip is pushed down, the tip of the nose is flattened.*

b. *If the tip of the nose is pushed forward to elongate the columella, the prolabium is shortened.*

deprived of its normal support from the septum (generally hypoplastic in bilateral clefts) (Fig. 23.11a).

We have learned from experience that the flattened nose can be corrected without repercussions on the prolabium if the wing of the nose is moved inward and attached to the nasal spine with a muscular suture, and the abnormal separation between the apices of the domes is rectified by suturing them together.

To guarantee a good end result, it is often advisable to reinforce the support of the nasal tip by grafting a small strip of cartilage excised from the septum (Fig. 23.11b). Towards the end of the growth phase, the cartilage can be replaced more beneficially by a bone graft (using the outer table of a rib).

In conclusion, the length gained during correction of the short columella is obtained by advancing tissue from either side rather than by taking it from the sagittal plane as originally taught. Since no undermining whatsoever is performed on the mucosa, which follows the cartilages as they are repositioned, the nostrils resume a normal shape. Their major axis now becomes antero-posterior rather than transverse (Fig. 23.12).

Technique

A midline columellar incision is made and extended slightly over the tip of the nose.

The alar cartilages are identified. This is not always easy, because they tend to be very thin and widely spaced in young infants.

The alar cartilage is freed by extensive undermining of the skin on its outer surface. It is striking

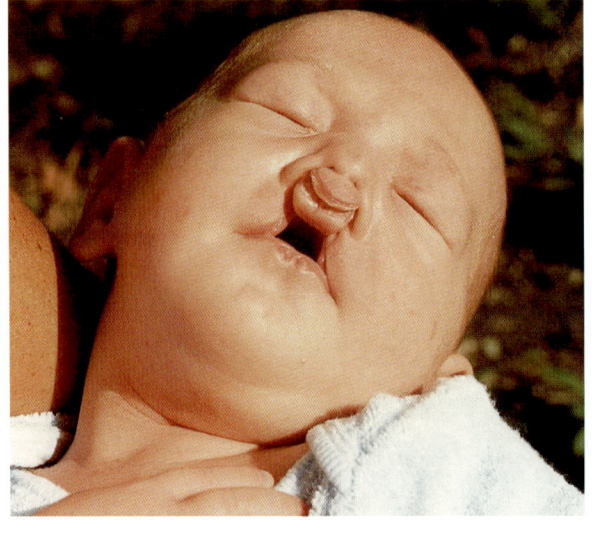

a

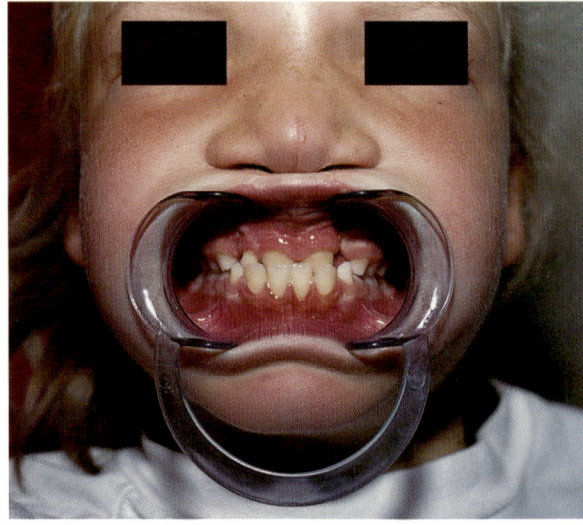

a

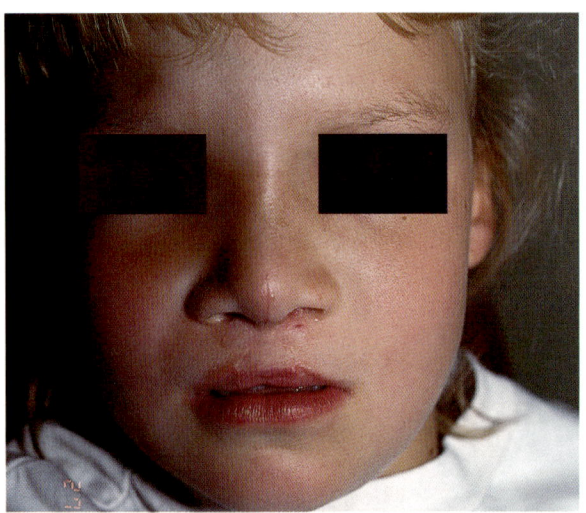

b

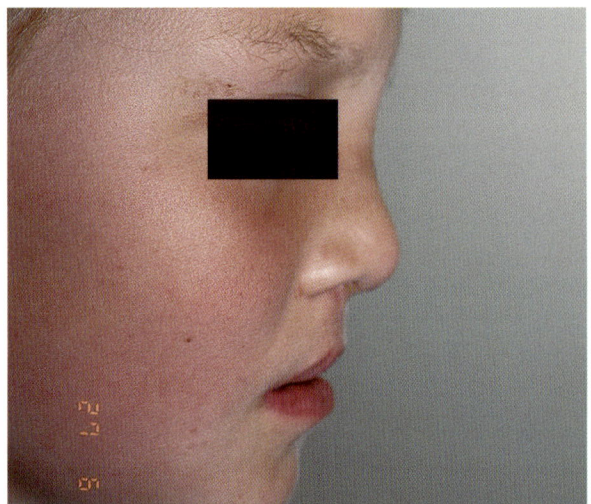

b

Fig. 23.12
a. Bilateral complete CLP.
b. Lip and nose result.

to see large, generally venous blood vessels exposed
on this level. They must be severed, since their loops
tend to maintain the shortness of the columella and
the curvature of the cartilages.

The septum is located and undermined on both
surfaces. In young children, when the septal cartilage
is sufficiently sturdy, a narrow rectangular graft is
removed (2 mm wide by 1–1.5 mm long) at a certain
depth so as to avoid further weakening of the free
border. The graft is fastened to the free border of the
septum with two or three nylon sutures in such a
position that it creates a good forward projection of
the nasal tip (Fig. 23.13).

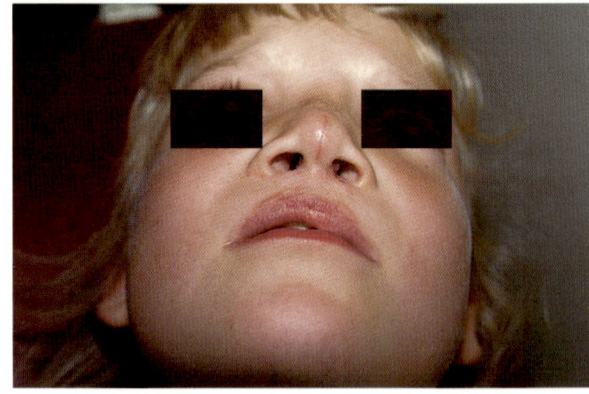

c

Fig. 23.13
a. Dental result.
b. Nasal tip with good forward projection.
c. The nostrils after early rhinoplasty.

The alar domes are sutured. Generally, one stitch suffices to anchor them to the extremity of the graft (Fig. 23.14).

Cutaneous suturing is carried out on two planes without resection. The septum is transfixed with an absorbable suture, which helps to encourage proper re-adhesion of the undermined mucosa.

When the patient has entered adolescence, if the sub-septal cartilage is flimsy, it is preferable to use a bone graft taken from a rib.

Removal of an outer rib table

A low thoracic incision (submammary in girls if breasts have developed), followed by incision of the muscle layer, exposes a rib.

The outer surface of the rib is denuded. Using a small chisel, it is easy to remove a rectangular graft of the desired size from the outer table only. This method provides a very slender but sturdy graft, which will not affect the thickness of the columella. It also avoids the pleural risk and post-operative pain connected with removing a cross-section of the whole rib.

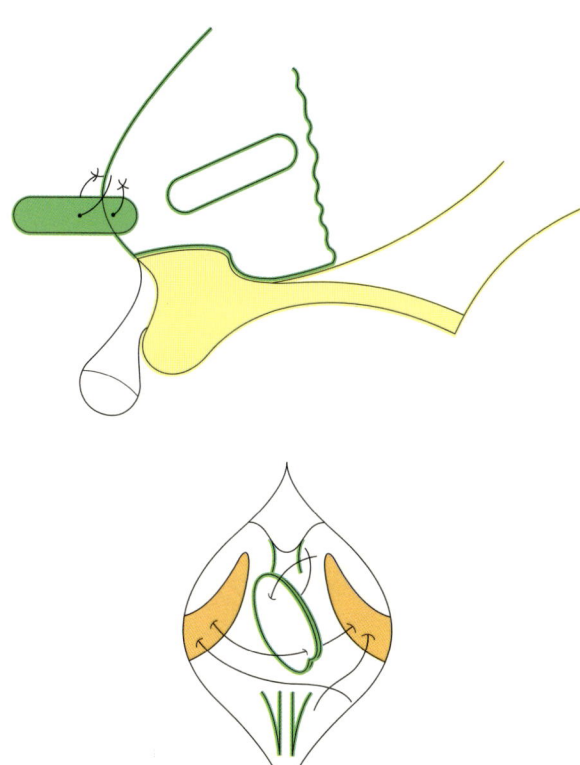

Fig. 23.14 *Cartilage graft from the septum.*

The base of the graft must be securely attached to the anterior nasal spine, which is first freshened and split through the incision in the columella.

The suture that unites the domes is fastened to the graft, in which a small notch has been excised to prevent slipping.

The surgeon must not be over-ambitious. When the graft is too long, perforation of the nasal tip may occur requiring secondary resection with a gouge. This does not generally cause infection or scarring, but does detract from the end result.

Lastly, during early rhinoplasty of bilateral clefts, there may be a need to correct the naso-vestibular fold on both sides.

LONG-TERM PHONETIC RESULTS OF EARLY PRIMARY PALATE REPAIR

This section was prepared with the collaboration of Chantal Trichet and Marie-Rose Mousset.

The method of early primary palate repair was first introduced 20 years ago, so we now have a valid perspective on its long-term results.

Originally, this technique was primarily aimed at improving osteo-dental results: we were disappointed with those obtained with 'classic' surgery using the method based on Veau's techniques and Petit's timing (cheiloplasty at 6 months, staphylorraphy at 18 months). This procedure involved elevation of the palatine mucoperiosteum.

The Schweckendieck method, described in 1944, seemed to produce encouraging skeletal results. However, postponing closure of the palatal cleft until the patient was well out of childhood (to avoid the iatrogenic risks arising from the elevation of the mucoperiosteum) did not seem conducive to satisfactory speech development. Our misgivings were confirmed by the poor phonetic results obtained.

With the early primary palate method, it was hoped that closure of the entire cleft with velar repair at a much earlier age might bring about an improvement not only in the bone structures, but also in the phonetic results.

Material and methods

Out of the total number who underwent early primary palate surgery, 112 of the oldest cases, treated between 1976 and 1982 (now between 15 and 22 years of age), were retained. These patients have been followed on a regular basis from the age of 12 months. Our speech pathologists have tested them every 6 months to monitor phonetic and articulatory evolution and to evaluate their speech and language skills.

Parental guidance, preliminary screening and orthophonic evaluations represent the various stages of this follow-up.

Parental guidance and preliminary screening from 1–4 years of age permit early action on the child's phonation, thanks to counselling of the parents. Thus, emergent speech development can be monitored and oriented according to an appropriate educational technique.

Objective assessments

Speech assessments proper are established from the age of 4 years and allow objective evaluation to take place over a long period.

The articulation of phonemes is routinely evaluated during sessions of repetition as well as free speech.

Velopharyngeal competence is tested to verify whether or not nasopharyngeal closure, thanks to simultaneous contraction of the soft palate and pharynx, is adequate.

Nasal air escape (termed velar insufficiency) can be heard, and is confirmed with a metallic mirror which mists when air passes through the nose. The mirror is placed beneath the child's nostrils (as soon as the child is willing to co-operate) during the production of isolated phonemes which he or she is asked to repeat. It is then used for connected syllables and sentences. If the mirror does not show mist during the repetition test for oral consonants (plosives of the [p/t/k] type), the closing mechanism is rated as efficient and it is assumed that the soft palate fulfills its normal function. If there is misting, the closing mechanism is considered inadequate and velar malfunction may be suspected as the cause.

The mirror test is a routine procedure. The results it shows are only thought to be significant for those oral phonemes that begin or end vocal emission.

It is also advisable to confirm patency of the nasal airway. This makes it possible to diagnose rhinolalia, which corresponds to an absence of the nasal air flow

normally produced when nasal consonants and vowels are pronounced.

Tests based on aural perception and on mirror misting are very simple and reliable for the experienced speech therapist, and are sufficient for our purposes. We have never felt the need for more sophisticated testing, which requires complex equipment as it is costly. Lateral X-ray does not show the isthmus. There is no doubt that nasal endoscopy (Pigott, 1969; Pigott *et al.*, 1982; Sinclair *et al.*, 1982) represents a revolution in the study of nasopharyngeal closing mechanisms, but it is not particularly helpful in orienting the therapeutic approach. The reason is simple: we believe that pharyngoplasty provides a unique means to combat velar insufficiency efficiently.

Thanks to the clinical findings, it is possible to classify the child's individual speech patterns under one of the headings of the system devised by Borel-Maisonny (see Chapter 14, reproduced by Mousset in Chapter 10).

A total of 112 case studies of complete labio-palatal clefts in patients who are now at least 15 years old have been retained. Those cases for which the follow-up was incomplete were automatically excluded, as were those where the patients presented associated disabilities that might interfere with phonation (cerebral palsy, mental disability, deafness, etc.). These 112 cases (73 boys and 39 girls) come under the following categories:

Complete left unilateral cleft	54
Right unilateral cleft	26
Bilateral cleft	32

As will be seen, the site of the cleft may have an effect on the results.

The results are furnished before and after pharyngoplasty in the event that surgery was required to correct a velar insufficiency that did not respond to speech therapy.

Results

To permit a comparison between our results, which are rated according to the Borel-Maisonny system of classification, and those of other schools, which apply different methods of treatment, we have attempted to align the criteria of our evaluations on those of

English-speaking authors. These are the most widely used in literature, and establish three levels:

1. Competence, which corresponds to satisfactory velar function. This covers our terms of phonation 1 (complete closure) and phonation 1/2 (where nasal escape is intermittent). Velar closure is possible under most circumstances.
2. Borderline, which seems to be the equivalent of phonation 2/1. The soft palate can be closed occasionally when special efforts are made for a drill, but air escape is almost consistently present during ordinary speech.
3. Incompetence, which corresponds to phonation 2 (permanent air escape), 2/3 (occasional substitution) and 3 (voice quality seriously distorted by glottal catches and hoarse aspirates; gross substitution errors).

Although this system of equivalence is somewhat arbitrary, it does enable us to work out a comparative evaluation of the results.

The 112 cases can be divided as follows:

Ph 1   55 cases
Ph 1/2   21 cases } = 76/112 competence: 67.85%
Ph 2/1   15 cases =   borderline: 13.40%
Ph 2   19 cases
Ph 2/3   2 cases } = 21/112 incompetence: 18.74%
Ph 3   0

Virtually no children presented glottal stop.

An analysis of the results according to anatomical type reveals interesting findings. In bilateral clefts, levels 1 and 1/2 (competence) represent only 62.51 per cent of the total. These statistics disprove the opinion of our predecessors and mentors, who thought that phonetic results were better for bilateral clefts. They believed that, since hypoplasia of the cavum was greater in these cases, the soft palate was more likely to achieve satisfactory closure.

In left unilateral clefts (the most common), 68.51 per cent are rated competent.

In right clefts, 73.07 per cent are rated competent.

Comparative evaluation

A comparative evaluation of results (before prospective pharyngoplasty) furnished the most significant information. A valid comparison can be made between these results and those obtained when we still followed the classic surgical schedule and techniques of Petit and his predecessor Veau.

At first glance the benefits are not self-evident for levels Ph 1 and 1/2, since the figure for the classic technique hovers around 62 per cent (although the percentage is higher for unilateral clefts in our experience). However, the 'classic' authors were less demanding since they also included speech level 2/1 under the general heading of 'satisfactory results'. Were we to do the same, the figure for our own 'satisfactory results' would rise from 62 to 81.25 per cent.

The figures are similar for our comparative statistics on Ph 2.

The improvement was far more striking, however, for 2/3 and 3 phonation. We had only two instances of Ph 2/3 with the early primary palate method and no cases of Ph 3, as opposed to 11 per cent of Ph 3 cases for the classic technique.

Glottal stops (phonation 3) were therefore practically eliminated, thanks to the early primary palate method.

Comparisons with other methods are more questionable since the surgeons, their techniques and their criteria differ. We will limit ourselves to a comparison with the results of the Schweckendieck method of delayed hard palate closure, as reported by Bardach *et al.* (1984) and Van Demark *et al* (1989). Bardach and colleagues have an objective point of view, since the authors themselves were not members of what is known as the Marburg team.

Van Demark, Gnoinski, Hotz, Perko and Nussbaumer devoted a very detailed analysis to the phonetic results of the Zurich School published in a later issue of the same journal. Perko applies the basic principles of the Schweckendieck method, but practices earlier closure of the palate between the ages of 5 and 6 years. Until this time, the child constantly wears a plate.

The Marburg results are for a total of 43 cases (which represents only a small group) involving patients who had undergone secondary hard palate closure. These figures speak for themselves:

Competence   18.6%
Borderline   34.8%
Incompetence   46.6%, with a considerable number of residual glottal stops.

		Veau	Marburg	Zurich	PP1
Competence	Phon 1 & 1/2	0.62	0.186	0.405	0.6786
Borderline	Phon 2/1	?	?	0.541	0.134
Incompetence	Phon 2	0.27	0.348		0.1874
	Phon 2/3				
	Phon 3 G-S +	0.11	0.466	0.054	0

Table 23.1 Comparison between the phonetic results published. We note the improvement with early and primary repair (PP1).

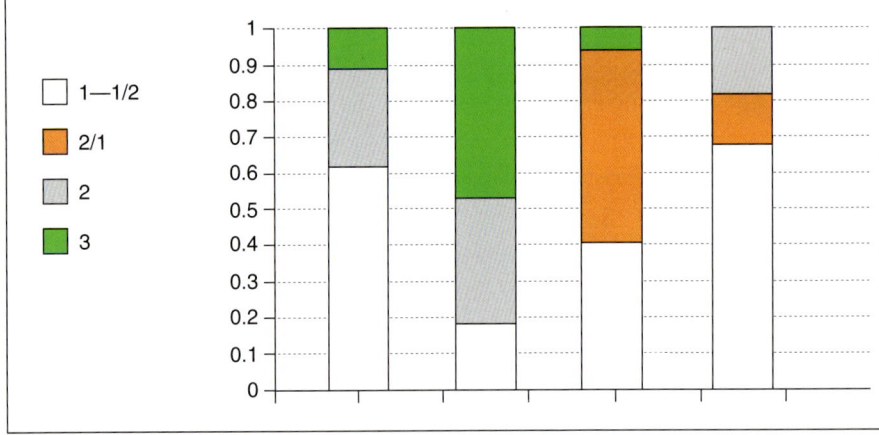

For the Zurich results, we have retained only those figures that concern the evaluation of velopharyngeal function:

Competence   40.5%
Borderline   54.1%
Incompetence   5.4%

It seems legitimate to draw the following conclusions:

First, the early primary palate technique produces a definite improvement in velar function with less velar incompetence (Table 23.1). This result can be explained as follows:

1. The existence of congenital hypoplasia of the palate is undeniable; it is consistently confirmed by clinical evidence because the soft palate seems short after repair.
2. If it is true that no specific act is performed to lengthen the velum (although the surgeon may have the impression that additional length has been gained after anterior disinsertion of the muscles during veloplasty), there is nonetheless a strong probability (but no way to prove it) that early repair leads to greater muscular development of the soft palate. It is thought that the velum develops more energetic contractions, which contribute to its actual lengthening during the growth process.
3. Lastly, veloplasty is performed at a stage where the bone structures are still very malleable. Hence, the fact that the skeletal elements of the lateral walls of the pharynx are brought closer together (a finding which we among others have confirmed on CT scans) should facilitate active closure of the nasopharynx once the sphincteric mechanism created by the levator palatini and the superior constrictor comes into play.

Secondly, a highly significant result of our experience lies in the virtual elimination of glottal stops. It is logical to attribute their disappearance to the fact that palatal repair is performed at a very young age. Indeed, patterns of speech are developed early in life. If the malformation is corrected before this stage, the child does not resort to compensatory patterns of misarticulation. These defects are extremely difficult to eradicate in patients operated on at a later age who have already become used to deviant neuromuscular circuits.

Thirdly, one of the major concerns in our experience lies in the problem of residual fistulae subsequent to primary surgery. The subject is developed in detail in the following sections. On a phonetic level, fistulae lead to anterior nasal air escape, which causes consonant production to lack clarity. The points of articulation may be shifted towards the back of the oral cavity.

Above all, velar function can be affected by a certain absence of reactivity, or 'laziness', which worsens as time goes by.

During the production of voiceless plosives [p/t/k], the role played by the soft palate can be described as follows. The pronunciation of plosives involves three phases:

1. Occlusion is produced by contact between the lips or between the tongue and a given zone within the oral cavity (point of articulation).
2. Impounding or the build-up of air pressure behind the zone of occlusion represents a very brief phase (a few tenths of a second). It should be totally silent.
3. Plosion or release of the impounded air when the lips are opened produces a characteristic sound which varies according to the point of articulation and should be clear and distinct.

In typical cases of velar insufficiency, the second phase (build-up of intra-buccal pressure) cannot be achieved anywhere within the oral cavity. The production of plosives is therefore a physical impossibility.

If velopharyngeal functioning is satisfactory but co-exists with anterior nasal air escape (as is the case with residual fistulae), the second phase of impounding cannot be obtained for the front plosives [p/t]. However, it remains possible for the back velar plosive [k], because the zone of occlusion closed by contact between the tongue and the soft palate is located behind the opening (Fig. 23.15).

Thus, in the presence of a fistula, clear and energetic production of the velar plosive [k] confirms satisfactory velar function although the front plosives are either non-existent or indistinct, accompanied by audible nasal air emission. This indicates that isolated closure of the fistula is the appropriate surgical treatment to correct the phonetic disorder concerned. If, however, the patient is incapable of producing the velar plosive [/k], then pharyngoplasty is called for.

Critical analysis of the criteria

To judge by present statistics, this criterion is reliable. In each case where we contended that velopharyngeal function was adequate, closure of the residual fistula resulted in phonation without a trace of nasal distortion (22 cases). However, the statistical study must be enlarged to cover a larger number of observations.

Surprisingly enough, in patients with extremely short soft palates, we are sometimes struck by production of [k,g] with no nasal distortion. The question arises as to whether the tongue participates in elevation of the soft palate: indeed, to produce [k,g], the entire dorsal portion of the tongue is mobilized upward and towards the back of the oral cavity. In two cases where this phenomenon was suspected, closure of the fistula confirmed proper velopharyngeal function. This hypothesis calls for confirmation based on further observations. A study of the soft palate under videofluoroscopy nasoendoscopy during the articulation of the syllables [ka/ko-/kou-] as opposed to [ta-/to-/tou-] should demonstrate whether the tongue does exert pressure on the velum to produce the velar plosive [ka-/ko-/kou-].

We have performed pharyngoplasties on 31 of our 112 patients. This figure may seem rather high, but it is justified by our new and very demanding standards.

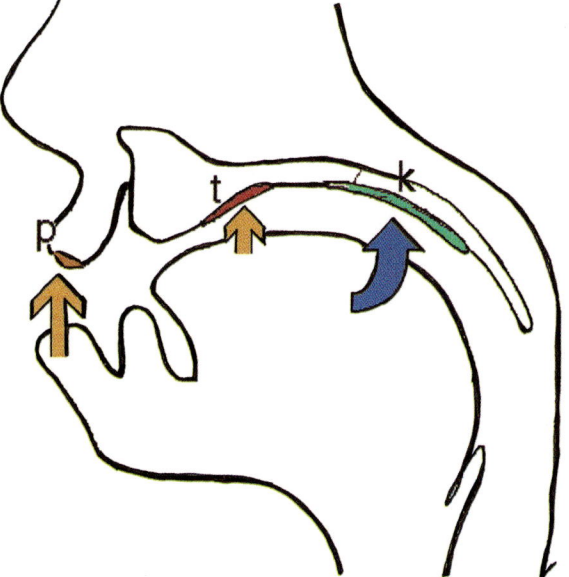

Fig. 23.15 *The contact zones for the different plosives during occlusion.*

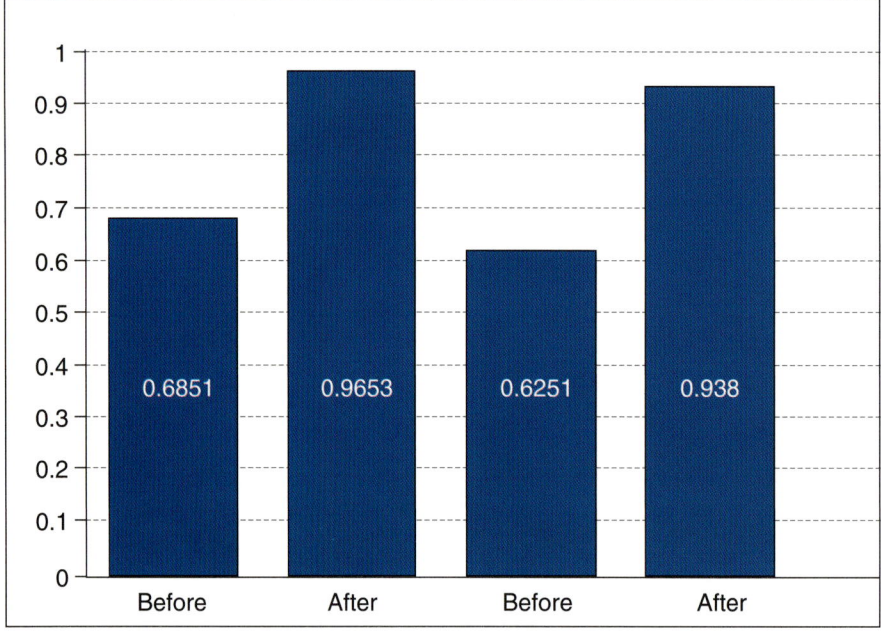

Unilateral clefts (10)		Bilateral clefts (15)	
Before	After	Before	After
0.6851	0.9653	0.6251	0.938

Table 23.2 The percentage of good results for Ph 1 and 1/2 can be improved further after pharyngoplasty.

These fulfill the expectations of the patients and their families, who are anxious to obtain satisfactory speech results of a permanent nature.

These considerations have led us to increase the number of proposed pharyngoplasties.

Before presenting the statistical data on our results, a few preliminary remarks are in order.

The technique of pharyngoplasty is described in Chapter 13. It consistently involves elevation of the palatine mucoperiosteum, an act that conflicts with the new principles adopted. This presents a risk for maxillo-dental development. Thus, there is indeed a dilemma.

In addition to those repercussions on growth which are of vascular origin (since the maxilla is deprived of a major source of blood supply normally provided by the posterior palatine vessels), the push-back of soft tissues leaves raw surfaces in the oral and nasal area which show a definite tendency to retract during the healing process. Consequently, there is a risk of causing displacements of the bone segments as well as growth disorders, which are detrimental to the skeletal results. Clearly, this is contrary to our aims, since these are precisely the results that the early primary palate method is intended to improve.

To reduce this danger of bone displacement, we consistently install a retainer plate, which is worn for at least 6 months, and has the additional advantage of protecting the fragile zones of the cleft, as well as any fresh sutures in these areas.

In the case of labio-palatal clefts, retro-displacement of the mucoperiosteum may cause the nasal layer to rupture, thus creating an anterior residual fistula. It is a fact that the tissues used for closure of the vault during early primary veloplasty are neither thick nor sturdy enough for the procedure to be totally risk-free.

Lastly, there is inevitable damage to the superior constrictor when the flap is elevated. Yet, as already stressed (Chapter 9), the mobility of this muscle is essential to satisfactory physiology in this region. The zone where the flap is dissected does not always heal altogether satisfactorily, and often develops an adhesion on the pre-vertebral level with a strand of fibrotic tissue which may pull the velum downward. This is detrimental to proper phonation.

There is another unpredictable factor in the long-term evolution of children who have undergone pharyngoplasty, particularly if the push-back was considerable. These children often suffer from pronounced snoring. A certain number of authors, by analogy with the pathology of snorers (roncopathies), have delved into its potential repercussions on the cardiovascular system.

It would be premature to express a definite opinion on the subject. What we can state is that, in the course of our experience of a good many years, we have yet to hear of such a disorder either among our own patients or among those of our predecessors on the same team who routinely performed pharyngoplasties. Naturally, during velar push-back we are cautious not to obstruct the choanae completely, which might cause rhinolalia. We have also reduced the dimensions of the pharyngeal flap.

The indications for pharyngoplasty must therefore be carefully assessed. In the early years it is possible that we may have proposed it a little too often. Naturally we were encouraged to do so by the favorable results of this operation, which is a reliable and relatively simple procedure. The results of our oldest patients are as follows (Table 23.2):

- In bilateral clefts, where we had 62.51 per cent of Ph 1 and 1/2, we obtained 93.8 per cent good results after 10 pharyngoplasties.
- In left unilateral clefts, we performed 15 pharyngoplasties for a total of 54 children (27.8 per cent). The statistics for Ph 1 and 1/2 rose from 68.5 to 96.3 per cent.
- In right clefts, the percentage increased from 73.07 to 96.2 per cent.

These phonetic results are therefore significantly better than those formerly obtained.

OSTEODENTAL RESULTS

This section was prepared with the collaboration of Hervé Martinez.

The osteo-dental results are of essential importance. This does not mean to imply that morphological and phonetic results are any less significant, but problems involving the bone structures are what originally convinced us to modify our methods and carry out the early primary palate experiment.

The pathology is characteristic. Throughout the period of growth, there is an intricate interaction between the effects of the embryonic lesions and the iatrogenic repercussions of the surgery intended to correct them. In the long run, it is extremely difficult to determine the respective responsibilities of the various factors.

We must stress the fact that it takes 15–20 years before the end results can be validly evaluated. Even if all the treatments termed 'secondary' (in time) play a significant part in the final outcome, we nonetheless remain convinced that success hinges essentially on the initial operations.

A truly valid comparison can be made between methods and operations if they are performed by the same surgeon. This eliminates any question of skill or technique.

Even though the historical perspective of 20 years is not really enough to permit a thorough assessment of our experience (the 40 years needed go beyond the work span of a single surgeon), the results we have obtained are sufficient both in number and in quality to justify the main choices we have made:

1. Inversion of the surgical protocol (soft palate first)
2. No elevation of the palatal mucoperiosteum, but total closure of the cleft.

The osteo-dental results can be analyzed on two levels: first, dental evolution of the upper arch itself and of its relationship with the lower teeth, particularly during the two phases of tooth development (mixed dentition and permanent dentition), and secondly, maxillary growth. This includes the relationship of maxilla to mandible and the occlusion of the upper and lower teeth based on cephalometric studies.

Dental results

Primary dentition (milk teeth)

Unilateral clefts

From the earliest days of our experiment we were struck, in the majority of cases, by the excellent spontaneous evolution of the upper arch and of the teeth, particularly the canine, which were located in a satisfactory position.

In these cases, there were no examples of lingual inclination. In addition, and this is a finding that contrasts with the classic method, we observed that infragnathia of the borders of the cleft or collapse of the arch was corrected (Figs 23.16, 23.17).

A supernumerary lateral incisor is often found in the area adjacent to the cleft; however, the existence of this extra tooth has no unfavorable repercussions. On the contrary, it helps to maintain a desirable width of space between the segments and contributes to satisfactory occlusion.

In 49.7 per cent of the cases of a supernumerary lateral deciduous tooth, there was no supernumerary permanent incisor. Within the context of permanent dentition, there were 17.8 per cent supernumerary lateral incisors for unilateral clefts and 19.4 per cent for bilateral clefts.

Lingual inclination of the canine (reference tooth) is not uncommon. This does not require any special attention since, generally speaking, orthodontic treatment is not applied to milk or primary dentition except when contact with the lower teeth causes a lateralization of the mandible. This contributes to a permanent deviation of the chin already described in Chapter 17.

Lingual inclination of the canine tooth often shows a spontaneous evolution in the right direction during the period of mixed dentition. Otherwise, if the arch itself is in a proper position, a short-term orthodontic treatment suffices to reposition the tooth in question and restore satisfactory occlusion (Fig. 23.18).

Bilateral clefts
As a rule, the spontaneous evolution is quite favorable. However great the original displacement of the premaxilla, it gradually recedes into its normal position. In our opinion, this is a foregone conclusion: the premaxilla retropositions itself satisfactorily without any need for pre- or post-operative appliances. It goes without saying that we take a firm stand against osteotomies of the premaxilla, which are difficult both to perform and maintain and which may result in complications, not to mention detrimental

Fig. 23.16 *Spontaneous situation of the canine in a large total cleft.*
a and b.   *Before surgery.*
c.   *5 years after surgery.*

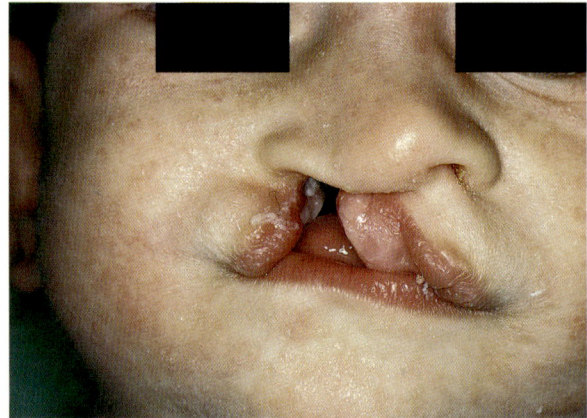

a

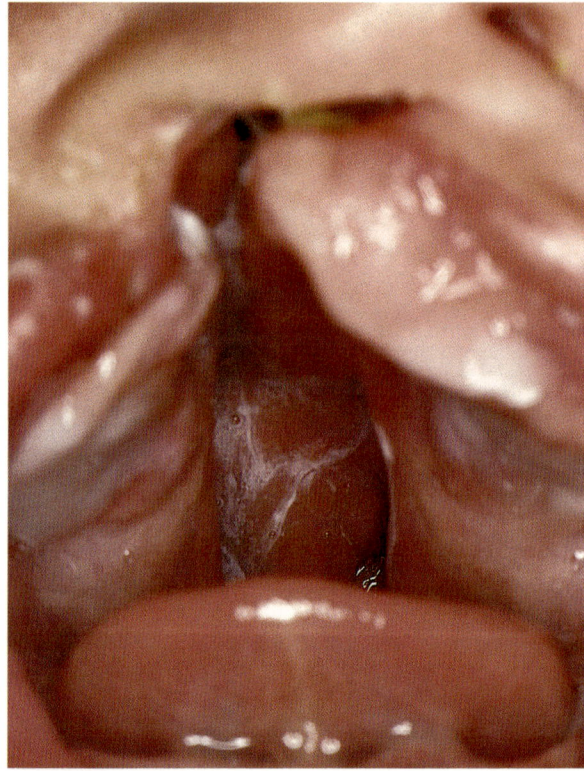

b

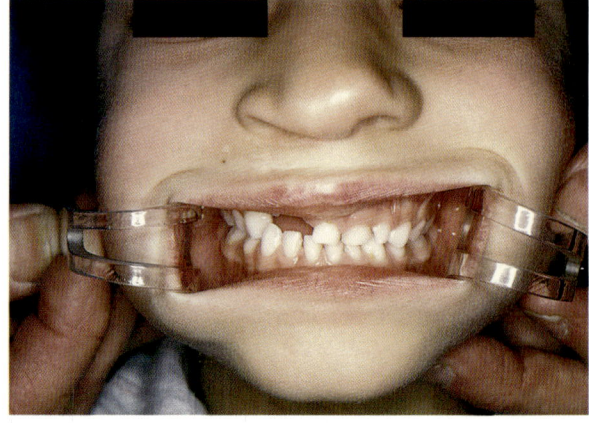

c

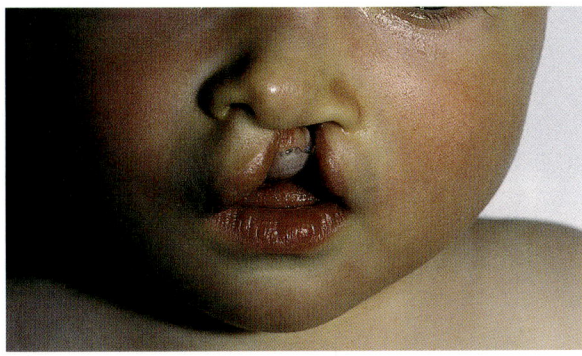

a

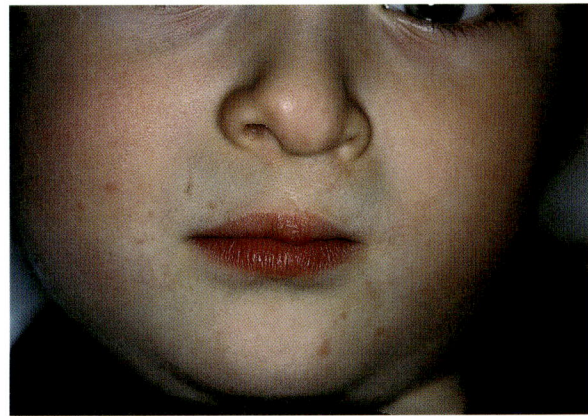

b

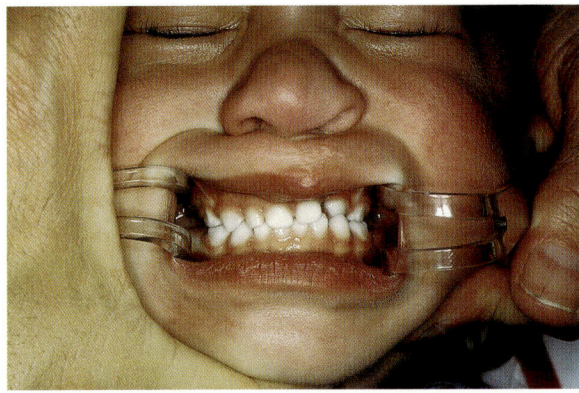

a

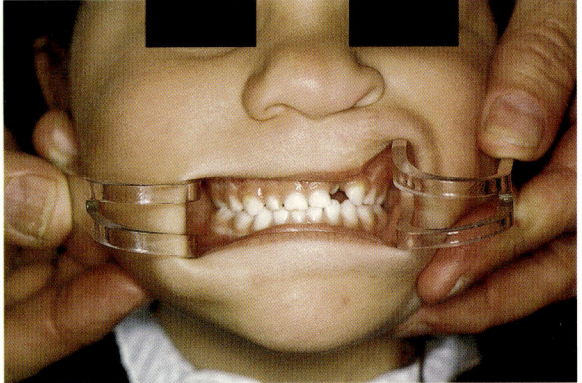

b

c

c

Fig. 23.17 *Spontaneous situation of the canine in a narrow form.*

a. Before surgery.

b. Morphological result.

c. 3 years after surgery.

Fig. 23.18 *Lingual inclination of the canine is easily corrected.*

a. At 3 months.

b. Before orthodontic treatment.

c. 2 years after.

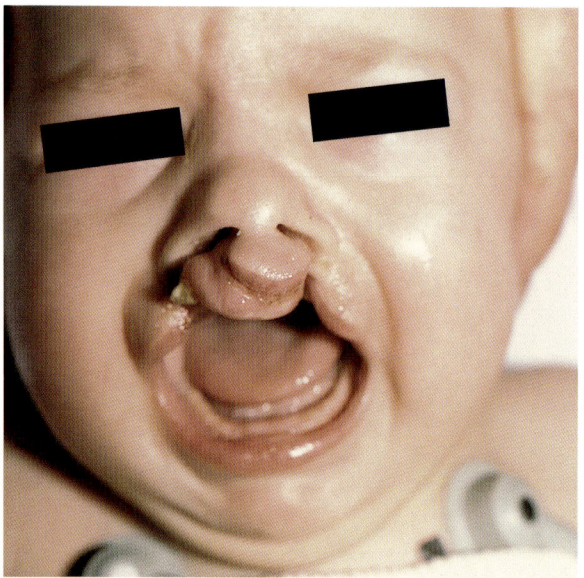

a

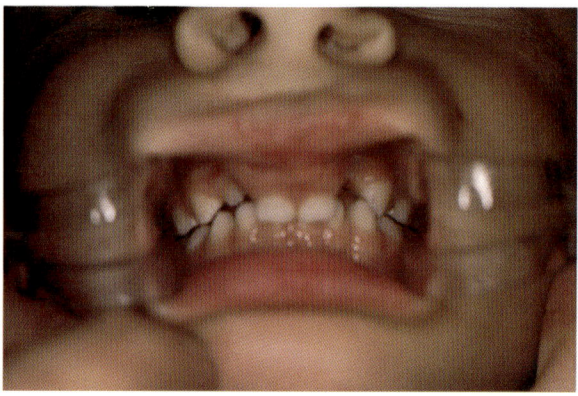

b

Fig. 23.19 *a and b. Spontaneous situation of the teeth in a bilateral case.*

permanent dentition. In unilateral clefts, the lateral incisor was missing in 22 per cent of our cases. In bilateral forms, it was missing in 20.9 per cent, with no prevailing rate for either side (Joseph, C.: Thesis, Paris 1999, based on 252 patients from our sample, including 185 unilateral clefts for 67 bilateral forms).

Permanent dentition

In order to permit a cross-comparison with other teams who apply the same criteria, we have retained the Goslon yardstick presented by Mars *et al.* in 1987. We have not evaluated those cases in which more than two orthodontists were involved.

The analysis of the three main criteria is based primarily on the following:

1. Antero-posterior relationships according to the relative positions of the upper and lower dental arches; retrognathism of the maxilla, mandibular prognathism (overjet and underjet).
2. Vertical position of the incisor teeth; vestibulocclusion, axial inclination of roots.
3. Transverse relationships; narrowness of the upper arch, canine and molar crossbites.

The assessments are ranked into three broad groups:

Group 1 (good): Requires no major orthodontic treatment
Group 2 (fair): Improvement can be obtained by orthopedic treatment
Group 3 (poor): Requires orthognathic surgery.

Basis of assessment: 92 unilateral clefts in patients over 15 years of age, repaired according to the early primary palate method between 1983 and 1988.

In 72.8 per cent of patients, the results were rated 'good' (1). These children, followed throughout the growth phase, did of course receive orthodontic treatment, but it was generally punctual and intended to simply correct dental alignment. Certain positions or inclinations of the teeth were obviously the consequence of surgical acts involving elevation of the flaps (such as rotation of the middle incisor, sometimes by as much as 90°). The canine on the small segment may also be located in a palatal position due to mucoperiosteal undermining or to the J-shaped

repercussions on growth. Yet, despite its many drawbacks, this practice still has some advocates.

Proper reinsertion of the muscle layer on the nasal spine and reconstruction of a medial vestibule cause the premaxilla to settle into a satisfactory position without scoliosis of the vomer (Fig. 23.19).

However, the results we have just presented on primary dentition do not predetermine the quality of permanent dentition; occlusion can be modified both by hypoplastic malformation, which may show up at a later date, and by the iatrogenic consequences of surgical acts.

There is also the problem of congenitally missing lateral incisors, which may involve both primary and

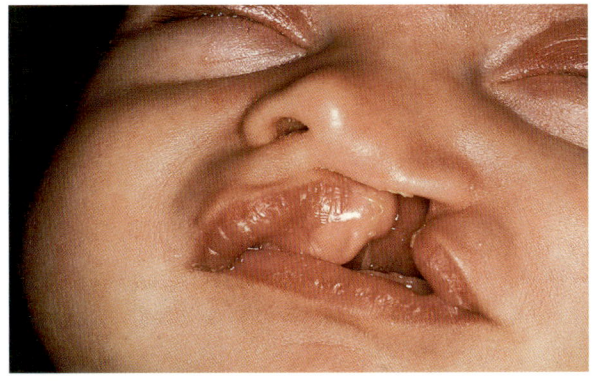

a

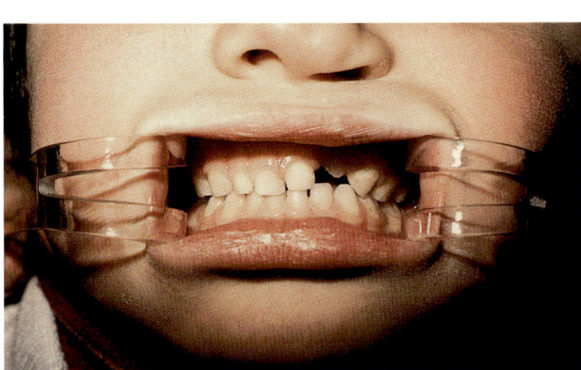

b

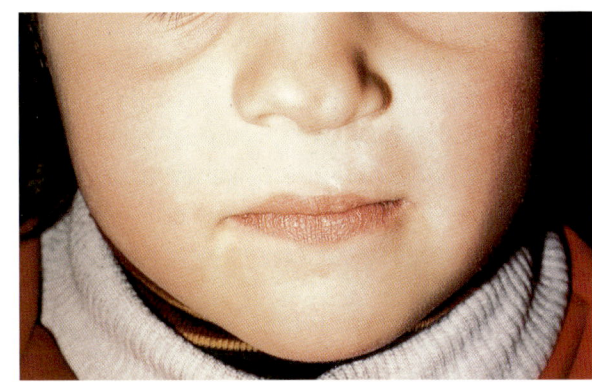

c

Fig. 23.20 *A large total case.*
a. At birth.
b. At 3 years.
c. Morphological result.

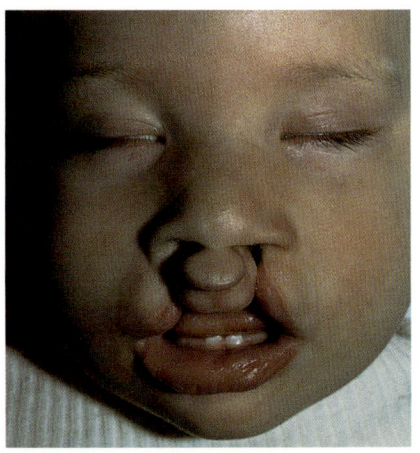

a

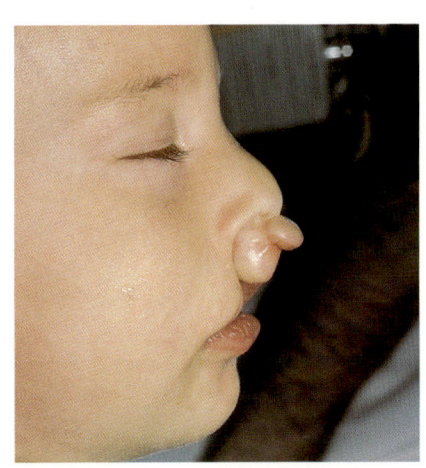

b

Fig. 23.21 *The permanent dentition obtained in a bilateral total case (Goslon 1).*
a and b. At 3 months.
c and d. At 17 years..

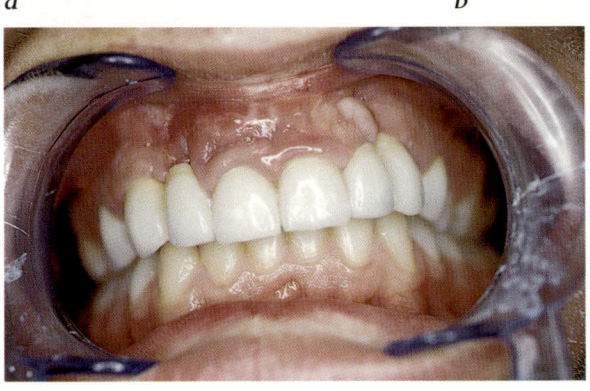

c

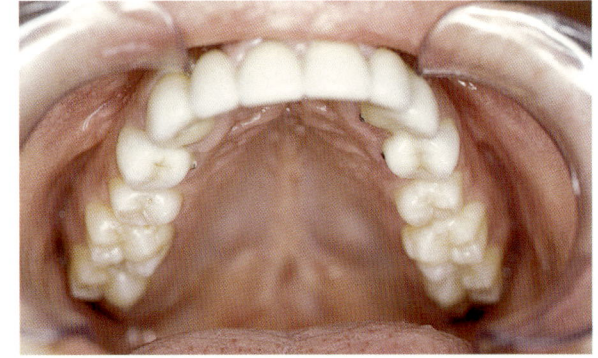

d

deformity described in Chapter 17, which can be linked to antero-posterior pressure from the divided muscle layer. Nonetheless, these cases were rated 'good' since orthodontic treatment sufficed to correct the inclination of the maxillary teeth or mild narrowing of the arch without resorting to long-term retention (Figs 23.20, 23.21, 23.22).

In 9.8 per cent of patients, results were rated 'fair' (2), therefore requiring complex orthopedic treatment to correct a tendency towards transverse narrowing thanks to the use of expansion appliances, and an unsatisfactory antero-posterior relationship requiring extra-oral traction based on headgear or chin caps, often worn permanently, palliated by marked dento-alveolar compensation (Fig. 23.23).

Lastly, 17.4 per cent of our results were 'poor' (3) and required surgery. Frequently, a fibromucosal elevation was carried out in secondary surgery. At one time,

our only solution was to await the age at which osteotomies could be performed (generally Lefort I). In the meanwhile, any orthodontic treatment undertaken was conditioned by the prospect of these future operations. At present, a certain number of specialists are experimenting with earlier surgery, as of the period of mixed dentition (expansion, maxillary distractions) (Fig. 23.24). These operations seem promising, but are not yet widespread. A harmless effect on the growth process has still to be proven.

In our opinion, these figures show considerable improvement over the results of the classic method although statistical studies were not then conducted as scientifically as they are nowadays. Nonetheless, we were able to make a valid analysis of the records of some 50 cases operated on by our team using the Veau–Petit method. We found 64 per cent of good or fair results (1 and 2) and 46 per cent of poor results (3).

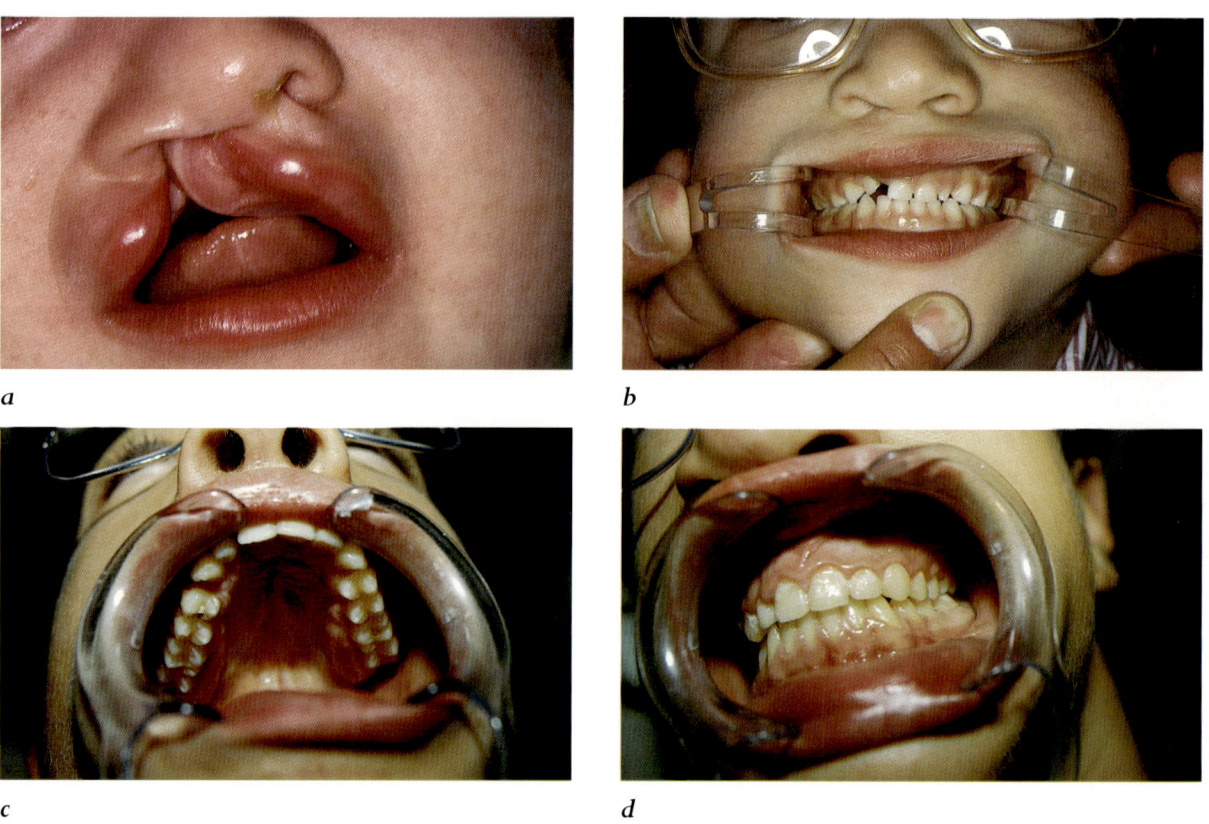

a

b

c

d

Fig. 23.22 *The permanent dentition in a narrow unilateral total cleft (Goslon 1).*
a. At birth.
b. The lacteal aspect.
c and d. At 15 years.

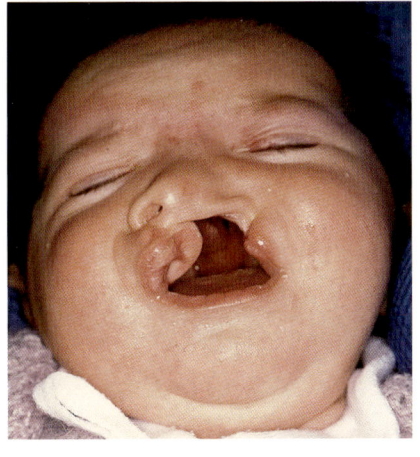

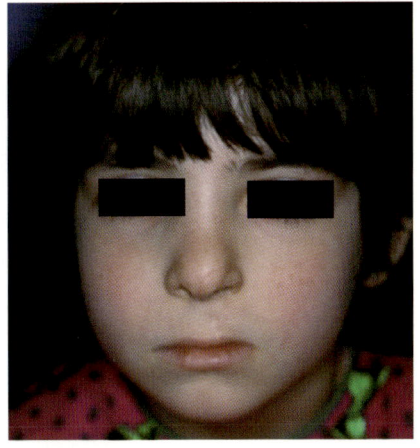

Fig. 23.23 A Goslon 2 case.
a. *Large gap at 3 months*
b. *Morphological result*
c. *Satisfactory lacteal dentition.*
d. *A major orthodontic treatment was necessary.*

a

b

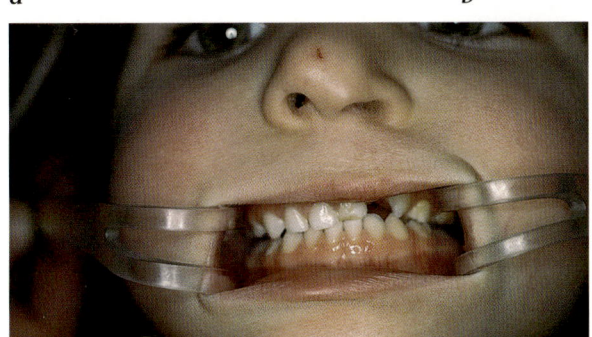

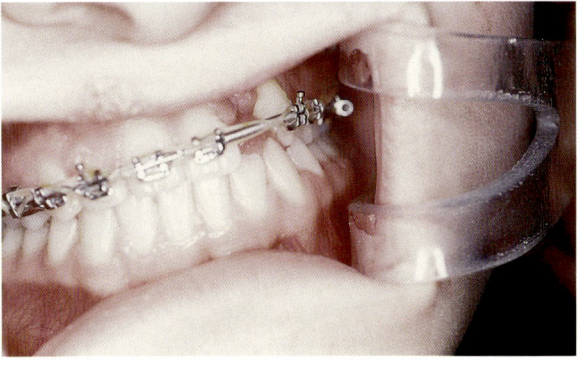

c

d

Two remarks are in order here:

1. Orthopedic treatment of the 'fair' results was often long-lasting and very demanding. The occlusion obtained was often merely tolerable with unsatisfactory dental compensations.
2. There was a very high rate of osteotomies (proposed for nearly 50 per cent of the cases, but sometimes refused by the patients) (Fig. 23.25).

It is difficult to compare these results with those published elsewhere in literature.

Bone grafting

We have already said (see Chapter 20) that we do not choose to use bone grafts in primary repair because we believe that it is unnecessary and creates a risk for the future.

A secondary graft at the age of mixed dentition is a possibility, but it was never performed as our orthodontist did not believe it would serve any purpose. Evolution of the teeth bordering the cleft

does not depend on the thickness of the bone. The migration of these teeth in a graft is satisfactory esthetically, but does not justify a further operation.

The use of a bone graft to stabilize the fragments in order to support a prosthetic bridge, however, may be used when growth stops, particularly when there is an important gap with absence of an incisor. This graft will also be useful in diminishing the height of the prosthesis. Covering the iliac graft is difficult, and sometimes requires the use of a Burian flap.

Growth and cephalometric findings

Thorough cephalometric studies are performed from 9 years of age, and are repeated at least once. We will not elaborate here on the method we use; it is derived from the Tweed technique which seems to be the most simple (Tweed, 1954).

On profile facial cephalometric radiographs, the SNA angle formed by a line traced from the center

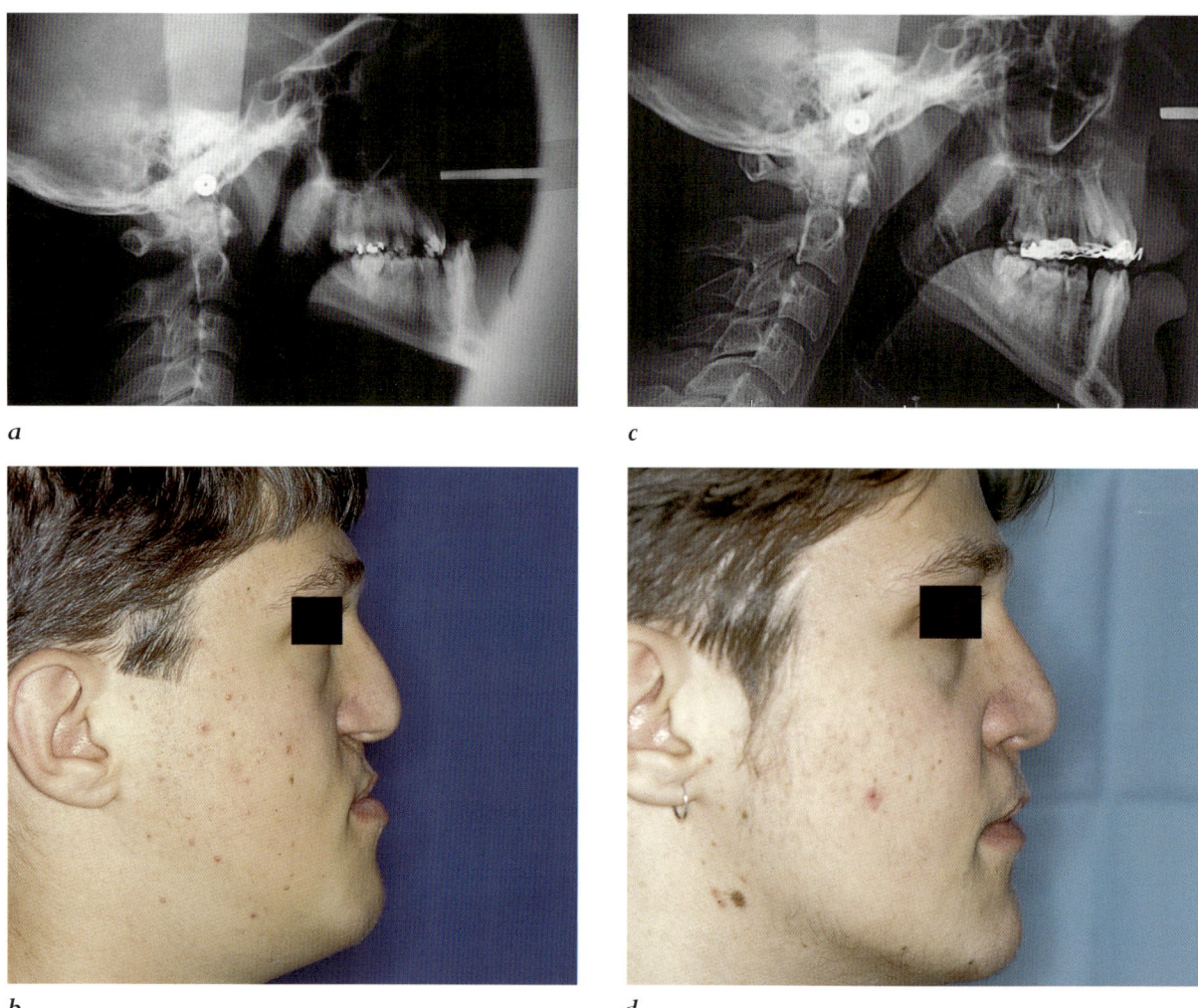

a

b

c

d

Fig. 23.24 *A Goslon 3 case which led to a maxillary distraction (Dr Oger).*
a and b. X-ray and clinical aspect before surgery.
c and d. After the operation.

of the sella turcica (S) to the base of the nose (N) and down to the base of the anterior nasal spine (A) is measured. This angle is used to assess the degree of retrognathism of the maxilla.

We also measure the ANB angle formed by a line drawn between points A and N and that which joins N to the deepest midline point on the mandible between the tip of the chin and the lower incisor tooth. This angle serves to evaluate the relationships and therefore the growth and balance between maxilla and mandible (Fig. 23.26).

The examination of cephalometric tracings for 92 patients presenting unilateral complete clefts with cleft palate (bilateral cases are more difficult to evaluate) and aged 15 years or older revealed

(Fig. 23.27):

Normal SNA	42%
SNA below normal	40%
SNA above normal	18%

When the SNA angle is below normal, which corresponds to retrognathism of the maxilla, the value of the ANB angle permits the following distinction (Fig. 23.28).

- 60 per cent of cases have an ANB angle ranging from 0–4° and show a satisfactory maxillo-mandibular balance.
- 24 per cent of cases have an ANB angle of over 4° and show retrognathism of the mandible.
- 16 per cent of cases have a negative ANB angle,

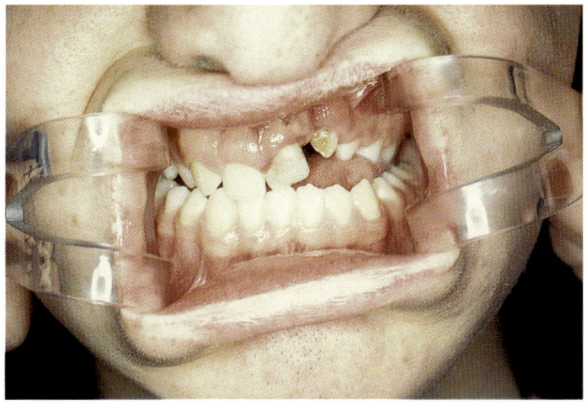

a

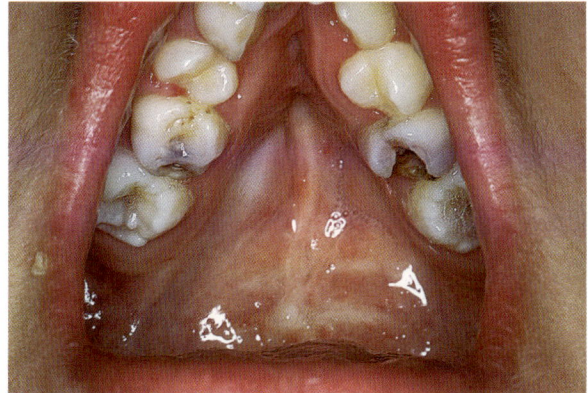

b

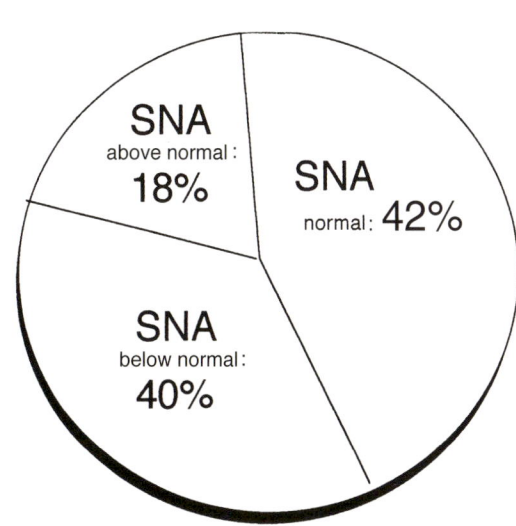

c

Fig. 23.25 *Poor results were frequent with the classic method.*

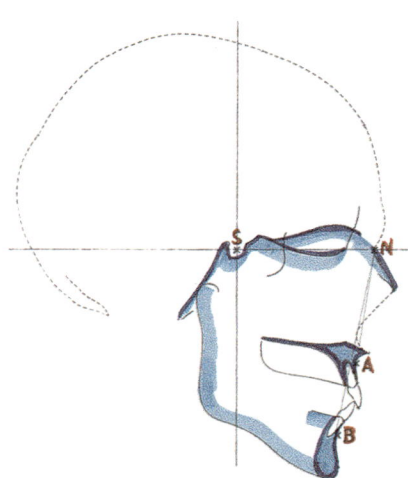

Fig. 23.26 *The situation of reference points in the cephalometric study.*

S. *center of the sella turcica*

N. *most anterior point of the frontonasal suture*

A. *deepest point of the contour of the upper alveolar arch*

B. *deepest point of the anterior contour of the mandibular arch.*

Fig. 23.27 *The value of SNA.*

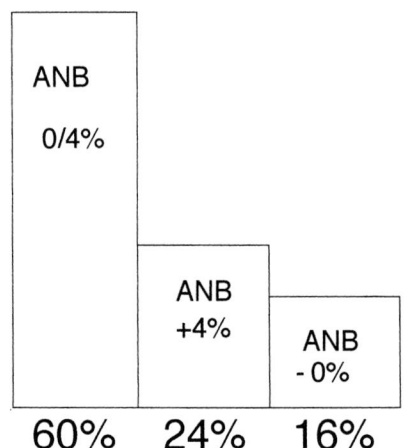

Fig. 23.28 When SNA is below normal, study of the ANB angle.

i.e. below 0°, and show major maxillo-mandibular imbalance.

As demonstrated by this study, the early surgery performed without elevating the palatine mucoperiosteum (at least during the first years of life) does not lead to disorders in maxillary growth.

Seeking an impartial opinion, we asked Bruce Ross of Toronto to examine our available sample of cephalometric radiographs using the same procedures employed in a previous multicenter study published in an issue of the *Cleft Palate Journal* (Ross, 1987). In this study, Ross had attempted to single out those factors that might influence osteo-dental results. He

was kind enough to oblige, and conducted a comparative analysis on our sample of 35 male patients (Ross, 1995). These are his conclusions:

> The Malek procedure for reconstruction of complete unilateral cleft lip and palate, performed by Professor Malek, results in excellent growth of the facial skeleton at 10 years of age

Conclusion

In conclusion, a parallel study, based on models and cephalometrics, of two samples of patients presenting approximately the same anatomical cleft form and treated by the same team throws sharp light on the highly detrimental effects produced on dental occlusion by elevation of the mucoperiosteum. This had already become a widely acknowledged fact following the work of Gillies and Schweckendieck.

Moreover, restoring the tongue to a more satisfactory position thanks to veloplasty *before* cheiloplasty represents a favorable factor as demonstrated by the reduced dimensions of the nasopharynx (seen in a CT scan).

The essential factor in accounting for better dental results seems to be re-establishment of the early moulding action of the tongue. While 50 per cent of the young patients treated by the classic method showed fair or poor occlusion, the new protocol produced only 27 per cent of fair to poor results.

Early closure of the entire cleft does not compromise facial growth, and it affords a major contribution to the prevention or reduction of functional disorders, primarily those connected with speech (Figs 23.29, 23.30, 23.31).

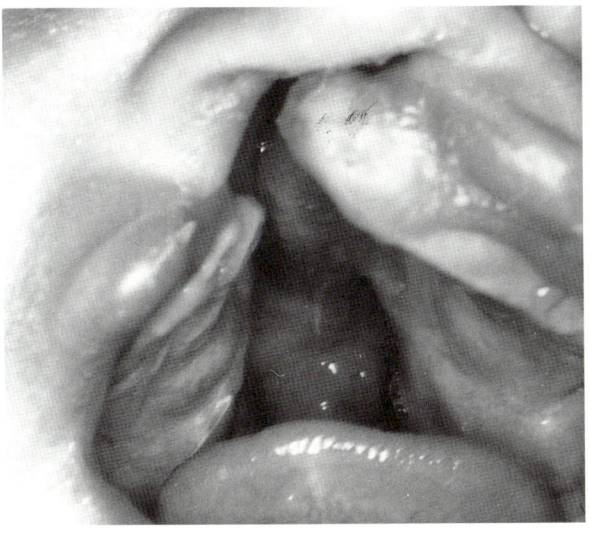

a

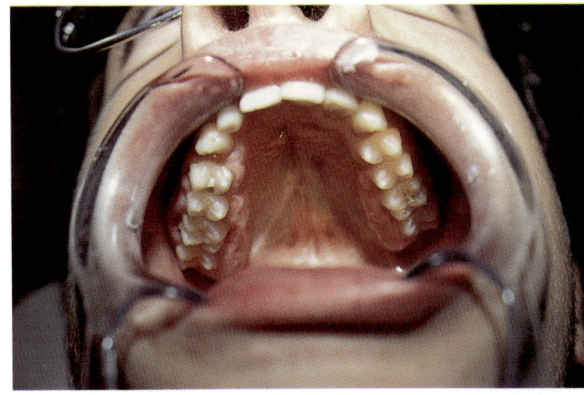

d

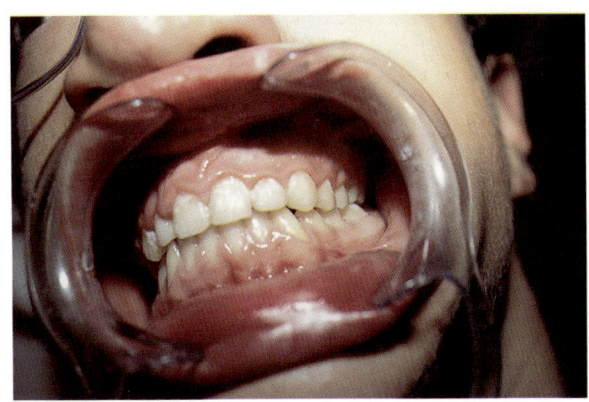

e

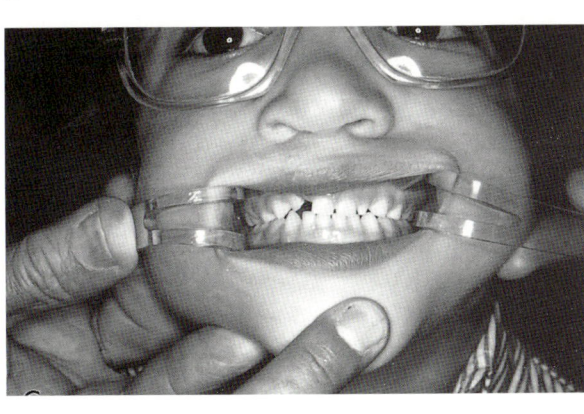

b

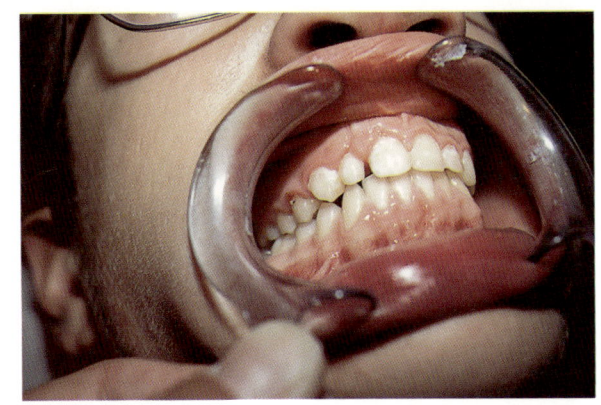

c

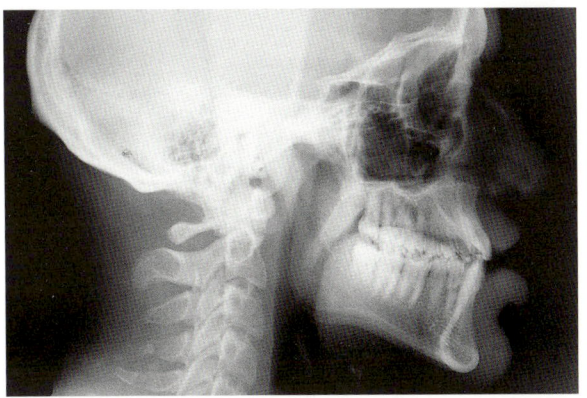

f

Fig. 23.29 *Example of long-term results in a complete cleft lip and palate with the early and primary method.*

a.   *Situation of the maxillary fragments and deformity of the nose.*

b.   *Morphological result.*

c.   *Dental result of the lacteal dentition.*

d, e and f. *Long-term result.*

g.   *X-ray.*

g

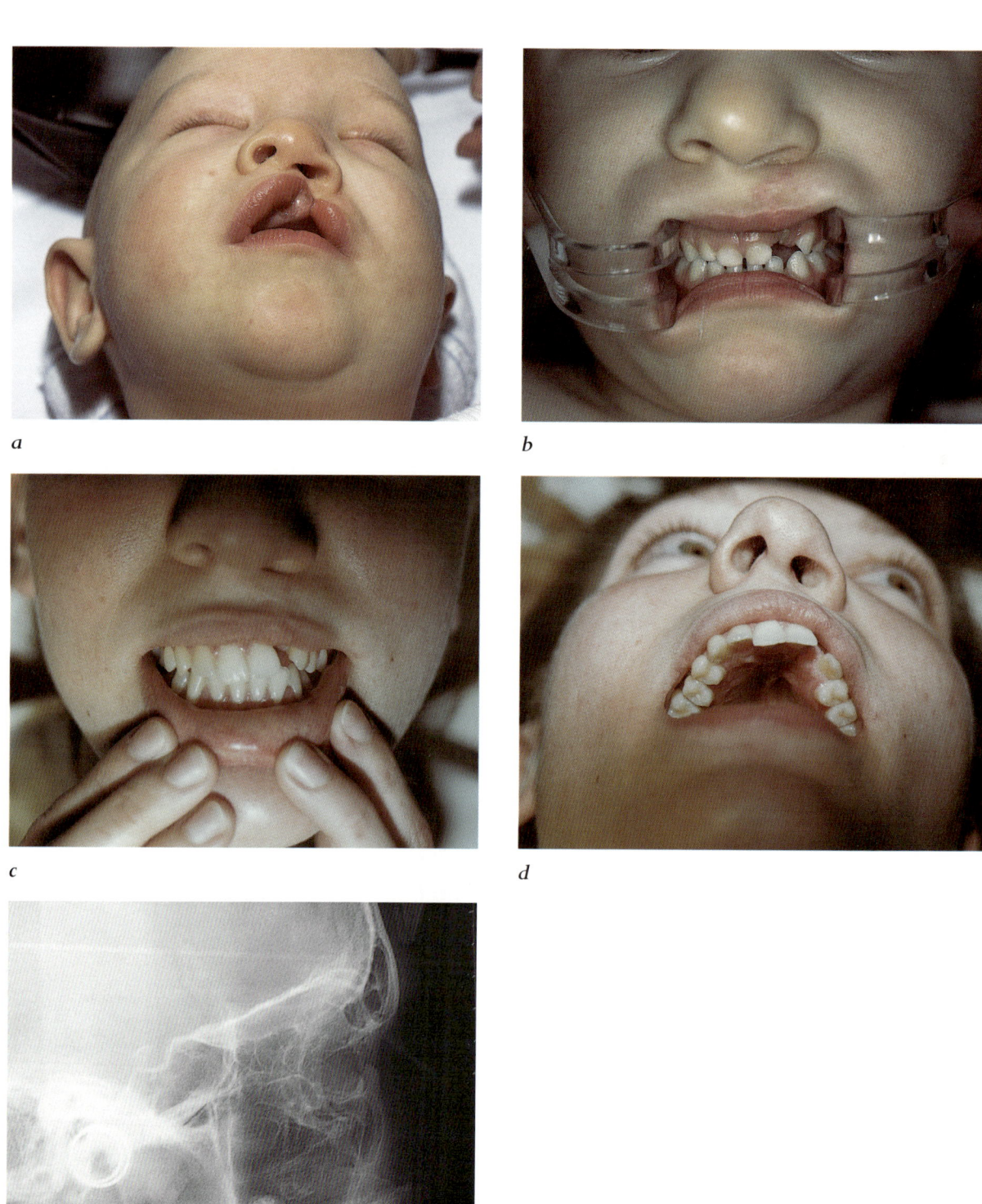

a

b

c

d

e

Fig. 23.30 *Another spontaneous long-term result in a narrow form.*

a.   *Before surgery.*

b.   *At 3 years.*

c and d. Permanent dentition at 15 years.

e.   *X-ray.*

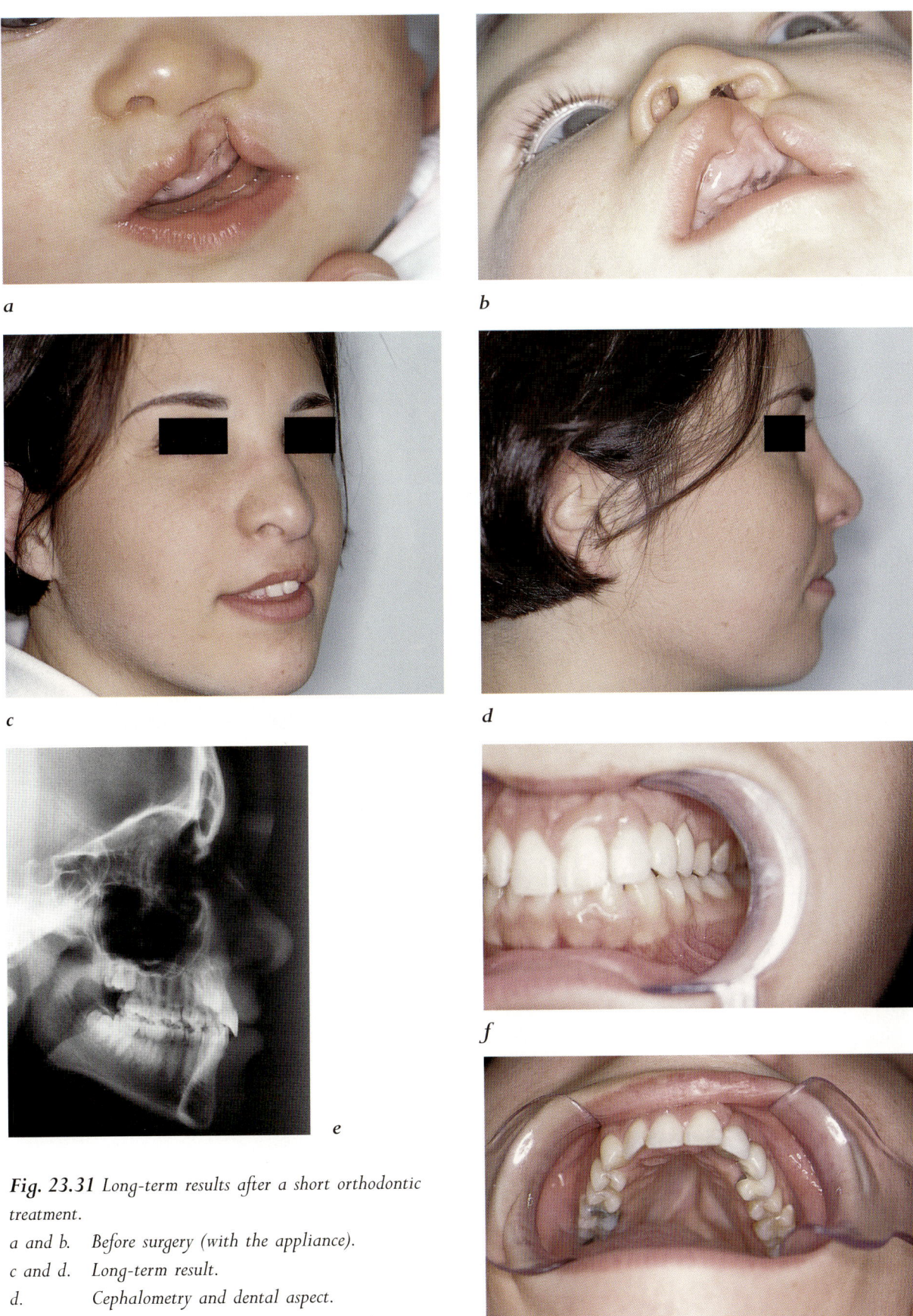

Fig. 23.31 *Long-term results after a short orthodontic treatment.*

a and b.   *Before surgery (with the appliance).*

c and d.   *Long-term result.*

d.   *Cephalometry and dental aspect.*

e.   *X-ray.*

f and g.   *Dental aspect.*

24. Complete forms without cleft palate

The study of embryology helps us to understand the lesions in this form, which is very specific but not uncommon since it accounts for about 10 per cent of the total number of cases. According to Veau, the proportion of uni- to bilateral forms is 63 per cent to 37 per cent.

The gap involves the lip, the alveolar ridge and the bony portion just behind it as far as the anterior palatine foramen. Thus, on the level of the bone structures, the cleft lies between the portion derived from the upper maxillary process (corresponding to the alveolar ridge) and that derived from the nasomedial process, which gives rise to the intermaxillary bone (premaxilla and primary palate). The palatal shelf is fused with its counterpart on the opposite side, but attachment of the vomer may vary.

With regard to the soft tissues, the cleft may be complete and correspond to the entire zone of non-fused bone, or it may be less extensive. Any uncertainty as to the simple or complete nature of the cleft is cleared up once the operation reveals whether or not there is, in fact, a gap in the bone (Fig. 24.1).

We have never had the opportunity to observe a complete form without cleft palate which involves a true bridge with an opening behind it.

UNILATERAL FORMS

Bone deformity, which is significant, can be easily explained by muscular imbalance (Fig. 24.2).

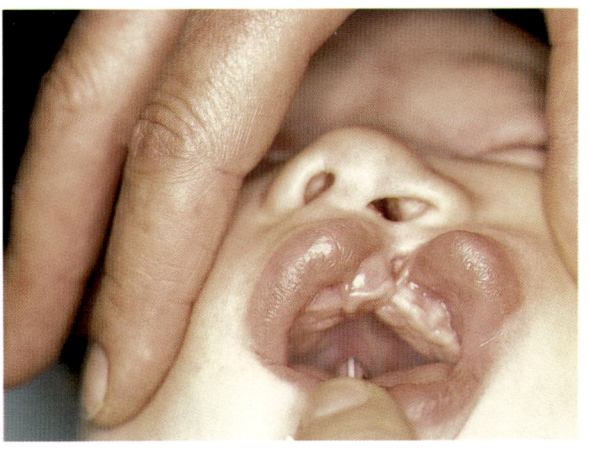

Fig. 24.1 Unilateral total cleft of the lip without cleft palate; discontinuity of the alveolar ridge is indicative of a total cleft.

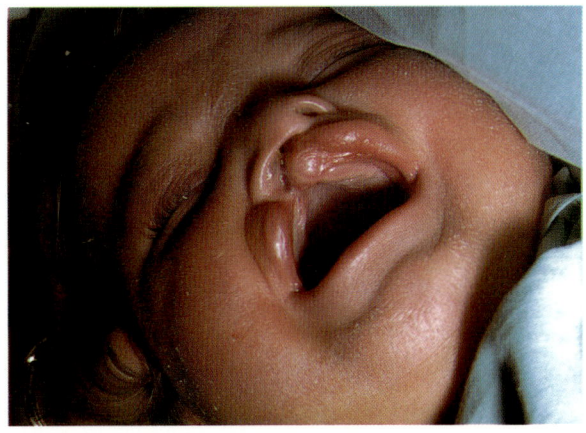

Fig. 24.2 The muscular imbalance explains the deformity and misalignment of the borders.

There is pronounced misalignment of the bony borders due to forward development of the premaxilla, which is no longer held in check by pressure from the orbicularis oris.

The maxilla is deformed into an oblique oval. This can be compared with a similar deformity that occurs in labio-maxillo-palatal clefts, with deflection of the anterior nasal spine towards the non-cleft side and deviation of the cartilaginous nasal septum.

The posterior portion of the septum and the vomer are neither deformed nor displaced, and the palatal vault is normal. The vomer in particular is properly inserted on the palatal shelves. The pharynx is also normal.

The nose shows considerable deformity, as in the complete form with cleft palate. Misalignment of the bone structures plays a major role here. The abnormal periosteal insertions of the facial muscles produce eversion of the wing of the nose, similar to that seen with cleft palate.

Surgical repair

Surgical repair is governed by the need to realign the two borders. The procedure required includes:

1. Elimination of the abnormal periosteal junction and an extensive vertical incision of the periosteum along the processus frontalis to facilitate forward displacement of the tissues (Fig. 24.3).
2. Reconstruction of the nostril floor, requiring a Z-plasty as described for labio-maxillo-palatal clefts with a flap of inner mucoperiosteum which is fitted into an outer incision in the mucoperiosteum of the alveolar border.

Suturing of the nasal layer must be painstaking to prevent formation of a residual fistula (Fig. 24.4). Once the cleft is repaired, the infant can keep his or her mouth tightly closed and is capable of producing high positive and negative pressure within the oral cavity.

The use of a flap of labial mucosa, which generally rules out any risk of leaving a fistula, is not automatically proposed. As discussed in Chapter 22, it presents a certain number of drawbacks (deep anchorage of the lip, shallow vestibule, interposition of tissues between the teeth).

After a few years, the arch is fully moulded and the dental result is excellent since there is no bone displacement.

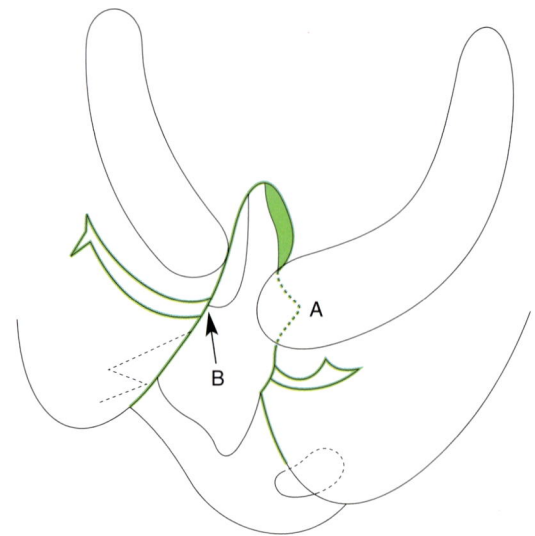

Fig. 24.3 *Operative view of complete form without cleft palate. The gap extends as far as the anterior palatine foramen. Mucoperiosteal incisions include dissection of a triangular flap behind the premaxilla (A) and a counter-incision along the processus frontalis to lodge the flap destined to correct the misalignment of the borders (B).*

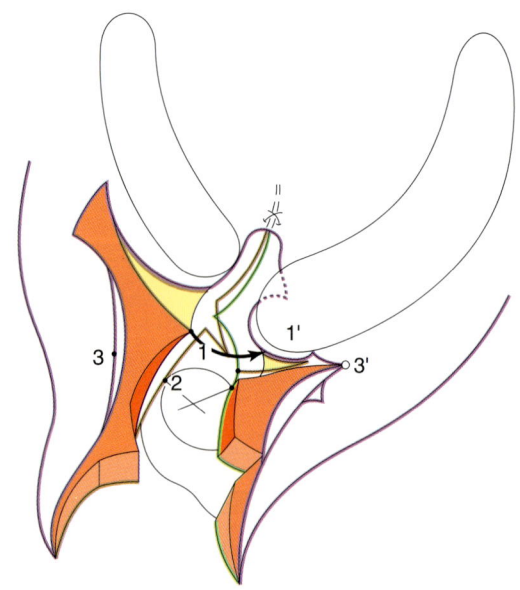

Fig. 24.4 *Closure of the alveolar region and primary palate in unilateral complete form without cleft palate.*
1→1' Reinsertion of muscles in periosteum of anterior nasal spine.
2 Reference points of nostril sill brought in line thanks to outer counter-incision.
3→3' Advancement of outer mucosa into bottom of vestibule after frenum of upper lip is sectioned.

BILATERAL FORMS

The lesions in this form present a very specific problem. Although the gap affects the primary palate as far as the anterior palatine foramen which, in this case, is absent, the intermaxillary bone shows no connection with the two palatal shelves (which are properly fused to one another). The lower border of the vomer seems to hang free above the shelves.

The premaxilla is extremely mobile. The anterior contour of the palatal shelves curves forward (Fig. 24.5).

In certain cases, there is a considerable degree of medial hypoplasia with a tiny, biconvex prolabium and a particularly flattened nasal tip. If the sub-septal cartilage is also underdeveloped, the aspect is that of an authentic Binder syndrome without cleft palate.

There is also a type of asymmetrical complete cleft without a palatal cleft on one side (Fig. 24.6).

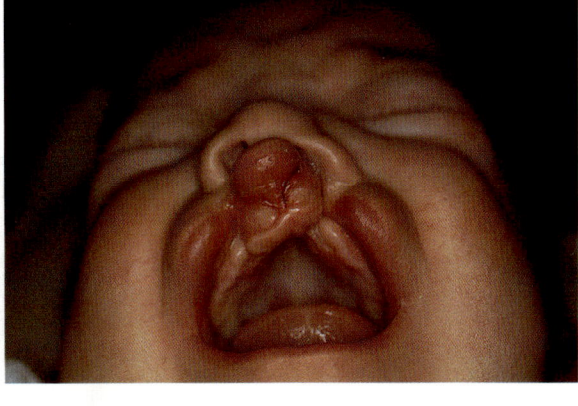

Fig. 24.6 *Example of asymmetrical bilateral complete form without cleft palate where vomer is attached to the palatal shelves.*

Surgical repair

Surgical repair involves a two-stage operation, as do all bilateral clefts for the reasons discussed earlier.

Reinsertion of the vomer may present a problem, particularly if its lower border is located in a significantly high position, at some distance from the palatal shelves (Fig. 24.7).

Thanks to the extensive exposure of the lateral skeleton and the septum during cheiloplasty it is possible to carry out suturing of a nasal layer, which is extended for a certain distance towards the rear. An attempt is made to apply it to the corresponding palatal shelf with a suture that takes a bite of oral mucosa anterior to the shelf. However, its chances of success are uncertain if not non-existent. Later on, when the second side is corrected, this fragile zone should not be tampered with. Since there is considerable misalignment of the bony borders, an extensive incision of the periosteum facing the maxillary processus frontalis is always necessary (Fig. 24.8).

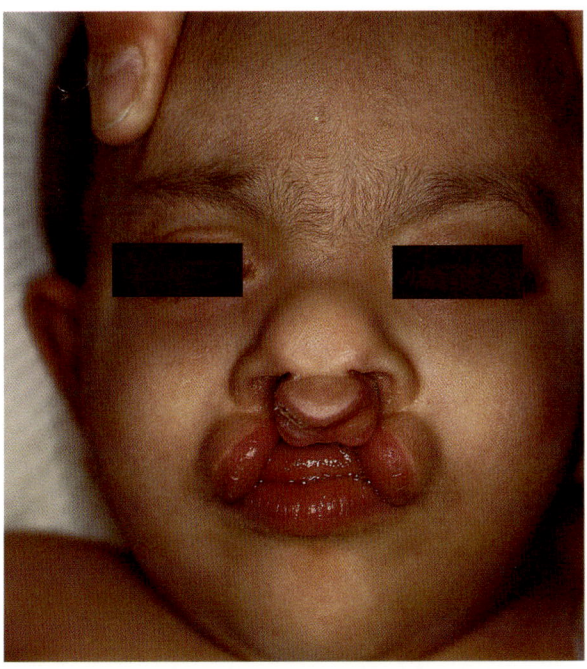

a

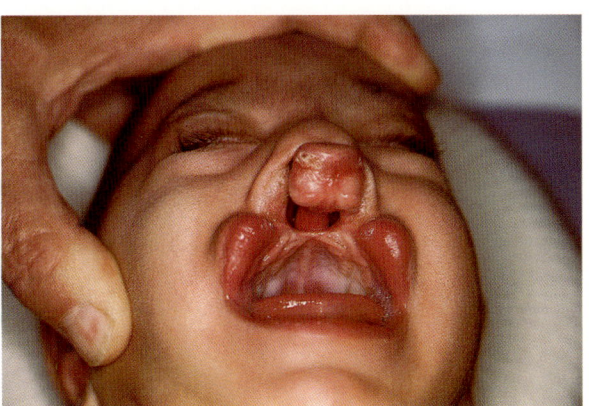

b

Fig. 24.5 *Bilateral complete cleft without cleft palate (symmetrical form) with vomer free of attachment to the palatal shelves.*
a. Curve of the ala
b. Important projection of the premaxilla.

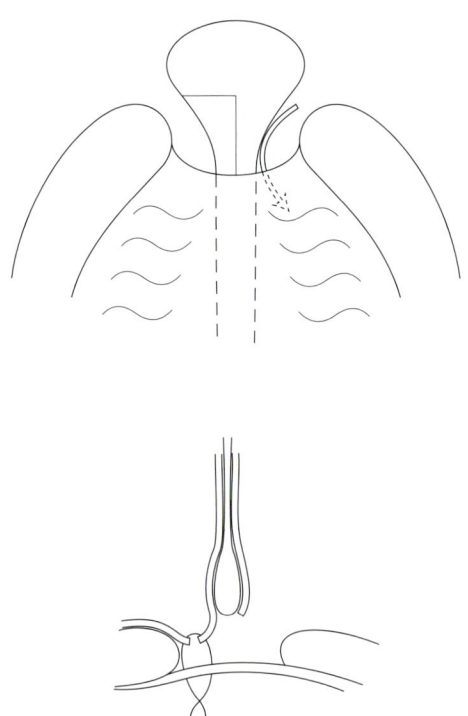

Fig. 24.7 *Where the vomer is not attached to the palatal shelves, suturing its mucosa to the nasal mucosa on one side does not suffice to prevent a fistula in the form of an antero-posterior canal. This layer must be carefully applied to the corresponding shelf.*

Despite its drawbacks, a flap of labial mucosa may be useful in these cases of complete clefts without cleft palate. When the end of the flap is sutured to the mucosa on the oral side, it helps to prevent the occurence of a small, antero-posterior fistula above the palatal shelf. In these bilateral forms, gingival mucosa is used to cover the premaxilla (Fig. 24.9).

It is important to bear in mind that specific technical problems are involved in the repair of these complete forms without cleft palate, although their prognosis is generally favorable.

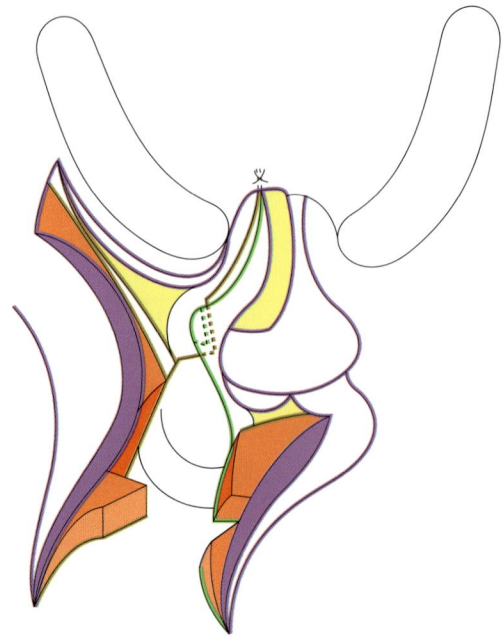

Fig. 24.8 *Reconstruction of layers during initial cheiloplasty.*

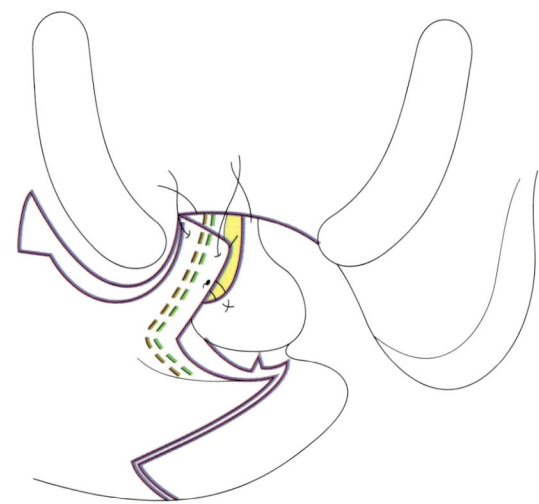

Fig. 24.9 *Use of a flap of labial mucosa to line the nasal layer.*

25. Conclusion

This study of labio-palatal clefts is based on 37 years of surgical experience and on thousands of operations by the same surgeon.

Although this is a long time span, the author found that it barely sufficed to acquire a knowledge of the complex lesions involved in this congenital deformity. The few full-length books on clefts tend to gloss over the description of these lesions, and the articles in print, however numerous, do not do them justice. At the same time, the functional disorders generated by the anomaly, even before birth, receive little or no attention.

We have attempted to address these problems as a whole. Thus, a therapeutic program was set up which took into account both the need to correct these anatomical and functional defects as well as the potential iatrogenic effects of the surgery involved.

To be worthy of credit, this new method had to stand the test of time. This is now the case, since our experiment covers a period in excess of 20 years.

It may arouse criticism or reservations and the younger generation of surgeons will form their own opinion after comparing these results with those of other methods. A consensus of opinion may not be reached at any time in the near future.

In the end, what really counts is the anatomical and physiological data. We only hope that we have served a worthwhile purpose in publishing it here.

Select bibliography

Aaronson SM, Fox DR, Cronin TD. The Cronin push-back palate repair with nasal mucosal flap. A speech evaluation. *Plast Reconstr Surg* 1985; **75**: 895.

Anderl H. Primary correction of the unilateral cleft lip nose: a preliminary report. In: Huddart AG, Ferguson MWJ, eds. *Cleft Lip and Palate*. Manchester University Press, 1990, 197–204.

Bardach J, Morris HL, Olin WH. Late results of primary veloplasty: the Marburg project. *Plast Reconstr Surg* 1984; **73**:207.

Berkeley WT. The cleft lip nose. *Plast Reconstr Surg* 1959; **23**: 567.

Berkeley WT. Correction of the unilateral cleft lip nasal deformity. In: Grabb WC, Rosenstein SW, Bzoch KR, eds. *Cleft Lip and Palate*. 1971, 227–42.

Beveridge ME. Laryngeal mask anaesthesia for repair of cleft palate. *Anaesthesia* 1989; **44**: 656.

Billroth T. Über uranoplastik. *Wien Klin Wochenschr* 1889; **2**: 241.

Blair VP. Nasal deformities associated with congenital clefts of the lip. *J Am Med Assoc* 1925; **84**: 185.

Blair VP, Brown JP. Mirault operations for single hare lip. *Surg Gyneco Obstet* 1930; 51–81.

Boorman JG, Sommerlad BC. Musculus uvulae and levator palatini: their anatomical and functional relationship in velopharyngeal closure. *Br J Plast Surg* 1985; **38**: 333.

Borde J, Bedouelle J, Malek R. Lambeau triangulaire équilatéral dans le traitement du bec de lièvre unilatéral. *Ann Chir Infant* 1961; **3**: 2.

Bosma JF, Lind J, Truby HH. Distortions of the upper respiratory tract and swallowing in infants with anomalies of the upper pharynx. *Acta Paed Scand* (Suppl.) 1965; **163**: 110.

Brain AIJ. The laryngeal mask: a new concept in airway management. *Br J Anaesth* 1983; **55** 801.

Braithwaite F. The importance of the levator palatini muscle in cleft palate closure. *Br J Plast Surg* 1968; **21**: 60.

Broomhead I. The nerve supply of the muscles of the soft palate. *Br J Plast Surg* 1951; **4**: 1.

Brophy M. Bone surgery essential in the treatment of complete cleft palate. *M Am Dent Ass* 1923; **1**.

Brunelle F, Oger P, Malek R. CT evaluation of CLP. The pterygo-mandibular index. Paper read at the 5th International Congress on Cleft Palate and Related Cranio-facial Anomalies, 1985.

Burian F. Chirurgie rozst-ep-u a patra. *Praha stathi zdzavotnické nake* 1954; 302.

Calnan J. The error of Gustav Passavant. *Plast Reconstr Surg* 1954; **13**: 275.

Calnan J. Congenital large pharynx. A new syndrome with report of 41 cases. *Br J Plast Surg* **24**: 263.

Caouette-Laberge L, Bayet B, Larocque Y. The Pierre Robin sequence: review of 125 cases and evolution of treatment modalities. *Plast Reconstr Surg* 1994; **93**: 934.

Changeux JP, Ricoeur P. *La Nature et la Règle*, Paris, O. Jacob, 1998.

Collis MH. The aesthetic treatment of harelip with a description of a new operation for more scientific remedy of the deformity. *Dublin J Med Sci* 1868; **45**: 292.

Copeland M. The effects of very early palatal repair on speech. *Br J Plast Surg*; **43**: 676.

Couly G, Cheron G, De Blic J, et al. Le syndrome de Pierre Robin. Classification et nouvelle approche thérapeutique. *Arch Fr Pediat* 1988; **45**: 553.

Cronin TD. Method of preventing raw area on nasal surface of soft palate in push-back surgery. *Plast Reconstr Surg* 1957; **20**: 474.

Delaire J. Considérations sur la croissance faciale. Déductions thérapeutiques. *Rev Stomatol* 1971; **72**: 57.

Delaire J. La cheilo-rhinoplastic primaire pour fente labio-maxillaire congénitale unilatérale. Essai de schématisation d'une technique. *Rev Stomatol* 1975; **76**: 193.

Delaire J. Influence du voile du palais sur la statique linguale et al croissance mandibulaire. Déductions thérapeutiques. *Rev Stomatol* 1976; **77**: 821.

Delaire J. The potential role of facial muscles in monitoring maxillary growth and morphogenesis. In: MacNamara, ed. *Monograph No. 8 Craniofacial Growth Series*. Ann Arbor: The University of Michigan Center for Human Growth and Development, 1978.

Delaire J. La cheilo-rhinoplastie fonctionnelle secondaire. *Chir Ped* 1983; **24**: 328.

Delaire J. Anatomie et physiologie velo-pharyngée. Incidences sur la croissance mandibulaire. Déductions thérapeutiques. *Actualités Odont Stomatol* 1988; **152**: 283.

Delorme R-P, Larocque Y, Caouette-Laberge L. Innovative surgical approach for the Pierre Robin anomalad: subperiosteal release of the floor of the mouth musculature. *Plast Reconstr Surg* 1989; **83**: 960.

De May A, VanHoot J, De Roy G, LeJour M. Anatomy of the oricularis oris muscle in cleft lip. *Br J Plast Surg* 1989; **42**: 710.

Desault PJ, Bichat X. Sur l'opération du bec de lièvre. *Oeuvres Chirurgicales ou exposé de la Doctrine et de la Pratique*, Paris: Mequignon, 1798.

Desai S. Primary cleft lip repair in newborn babies. In: Ely, JF, ed. *Transactions of the 7th International Congress of Plastic and Reconstructive Surgery*. Rio de Janeiro: Sociedade Brasileira de Cirurgia Plastica, 1980, 309.

Di George AM. *Congenital Absence of the Thymus and its Immunologic Consequences*. New York: The National Foundation-March of Dimes, New York City, 1968, 116.

Douglas B. The treatment of micrognathia associated with obstruction by a plastic procedure. *Plast Reconstr Surg* 1946; **1**: 300.

Dorf DS, Curtin JW. Early cleft palate repair and speech outcome. *Plast Reconstr Surg* 1982; **70**: 74.

Dorrance GM. Lengthening the soft palate in cleft palate operations. *Ann Surg* 1925; **82**: 208.

Dorrance GM. *The Operative Story of Cleft Palate*. Philadelphia: WB Saunders, 1933.

Dursy E. *Zur Entwicklungsgeschite des Kopfes des Menschen und der Höhern Wiebelthiere*. Tübingen, Verlag der H. Lauppschen Buchlandlung, 1869, 99.

Edgerton MT. The island flap pushback and the suspensory pharyngeal flap in surgical treatment of the cleft palate patient. *Plast Reconstr Surg* 1965; **36**: 591.

Eley, Cannon and Farber (1930) Hypoplasia of the mandible (micrognathy). *Am J Dis Child* 1930; **39**: 1167.

Enlow DH. *Handbook of Facial Growth*. Philadelphia, London, Toronto: WB Saunders, 1975.

Epois V. Anatomie et évolution du squelette facial dans les fentes labio-maxillo-palatines. *Chir Pediatr* 1983; **24**: 240.

Fara M. Musculus orbicularis oris in clefts. Thesis; Charles University, Prague, 1966.

Fara M. Anatomy and arteriography of cleft lip in stillborn children. *Plast Reconstr Surg* 1968; **4**: 225.

Fara M. and Dvorak J. Abnormal anatomy of the muscles of palato-pharyngeal closure in cleft palates. *Plast Reconstr Surg* 1970; **44**: 488.

Friede H, Johanson B. Adolescent facial morphology of early bone grafted cleft lip and palate patients. *Scand J Plast Reconstr Surg* 1982; **16**: 41.

Furlow LT Jr. Cleft palate repair by double opposing Z-plasty. *J Plast Reconstr Surg* 1986; **78**: 724.

Gianoli GG, Miller RH, Lindhe Guarisco J. Tracheostomy in the first year of life. *Ann Otol Rhinol Laryngol* 1990; **99**: 896.

Gibson T. Pierre-Joseph Cecilien Simonart (1816–1846) and his intra-uterine bands. *Br J Plast Surg* 1977; **30**: 261.

Gibson T, Gustav S. (1824–1846). Simonart (s) (z) of the band? *Br J Plast Surg* 1977; **30**: 255.

Gillies HD, Kelsey-Fry W. A new principle in the surgical management of congenital cleft palate and its mechanical counterpart. *Br Med J* 1921; **1**: 339.

Grabb WC, Rosenstein S, Bzoch KR. *Cleft Lip and Palate; Surgical, Dental and Speech Aspects*. Boston: Little Browne and Co., 1971.

Hagedorn W. Über eine Modifikation der Hagen charten Operation. *Centralbl Chir* 1884; **11**: 756.

Hamilton WJ, Boyd JD, Mossman HW. *Human Embryology*, 3rd edn. Cambridge: W. Heffer and Sons Ltd, 1964.

Herfert O. Fundamental investigations into problems related to cleft palate surgery. *Br J Plast Surg* 1958; **11**: 97.

Hinrichsen WJ, Storey E. The effect of force on bone and bones. *Angle Othod* 1963; **38**: 155.

His, W. *Unsere Koerperform und des Physiologische Problem ihrer Enstehung*. Leipzig: Verlag con F.C.W. Vogel, 1874, 87.

Hochstetter F. Über die Art und Weise, in welcher sich bei Sandgertieren und beim Meuschen aus der sugennausen Riezch grube die nasenhöhle ent wickelt. *Zeis Anat Entw* 1944; **113**: 105–144.

Hotz M, Gnoinski W, Perko M *et al*. eds. *Early Treatment of Cleft Lip and Palate*. Proceedings of the third International Symposium. Zurich 27–29 Sept 1984. Bern: Hans Huber Publishers, 1986.

Huddart AG, Ferguson MWJ. *Cleft Lip and Palate. Long-term Results and Future Prospects*. Manchester and New York: Manchester University Press, 1990.

Huffman WC, Lierle DM. Studies on pathological anatomy of unilateral hare lip nose. *Plast Reconstr Surg* 1949; **4**: 225.

Hynes W. Pharyngoplasty by muscle transplantation. *Br J Plast Surg* 1950; **3**: 128.

Ivy RH. Prolabium – Editorial. *Plast Reconstr Surg* 1962; **29**: 611.

Jalaguier A. Traitement du bec de lièvre unilatral simple. *Presse Med* 1910; **11**.

Kaplan EN. Cleft palate repair at three months? *Ann Plast Surg* 1981; **77**: 179.

Kremenak CR, Huffman WC, Olin WH. Growth of maxilla in dogs after palatal surgery: I. *Cleft Palate J* 1967; **4**: 6.

Kremenak CR, Huffman WC, Olin WH. Growth of maxilla in dogs after palate surgery: II. *Cleft Palate J* 1970a; **9**: 719.

Kremenak CR, Huffman WC, Olin WH. Maxillary growth inhibition by mucoperiosteal denudation of palatal shelf bone in non-cleft beagles. *Cleft Palate J* 1970b; **7**: 718.

Kriens OB. An anatomical approach to veloplasty. *Plast Reconstr Surg* 1969; **43**: 29.

Kriens OB. Anatomy of the velopharyngeal area in cleft palate. *Clin Plast Surg* 1975; **2**: 261.

Larsen LJ et al. Multiple congenital dislocations associated with characteristic facial abnormality. *J Pediatr* 1950; **37**: 574.

Latham RA, Deaton TG. The structural basis of the philtrum and the contour of the vermilion border: a study of the musculature of the upper lip. *J Anat* 1976; **121**: 151.

Legent F, Perlemuter L, Vandenbrouck C. *Cahiers d'Anatomie O.R.L.* Paris: Masson et Cie, 1986.

Le Mesurier AB. A method of cutting and suturing the lip in the treatment of complete unilateral clefts. *Plast Reconstr Surg* 1949; **4**: 1.

Lespargot A. Carrefour aéro-digestif. Anatomie fonctionnelle. *Motricité Cérébrale* 1987; **7**: 1.

Levret P. (1772) De nouvelles observations sur l'allaitement des enfants. *J Med Chir Pharm Paris* 1772; **37**: 233.

McComb H. Treatment of the unilateral cleft lip nose. *Plast Reconstr Surg* 1975; **55**: 196–601.

Malek R. Traitement initial des fentes labio-palatines. *Chir Ped* 1983; **24**: 256.

Malek R, Grossman JAI. Cleft lip repair by a systematic Z-plasty. *Clin Plast Surg* 1984; **24**: 286.

Malek R, Oger P. Must the soft palate be lengthened during primary repair of the cleft palate? *Third International Congress on the Cleft Palate*, Toronto, 1981, 6–1977.

Malek R, Psaume J. Nouvelle conception de la chronologie et de la technique chirurgicale du traitement des fentes labio-palatines. *Ann Chir Plast* 1983; **28**: 237.

Malek R, Martinez H, Mousset M-R, Trichet C. Multidisciplinary management of cleft lip and palate in Paris, France. In: Bardach J, Morris HL, eds. *Multidisciplinary Management of Cleft Lip and Palate*. Philadelphia: WB Saunders, 1990, 1–10.

Malek R, Oger P, Martinez H, Mousset M-R, Trichet C. Early palatal closure and reverse surgery in complete CLP. Late results of 700 cases experience. Paper presented at the 7th International Congress on Cleft Palate and Related Cranio-Facial Anomalies. Broadbeach, Queensland, Australia, 1993.

Malgaigne JF. *Manuel de Médecine Opératoire*, 7th edn. Paris: Germer Ballière, 1861.

Marcks KM, Trevaskis AE, De Costa A. Further observations in cleft lip repair. *Plast Reconstr Surg* 1966; **38**: 444.

Mars M, Plint DA, Houston WJB, Bergland O, Semb G. The Goslon yardstick: a new system of assessing dental arch relationships in children with unilateral clefts of the lip and palate. *Cleft Palate J* 1987; **24**; 314–22.

Marsh JL, Grames LM, Holtman B. Intravelar veloplasty: a prospective study. In: Bardach J, Morris HL, eds. *Multidisciplinary Management of Cleft Lip and Palate*. Philadelphia: W.B. Saunders, 1990.

Martin C, Morgon A. Physiologie du voile du palais. In: Uziel A, Gurrier Y, eds. *Physiologie des Voies Aéro-digestives Supérieures*. Paris: Masson et Cie, 1984.

Millard DR. A radical rotation in single hare lip. *Am J Surg* 1958; **9**: 318.

Millard DR Jr. Wide and/or short cleft palate. *J Plast Reconstr Surg* 1962; **29**: 40.

Millard DR Jr. The island flap in cleft palate surgery. *SGO* 1963; **116**: 297.

Millard DR. Refinements in rotation–advancement cleft lip technique. *Plast Reconstr Surg* 1964; **33**: 26.

Millard DR Jr, Batstone, JH, Heycock MH, Benson JF. Ten years with the palatal island flap. *Plast Reconstr Surg* 1970; **46**: 540.

Millard DR. *Cleft Craft*. Boston: Little Browne and Co., 1976.

Millard DR Jr. *Cleft Craft*, Vol. 3. Boston: Little Browne and Co., 1980.

Mirault G. Deux lettres sur l'opération du bec de lièvre considéré dans ses divers états de simplicité. *J Chir* 1844; **2**; 275.

Morel-Fatio D, Lalardrie P. External nasal approach in the correction of major morphologic sequelae of the cleft lip nose. *Plast Reconstr Surg* 1966; **38**: 116.

Morley ME. *Cleft Palate and Speech*, 4th edn. Edinburgh and London: E & S Livingston, 1958.

Mousset M-R. L'acquisition du langage par l'enfant porteur d'une fente palatine. Thesis, Université Paris-III-Sorbonne Nouvelle, Paris, 1989.

Murison MSC, Pigott RW. Medial Langenbeck: experience of a modified von Langebeck repair of the cleft palate. A preliminary report. *Br J Plast Surg* 1992; **45**: 454.

Myrrhen A. Uvulae abortu defectum resarciunt vicinae partes, sine incommodo. In: Mangetti JJ, ed. *Bibliotheca Chirurgica*. Geneva: Gabrieli de Tournes and Sons, 1721, 352.

Nicolau PJ. The orbicularis oris muscle: a functional approach to its repair in the cleft lip. *Br J Plast Surg* 1983; **36**: 141.

Oblak P. New concept of morphogenesis of clefts in the lip, alveolus and palate. *J Max-Fac Surg*. 1975a; **3**: 182.

Oblak P. New guiding principles in the treatment of clefts. *J Max-Fac Surg* 1975b **3**: 231.

Oger P. Étude critique du traitement de 2000 divisions palatines congénitales. Paris: Thèse de Médecine, 1976.

Orticochea M. Construction of a dynamic muscle sphincter operation. *Plast Reconstr Surg* 1968; **41**: 4.

Orticochea M. Results of the dynamic muscle sphincter operation. *Br J Plast Surg* 1970; **23**: 108.

Paré A. *Les Oeuvres de Mr Ambroise Paré*. Paris, G Bruon, 1575.

Passavant G. Über die Verschliessrug des Schlundes beim sprechen. *Wirchow's Arch Path Anat Physiol Klin Med* 1869; **46**: 1.

Passavant G. Über die operation der angeboren spaltn des Harten Gaumens und der damit complicierten. *Hasenscharten Arch Ohr Nas Kehlkoptheilk* 1882; **3**: 93.

Perko M. In quest for a non-traumatic surgical technique in treatment of cleft lip and palate.

Prevention of maxillary growth disturbance. In: Kehrer B, Slongo T, Graf B, Bettex M, eds. *Long-term Treatment in Cleft Lip and Palate*. Bern: Hans Huber Publ., 1981.

Petit P, Psaume J. A quel âge convient-il d'opérer le bec de lièvre? *Semaine des Hôpital* 1956; **31**: 64.

Petit P, Psaume J. *Le Traitement du Bec de Lièvre*. Paris: Masson et Cie, 1962.

Petit P, Borel-Maisonny S, Psaume J. Apropos des insuffisances vélaires et leur traitement par pharyngoplasties. *Ann Chir Plast* 1956; **1**: 257.

Peyton WT. Dimensions and growth of the palate in normal infant and in the infant with gross maldevelopment of the upper lip and palate. *Arch Surg* 1931; **22**: 104.

Piggott RW. The naso-endoscopic appearance of the normal palatopharyngeal valve. *Plast Reconstr Surg* 1969; **43**: 19.

Piggott RW, Makepeace AP. Some characteristics of endoscopic and radiological systems used in elaboration of the diagnosis of velopharyngeal incompetence. *Br J Plast Surg* 1982; **35**: 19.

Pruzansky S. Longitudinal growth studies of cranio-facial anomalies 1949–1983; what have we learned? In: Huddart AG, Ferguson MWJ, eds. *Cleft Lip and Palate, Long-term Results and Future*. Manchester: Manchester University Press, 1990.

Pruzansky S, Richmond JB. Growth of the mandible in infants with micrognathia. Clinical implications. *Am J Dis Child* 1954; **88**: 42.

Psaume J. Contribution à l'étude des déformations osseuses du bec de lièvre non opéré. Thesis, Paris, 1950.

Psaume J, Martin M. Déformation oblique ovalaire de l'arcade supérieure et déviation arciforme de la face des fentes unilatérales. *Rev Stomat* 1975; **76**: 535.

Psaume J. Les deformations osseuses précoces dans les fentes faciales unilaterales. *Ann Chir Plast* 1975; **20**: 299.

Psaume J, Malek R, Mousset M-R, Trichet C, Martinez H. Early surgical technique for cleft palate and results. *Folia Phoniatr.* 1986; **38**: 176.

Randall P. A triangular flap operation for the primary repair of unilateral clefts of the lip. *Plast Reconstr Surg* 1959; **23**: 31.

Randall P. A lip adhesion operation in cleft lip surgery. *Plast Reconstr Surg* 1965; **35**: 371.

Randall P, Krugman WM, Janina S. Pierre Robin and the syndrome that bears his name. *Cleft Palate J* 1965; **2**: 237.

Randall P, La Rossa DD, Fakhraee SM, Cohen MA. Cleft palate closure at 3 to 7 months of age: a preliminary report. *Plast Reconstr Surg* 1983; **71**: 624.

Rees TD, Swinyard CA, Converse JM. The prolabium in the bilateral cleft lip. *Plast Reconstr Surg* 1962; **30**: 651.

Robin P. La chute de la base de la langue considérée comme une nouvelle cause de gêne dans la respiration nasopharyngienne. *Bull Acad Nat Med* 1923; **89**: 37.

Robin P. *La Glossoptose*. Paris: Doin Eds, 1928.

Robin P. Glossoptosis due to atresia and hypotrophy of the mandible. *Am J Dis Child* 1934; **48**: 541.

Rogers BO. History of cleft lip and palate surgery. In: Grabb et al., eds. *Cleft Lip and Palate*. Boston: Little Browne and Co., 1971, 142.

Rose W. *Harelip and Cleft Palate*. London: HK Lewis and Co. Ltd, 1891.

Rosenthal W. Zur Frage der Gaumenplastik. *Zbl Chir* 1924; **51**: 1621.

Ross RB. Treatment variables affecting facial growth in complete unilateral cleft lip and palate. *Cleft Palate J* 1987; **24**: 5–71.

Ross RB. Growth of the facial skeleton following the Malek repair for unilateral cleft lip and palate. *Cleft Palate-Cranio-Facial J* 1995; **32**: 194.

Routledge RT. The Pierre Robin Syndrome: a surgical emergency in the neonatal period. *Br J Plast Surg* 1960; **13**: 204.

Rouviere H. *Anatomie Humaine. Descriptive et Topographique*. Paris: Masson et Cie, 1943.

Roux PJ. Observation sur une division congenitale du voile du palais et de la luette guérie au moyen d'une opération analogue à celle du bec de lièvre. *J Univ Sci Med* 1819; **15**; 356.

Ruding R. Cleft palate, anatomical and surgical considerations. *Plast Reconstr Surg* 1964; **33**: 132.

San Venero-Rosselli GL. *Les Palatoplasties, les Pharyngoplasties et la Voix*. Paris: Maloine, 1953.

San Venero-Rosselli GL. Verschluss von Gaumenspalten under Verwendung von

Pharynxlappen. *Fortschr Kiefer- und Gesichtschir* 1955; **1**: 65.

Schweckendieck H. Ergenbisse bei Lipen-Kiefer-Gaumans Palatoperationen mit der Primaren Veloplastik. *Fortsch Kiefer Gesicht Chi* 1958; **4**: 167.

Schweckendieck H. Primary veloplasty. Long-term results without maxillary deformity. A 25-year report. *Cleft Palate J* 1978; **15**: 268.

Schweckendieck W. Two-stage closure of the palate: rationale for its use. Speech development after two-stage closure of the palate. In: Kehrer B, Slongo T, Graf B, Bettex M, eds. *Long-term Treatment in Cleft Lip and Palate*. Bern: Hans Huber Pujbl., 1981.

Scrudde J, Stellmarch R. Primäre osteoplastik und kieferbogenformund bei Lippen-Kiefer-Gaumenspalten. In: Schuchardt K, ed. *Forstschr Kiefer-Gaumenspalten* 1959; 5-247.

Sher AE. Mechanisms of airway obstruction in Robin sequence: implications for treatment. *Cleft Palate-Cranio-Facial J* 1992; **29**: 224.

Schprintzen RJ. The implications of the diagnosis of Robin sequence. *Cleft Palate-Cranio-Facial J* 1992; **29**: 205.

Schprintzen RJ, Goldberg RB, Lewin ML, et al. A new syndrome involving cleft palate, cardiac anomalies, typical facies and learning disabilities: velocariofacial syndrome. *Cleft Palate J* 1978; **15**: 56.

Silva Filho OGB, Cristovao RM, Semb G. Prevalence of soft tissue ridge in a sample of 2014 patients with complete unilateral clefts of the lip and palate. *Cleft Palate J* 1994; **31**: 122.

Sinclair SW, Davies DM, Bracka A. Comparative reliability of nasal pharyngoscopy and video-fluorography in the assessment of velo pharyngeal incompetence. *Br Jr Plast Surg* 1982; **35**: 113.

Skoog T. A design for the repair of unilateral cleft lips. *Am J Surg* 1958; **95**: 223.

Skoog T. Repair of unilateral cleft lip deformity: maxilla, nose and lip. *Scand J Plast Reconstr Surg* 1969; **3**: 109.

Skoog T. *Plastic Surgery, New Methods and Refinements*. Stockholm: Almquist & Wiksell International, 1974a.

Skoog T. *Plastic Surgery. New Methods and Refinements*. Stuttgart: Georg Thieme Verlag, 1974b.

Slaughter WB, Brodie AG. Velar closure. In: Grabb WC, Rosenstein SW, Bzoch KR, eds. *Cleft Lip and Palate*. Boston: Little Browne, 1971.

Slaughter WB, Pruzansky S. The rationale for velar closure as a primary procedure in the repair of cleft palate defects. *Plast Reconstr Surg* 1954; **13**: 341.

Stark RB. Embryology of cleft lip and palate. In: Converse JM, ed. *Reconstructive Plastic Surgery*. Philadelphia and London: WB Saunders, 1964.

Stark RB, Dehaan CR. The addition of a pharyngeal flap to primary palatoplasty. *Plast Reconstr Surg* 1960; **26**: 378.

Stellmach R, Langenbecks' Archiv für klinische Chirugie, vol 292. Berlin: Springer Verlag, 1959.

Stickler GB, Belau PG, Farrell FJ et al. Hereditary progressive arthro-ophthalmopathy. *Mayo Clin Proc* 1965; **40**: 433.

Stricker M, Raphael B. Le périoste dans les fentes labio-palatines. *Chir Pediat* 1983; **24**: 274.

Subtelny JD. Width of the nasopharynx and related anatomic structures in normal and unoperated cleft palate children. *Am J Orthodont* 1955; **41**: 889.

Tagliacozzi G. *De Curtorum Chirurgica per Insitionem*. Venice: Gaspar Bindonus Jr, 1597.

Tennison CW. The repair of unilateral cleft lip by the stencil method. *Plast Reconstr Surg* 1952; **9**: 115.

Thomson JE. An artistic and mathematically accurate method of repairing the defect in case of harelip. *Surg Gynec Obstet* 1912; **14**: 498.

Trauner R. Die operation der lippenspalte. *Fortschr Kiefer Gesichts Chir* 1955; **1**: 16.

Trauner R. Korrectur operationen an lippe und nase bei lippenspalten. *Fortschr Kiefer Gesichts Chir* 1959; Bd. 294.

Tweed CH. The Francfort mandibular plane angle (FNIA) in orthodontics diagnosis, treatment, planning and prognosis. *Angl Orthodont* 1954; **24**: 121–69.

Van Demark DR, Gnoinski W, Hotz M-M, Perko M, Nussbaumer H. Speech results of the Zurich approach in the treatment of unilateral cleft lip and palate. *Plast Reconstr Surg* 1989; **83**: 605.

Veau V. Division Palatine. Anatomie, Chirurgie, Phonétique. Paris: Masson et Cie, 1931.

Veau V. *Bec de lièvre*. Paris: Masson et Cie, 1938.

Veau V, Politzer G. Embryologie du bec de liévre. *Ann Anat Path* 1936; **13**: 275.

von Graefe CF. Kurze Nachrichten und Auszuge. *J Pract Arrnek Wundarzk* 1817; **4**: 116.

Von Graefe CF. Die Gaumennath ein neuentdecktes mittel gegen angeborene Fehler der sprache. *J Chir Augenh* 1820; **1**: 1.

Von Langenbeck B. Die uranoplastik mittelst Ablosung des muco-periostalen Gaumentuberzuges. *Arch Klin Chir* 1862; **2**: 205.

Von Roonhuyse H. *Historicher Heilcurren in zwei Theile verfassete Anmerckungen*. Nürnberg, Michael and Johann Frederich Endtern, 1674.

Wallace AB. Some early and recent studies in Edinburgh in relation to causes of cleft lip and palate. In: Longacre JJ, ed. *Cranio-Facial Anomalies. Pathogenesis and Repair*. Philadelphia: JP Lippincott Co., 1968.

Wardill WEM. Cleft palate. *Br J Surg* 1928; **26**; 127.

Wardill WEM. The technique of operation for cleft palate. *Br J Surg* 1961; **28**: 282.

Warren JM. On an operation for the cure of natural fissure of the soft palate. *Am J Med Sci* 1828; **1**: 1.

Warren JM. *Surgical Observations with Cases and Operations*. Boston: Ticknor and Fields, 1867.

Whillis J. A note on the muscles of the palate and the superior constrictor. *J Anat Phys* 1930; **65**: 92.

Wynn SK. Further advances in the lateral flap cleft lip. *Plast Reconstr Surg* 1965; **35**: 613.

Yperman J, quoted by Carolus JMF. *La Chirurgie de Maître Yperman* F & E Gyselynck Gand, 1854.

Index